The Crystal Clear Guide to

Guide to

SIGHT FOR LIFE

Johnny L. Gayton, M.D.
Jan Roadarmel Ledford

The Crystal Clear Guide to
SIGHT FOR LIFE

Johnny L. Gayton, M.D.
Jan Roadarmel Ledford

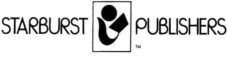
STARBURST PUBLISHERS

P.O. Box 4123, Lancaster, Pennsylvania 17604

To schedule Author appearances write:
Author Appearances, Starburst Promotions, P.O. Box 4123,
Lancaster, Pennsylvania 17604 or call (717) 293-0939

The Publisher and its representatives take no responsibility for
the validity of any material contained in this book. There are no
warranties which extend beyond the educational nature of this
book. Therefore, the Publisher shall have neither liability nor
responsibility to any person with respect to any loss or damage
alleged to be caused, directly or indirectly, by the information
contained in this book.

Credits:
Cover art by Terry Dugan Design

First Printing, April, 1996

ISBN: 0-914984-68-3
Library of Congress Catalog Number 95-069730
Printed in the United States of America.

IMPORTANT NOTICE

This book is not meant to take the place of an eye-care professional. Please consult your doctor if you have problems, and always have regular eye exams.

The Authors and Publisher do not accept responsibility for problems, medical or otherwise, arising from the use or misuse of any information found in this book.

MEET THE AUTHORS

A UTHORS Johnny Gayton and Jan Ledford both feel that their careers as eye care professionals are more than just jobs . . . they're opportunities for service. This team has been working together since 1985. With Dr. Gayton as the physician and surgeon, and Mrs. Ledford as the ophthalmic medical technologist and writer, they have co-authored numerous articles both for the public and the medical profession. They both rate this book, though, as their most significant published work to date because of its potential to help so many people.

Johnny L. Gayton (his name is *not* "John"!) was born and raised in Georgia. Believe it or not, he got into ophthalmology because his hands are small. "I wanted to be a weight lifter, but my hands are too small to grasp the bar used in competition," he says. He decided to become a doctor instead. For several years after graduating from the Medical College of Georgia in 1983, he was the youngest ophthalmologist in the United States. He established a practice in Warner Robins, GA, that has grown to a multi-physician medical practice with several satellite offices in south Georgia towns.

Gayton wrote several award-winning papers during his college days, but didn't have much time to write during the early years of his practice. He was busy, especially in surgery, trying to find better ways to do things. He began to surround himself with people who had the time and skill to write for him. His technique for helping claustrophobic patients tolerate surgery was published in 1990. That year started a flood of publishing, lecturing, and research that hasn't stopped yet. Johnny's innovations have benefited those with glaucoma, cataracts, nearsightedness, and astigmatism, to name a few.

It's impossible to know Johnny Gayton without realizing that he loves his kids. He and his wife Faye have seven children: Christopher, Amanda, Amy, Mary, Stephen, Allan, and Elisabeth. In his spare time he enjoys music, tinkering with electronics, and weight-lifting.

Jan Roadarmel Ledford grew up in Middle Georgia. She began working in ophthalmology in 1982. "When I decided to answer the newspaper ad for an ophthalmic assistant, I had to look up *ophthalmologist* in the dictionary. I had no idea what it was!" she confesses. By 1988 she had risen to the top of her profession by becoming certified as an ophthalmic medical technologist.

But Jan also had another dream. She wanted to be a writer. She had written poems and stories since she was eight. At seventeen she self-published a collection of them. "I didn't think you could earn a living by writing, so I gave it up when I went to college," she says. But the desire never died. In 1985 her first ophthalmic article was published, and she hasn't stopped writing since. She's produced dozens of articles, brochures, audio tapes, TV and radio scripts, and two books (this is her third). Her work has appeared in the *Journal of the Southern Medical Association,* and *Annals of Ophthalmology,* among others. She says, "All but that very first article and a few brochures have been written since I joined Dr. Gayton's staff. He's played a huge role in my writing career by encouraging me. (And giving me writing jobs!)" She now writes almost full time, but still sees patients in the eye clinic several days a month.

She married Jim Ledford, a native Georgian, in 1976. They have two boys, T. J. and Collin. Jim is a Physician's Assistant. They are in the process of moving to Franklin, NC. Jan enjoys reading, music, and bowling. She is also writing a novel.

Of this eye care volume, she states, "A lot of prayer has gone into this book from the beginning. It is our hope that you will find the information that you need, written in a way that speaks to you."

DEDICATION

This work is dedicated to the two men who have had the most influence on my life. First, to the memory of my father, Willard F. (Bud) Roadarmel, a brave man who taught me to always do my best. Second, to my husband, Jim: my life-friend, protector, lover, and so much more that is good and simply wonderful.

Jan Roadarmel Ledford

Dedications are very difficult. So many people have meant so much in my "Horatio Alger" life. I thank them all. I would like to dedicate this work to the memory of my maternal grandfather, Gilbert Brand, and my paternal grandmother, Alma Gayton. While limited in their own educational experience, they encouraged the pursuit of mine. Thanks Grandaddy and Nana. Enjoy your rest . . . you deserve it.

J. L. Gayton

THE *Crystal Clear Guide to Sight for Life* is exactly that. Oh, if I had had such an encyclopedia of eye care in my younger years! (Perhaps I wouldn't have resorted to all the subterfuge I did, thinking to preserve and protect this priceless sight of mine and avoided the subsequent guilt!). I am most certainly unable to write what I'd consider a creditable foreword for such a wonderful book. Here, at least, is a short introduction which tries to express how important the sense of eyesight is to me.

All my life I dreamed of being a fighter pilot. (My mother told me I vowed to her, at age four, that this was my chosen profession.) And thank the Lord, I did realize my ambition. I must also thank Him for good eyesight. My eyes have been the windows of my world, my treasures. 20/20 was the key to all my dreams. As far back as my first eye exam I memorized the 20/20 line on the eye charts . . .

At West Point both my roommates had already been to college, yet they always seemed to be studying. So much so that I was sure they endangered their eyesight. I decided to protect my eyes, no matter what. So I studied just enough to barely pass. If I felt the slightest fatigue, I'd stop reading and rest my eyes. Sitting on my bed (forbidden before Tattoo!), I would lean back against my folded mattress and cover my eyes with the red comforter.

Periodically, though, the Tactical Officer would arrive for his routine inspection. (In Kaydet lingo we called him the Tac.)

"Mr. Scott," he said, "What the . . . ! Are you so smart you don't have to study like your roommates?"

"Oh, no Sir," I replied, "they're smarter than I'll ever be! They've already been to regular colleges. Sir, I'm saving my eyes so I can pass the vision exam for the Army Air Corps."

Couldn't he understand that all my plans would be shot down if my vision wasn't perfect?

The Tac just shook his head as he wrote my name on his Skin-List ("Mr. Scott, R.L.—In bed before Tattoo"). Then he added, "I hardly think you'll get that far." But he was wrong. I did graduate (still with 20/20 eyesight), and my silver wings were pinned on at Kelly Field many years ago.

It turned out that memorizing the letters and barely studying weren't really necessary after all. (Dr. Gayton and Jan tell me that *using* my eyes won't make them weaker!) But I wanted to protect my precious eyesight. I still do. This book will help you do the same. Interesting and easy to understand, you will find yourself referring to it again and again. Whether you've been told you have a specific eye condition, are undergoing treatment, or are noticing symptoms of some sort, this book will answer your questions.

Good vision is always important, regardless of age. Old as I am, they still let me fly the fastest fighter jets. And do you know, I can still read the fine print in the Bible if I squint *just* a little!

Robert L. Scott
B/Gen., USAF
Vision: 20/20

MAJOR DIVISIONS

TABLE OF CONTENTS

INTRODUCTION

ONE Monday morning, Sharon Watson thought she noticed a fly buzzing around her head. "Now how did he get in the house?" she wondered as she swatted at it. By lunch time she realized that it wasn't a fly. It was a spot in the vision of her right eye. That night when she went to bed, she noticed neon-bright jags of flashing lights every time she moved her eyes from side to side. "It'll probably be gone in the morning," she told herself. It wasn't gone the next morning. Or the next week. But she was busy with family and vacation.

Three weeks later, Sharon noticed that the spot was much larger. When she looked out her window at her flower garden and covered her right eye, all was clear. When she covered her left eye, she was shocked to find that in addition to the spot, the view was hazy. She called her ophthalmologist's office, expecting an appointment in a few weeks. But when she told the secretary what her symptoms were, she was given an appointment for that morning. Now she wondered if her problem was more significant than she had thought.

"I'm afraid this is a rather serious problem," Dr. Soper said. "You've had a retinal detachment. When did you first notice the spot and the lights?"

"About three weeks ago." The doctor's voice seemed to be coming from far away. Retinal detachment! Thoughts of blindness flooded her mind.

". . . and you didn't do anything to cause this to happen," Dr. Soper was saying, "but I wish that you had called me right away, when you first noticed the spot. At that point your retina had just begun to detach. Since then, you've also developed a large retinal tear. We'll need to do surgery . . ."

Two months later, Sharon was having tea with a friend. "The surgery wasn't too bad, but my vision will never completely recover. Dr. Soper said that if the retina had only detached part way and not torn, things would have been a lot better. I wish I had called him when I first noticed that spot. I just didn't realize how serious spots and light flashes were!"

Spots and light flashes. Halos around lights at night. Foggy vision that comes and goes. These symptoms and many others are more likely to occur after age forty. How serious are they? This book was written to help you find out. Not so you can diagnose yourself, but so you will be aware of how crucial your symptoms may be. So you will know when you need help.

This book is not only meant to warn you about what happens when things go wrong. We have carefully explained various eye diseases and their treatment. Some problems may have more than one therapy choice. We explore the various methods so that you can understand what your doctor is recommending, why, and what you can expect. This will be a volume that you will refer to again and again.

The situations depicted in this book are real, but names have been changed to protect the privacy of our patients. Physician names are fictionalized as well.

CHAPTER 1

About the Eye

THERE is no doubt that the eye is one of the most intricate and specialized organs of the body. Even Charles Darwin, author of evolution, admitted that the development of the eye was not explainable by his theory.

Lids

The eyelids protect the eye from physical damage and from dryness. The blink reflex helps to guard the eye from injury. Blinking swabs tears over the eye to keep the eye moist. The eyelashes catch dust and debris, reducing damage and irritation.

Conjunctiva

The inside of the lids is lined with a membrane called conjunctiva. The conjunctiva folds over on itself to also cover the sclera (white of the eye). Thus a "pocket" is formed around the whole eye. The conjunctiva contains small tear glands and blood vessels.

Sclera and Episclera

The sclera is a tough fibrous tissue that protects the delicate inner structures of the eye. The muscles that move the eye attach to the sclera in various places. Sandwiched between the conjunctiva

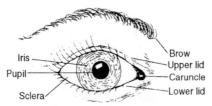

Figure 1-A The external eye.

and sclera is the episclera. The episclera is rich in blood vessels that nourish the sclera.

External muscles

There are six muscles for eye movement attached to each eye (see Figure 1-B). The muscle on each side of the eye pulls the eye to the left or right. Of the other four muscles, two are attached at the top and two at the bottom of the eyeball. They are placed in such a way that they act to turn the eye up and down as well as to various angles. A weakness in any muscle (or a palsy in a nerve that runs to any muscle) can result in crossed eyes and/or double vision.

The Pathway of Light

The eye works much like a camera (see Figure 1-C). Light enters the camera and passes through several lenses and empty spaces. The image is focused and projected on the film. In a similar manner, light entering the eye must also cross numerous structures in order for us to see (see Figure 1-D).

Tears

First, light must pass through the tear film. The tears are made up of three parts: water, oil, and mucus. The watery part of the tear film is made by the tear glands. The main and largest of these, the lacrimal gland, lies under the brow bone. The oil and mucus portions are secreted by glands in the lids and conjunctiva. The water, oil, and mucus portions of the tears are each important, and must be present in the right combination.

Every time the eye blinks, tears are washed over the eye. The

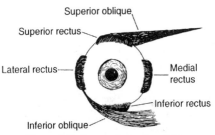

Figure 1-B External muscles of the eye.

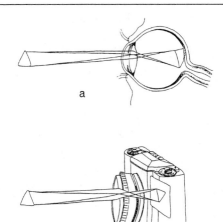

Figure 1-C The optical system of the (a) eye compared to the (b) camera.

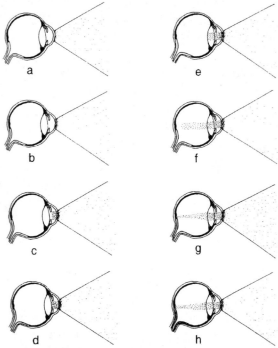

Figure 1-D The pathway of light as it passes through: (a) the tear film, (b) the cornea, (c) the aqueous, (d) the pupil, (e) the lens, (f) the vitreous, (g) the retina and (h) the optic nerve.

tears serve to keep the eye moist and to wash away dirt and other debris. The tears create a smooth surface over the eye, much like the coating on the surface of a mirror. If the tear film is clouded by ointment or matter, then vision will be unclear.

Cornea

Next, incoming light passes through the cornea. The cornea is the clear window-like covering over the iris (colored part of the eye). The cornea is actually a type of lens, and helps to focus the light. A clear cornea allows light to pass through unhindered. However if there are scars, cloudy patches, or growths on the cornea, vision is hampered.

Aqueous

After the cornea, the light travels through two chambers. The anterior chamber is between the cornea and iris. The posterior chamber lies between the iris and the lens. Both chambers are filled with a clear watery fluid called aqueous (or aqueous humor). The aqueous is formed by a structure called the ciliary body (located on the back side of the iris), then circulated inside the front portion of the eye. It drains out through a network of canals, called the trabecular meshwork, in an interior area known as the angle. Because the aqueous is constantly being formed, there is pressure inside the eye (intraocular pressure, or IOP). If the aqueous is not clear, it is like trying to see through muddy water.

Pupil and Iris

The fourth item that light crosses is the pupil. The pupil is actually a hole . . . an opening in the iris or colored part of the eye. The iris contains two muscles: one acts to open the pupil wider and the other causes the pupil to close. This controls the amount of light that enters the eye. An abnormally large or small pupil can make it difficult to see.

Lens

The lens is the next structure that light must pass through. The lens lies behind the pupil and, like the lens of a camera, focuses the light coming into the eye. The lens must also be clear. Any cloudiness of the lens is called a cataract (we'll talk more about cataracts in Chapter 11). Vision through a cataract is blurred, like looking through waxed paper or frosted glass.

Vitreous and Retina

After the lens, the focused light travels through a jelly-like substance known as vitreous (or vitreous humor). The vitreous fills the back portion of the eye, aptly named the vitreous cavity. The vitreous, too, must be clear.

Finally, the light reaches its destination at the back of the eye: the retina. The retina is like the film in a camera. It is made up of light-sensitive cells called rods and cones. These cells gather the incoming light before it is transmitted to the brain. The rod cells are scattered over the entire retina, and are responsible for vision in dim light. The cone cells provide finely detailed and color vision. The cones are concentrated in the area of central vision, the macula. A small pit in the macula, the fovea, has only cones and no rods (see Figure 1-E).

Think about the camera comparison again. Suppose you had a very expensive camera and a fancy lens system. Now imagine that the film in your camera is no good. Will you get good pictures with your costly camera? Of course not. It's the same with the eye. If the retina is diseased the vision will be decreased, even if the rest of the eye is healthy.

Once the light is gathered by the retina, it travels to the brain through the optic nerve. The optic nerve is at the back of the eye, and contains nerve fibers and blood vessels. (There are no rod or cone cells in the optic nerve, making it the "blind spot".) Light signals from the retina travel through the optic nerve to the brain.

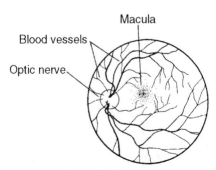

Figure 1-E The fundus.

The brain then interprets what is seen.

Binocular Vision

You can see from this discussion that each part of the eye is important in order to have clear vision. The eyes must also work together for the visual system to be most effective.

One of the advantages of having two healthy eyes is binocular vision. (Binocular refers to "two eyes.") Here's how it works: Each eye sees an object from a slightly different angle. The brain fuses these different perspectives into a three-dimensional picture. This gives us a sense of where objects are in relation to ourselves and other objects (depth perception).

Peripheral (side) vision is another area where it's advantageous to have two eyes. The peripheral vision of each eye overlaps in front of your body. This helps with binocular vision. But on the outer side, the opposite occurs. That is, the left eye gives you side vision farther to the left than the right eye alone. And the right eye sees more to the right.

Now that you understand more about the eye, you need to know about the professionals who care for this amazing organ, the subject of the next chapter.

CHAPTER 2

ChoosingYour Eye Care Physician
(And Relating to the Office Personnel)

L EE Rhodes was fishing when he first noticed that the vision in his right eye was not what it should be. Startled, he reeled in his line and trudged up to the cabin. As Mr. Rhodes thumbed through the yellow pages to find an eye doctor, he began to wonder: *Just who should I call?* An optician? Optometrist? Ophthalmologist? He noticed an ad for an ocularist. *What in the world is that?*

There are many symptoms and conditions involving the eye. Different eye care specialists stand ready to meet the needs created by these problems. But how do you know which one to go to for help? In this chapter we will talk about the different occupations in eye care. We'll also look at how to choose a physician, how to change doctors, and second opinions. Plus, there are tidbits on how to get what you want and need from the office staff.

Doctors

Title: **Optometrist (O.D.)**
Function: Optometrists are licensed to perform eye exams and pre-scribe glasses and contacts. They are very knowledgeable about meas-uring and prescribing lenses. Special testing such as visual fields, and visual training are also done by optometrists.

These important eye care physicians can diagnose and treat most eye diseases and injuries, then refer for further treatment when necessary. In most states, they are allowed to prescribe medications to treat eye infections and other conditions.

Most optometrists have an optical shop. An optometrist may employ an optician, or do the lens grinding and spectacle fitting him/herself. Many have their own offices. Some work for chain stores or in a clinic.

Training: The candidate for optometry school usually gets a four year college degree before starting the program. He/she then goes to school for an additional four years to earn the diploma. After that, he/she must take a licensing examination in order to practice.

Title: **Ophthalmologist (M.D.)**
Other Title(s): Oculist
Function: An ophthalmologist is a medical doctor (M.D.) who is licensed to diagnose and treat diseases and conditions of the eye. This includes performing eye surgery. He/she can give eye exams and prescribe medications, glasses, and contacts. Some fit contacts as well. An ophthalmologist may have his/her own office, or work in a group or clinic. If there is an optical shop in the office, an ophthalmologist often hires an optician (explained below) to help.
Training: After getting a four year college degree, the ophthalmologist-to-be must go through four years of medical school. (This is the same "medical school" that every medical doctor attends.) He/she then generally serves a one year rotating internship, followed by three years as a resident in ophthalmology. He/she often puts in an additional year or two to earn a Fellowship in a special area of ophthalmology.
Specialists: Some ophthalmologists work exclusively with a certain part of the eye, or a particular condition. The following list covers most areas:

- Geriatrics—cares for the elderly.
- Pediatrics—cares for children.
- General—cares for all ages, does most types of eye surgery.
- Plastics—involved in plastic surgery of the eyes, eyelids, and eye brows. This includes repair, reconstruction, and cosmetic surgery. He/she also removes growths and cancers.
- Neurology—evaluates the optic nerve, brain, and nerves that move the eyes.
- Retina—examines and treats the retina (inside lining of the eye).
- Cornea—examines and treats the cornea (clear covering over the front of the eye). Fits contact lenses in special cases.
- Glaucoma—specializes in caring for patients with glaucoma including medication, laser, and surgery.

Other Eye Specialists

Title: **Ocularist**
Function: The ocularist is a specialist in prostheses (artificial eyes). He/she is an expert in finding the right size and shape of eye for each

patient. Prosthesis fitting is very much an art. (Did you ever realize that there are many different shades of white?) Careful attention to detail is needed in order to fashion an artificial eye that matches the remaining eye as closely as possible. Some ocularists have an office of their own. Others travel, visiting various eye care offices so that more people can be served.

Training: To become a board certified ocularist (B.C.O.), one must spend 10,000 hours in hands-on training, get 750 credit hours of instruction, then pass written and practical examinations. In order to remain certified, continuing education credit is required.

Title: **Optician**

Function: In the most basic sense, the optician makes lenses and dispenses eye glasses. He/she is involved with helping you choose a frame that is correct for your face, complexion, occupation, hobbies, and budget. He/she also makes suggestions regarding the lenses, such as shape, size, segment (bifocal or trifocal), and material (glass or plastic). The optician prepares the lenses including grinding, tinting, coating, and shaping. He/she then inserts them into the frame. Frames are adjusted and repaired as needed. Many opticians also dispense contact lenses, and some fit prosthesis (artificial eyes). They often have shops of their own, although some work in chain stores, or in eye doctors' offices.

Training: Many are trained on the job. Other serve several years (usually 2–4) in an apprentice program. Two-year college programs are also available. Some states require a license. In this case, the candidate must have met educational and training standards, then pass a written and/or practical exam.

Title: **Orthoptist**

Function: An orthoptist in involved in working with diagnosing and managing lazy and/or crossed eyes. Because these conditions are best treated early, orthoptists usually treat children. However, they might assist adults who have developed eye muscle imbalances. Orthoptists are auxiliary personnel, and must work under the supervision of an ophthalmologist. That is to say, they may not have a private office of their own.

Training: An orthoptist takes two years of postgraduate training and must pass a certification exam.

Title: **Ophthalmic Registered Nurse**

Function: Ophthalmic RNs are nurses who specialize in ophthalmology. They must work with the doctor, and may not set up an office of their own. They assist with patient care in the office and during surgery.

Training: Any licensed RN may work in ophthalmology. However, there is a special certification which is optional. A two or four year RN degree is followed by two years' experience in eye care. Then the candidate must pass an examination.

Title: **Physician Assistant (P.A.)**

Function: A physician assistant can work in any area of medicine. The duties of an ophthalmic PA might include minor surgery, surgical assisting, physical exams, post operative evaluation, routine eye exams, anesthesia, and emergencies. Laws governing their duties vary from state to state. They must work with a physician and cannot set up their own practice.

Training: This college program is generally four to five years long. They must pass a national board exam and become licensed.

Title: **Optometric Assistant**

Function: The optometric assistant helps the optometrist by performing eye screening exams and assisting in frame selection.

Training: Most are job trained. There are 1 year programs available at technical schools, community colleges, and colleges of optometry.

Title: **Ophthalmic Medical Personnel (O.M.P.'s)**

Function: These auxiliary personnel assist the ophthalmologist. Common duties include screening during routine eye exams and performing special measurements and tests.

Training: There are a dozen or so formal training programs in the United States, but most OMP's are job-trained. There are three levels of certification: Assistant, Technician, and Medical Technologist. An OMP can also specialize and become certified in photography, ultrasound, surgical assisting, and contact lens fitting. Certification is not required.

Which Type of Practice is Best for Your Eye Care Needs?

Should you go to a private office or a university? What about a private practice clinic? Here's a brief outline of your options:

Practice Type: **Private practice**
Advantages: Probably close to home. You will always see the same doctor, so a relationship can be developed.
Disadvantages: Equipment may not be state-of-the-art. Must refer special cases. If your doctor is unavailable during an emergency, you will have to see a doctor you don't know.

Practice Type: **Private clinic**
Advantages: May be better equipped. Practice may include specialists so you do not have to be referred out-of-house. If your doctor is unavailable during an emergency, other doctors in the practice still have access to your records.
Disadvantages: May be a distance from home.

Practice Type: **University clinic**
Advantages: State-of-the-art equipment. Involved in studies and treatments unavailable in the private sector. Your participation in such a program can provide valuable information that is used to help others.
Disadvantages: May be a distance from home. Doctors (residents) come and go.

General Care vs. Specialist

Should you start out in general care (with an optometrist or general ophthalmologist) or with a specialist? It all depends. If you suspect you have a problem, general care is a good place to start. If an optometrist finds an eye problem needing surgical treatment, you will be referred to an ophthalmologist. A general ophthalmologist also makes referrals if a specialist is necessary.

On the other hand, if you have been told in the past that you have a specific condition, then you might seek a specialist in that field. Some specialists only see patients that are referred by another doctor. If you are trying to get an appointment on your own, be sure and explain that a doctor has previously diagnosed the problem.

For suggestions on who to see for what refer to Table 2-1.

Choosing an Eye Physician and Practice

Selecting an eye care specialist is an important step. How can you find the physician of your dreams? Well, no one is perfect, but we'll discuss some things that might help you select someone who's right for you.

First, ask your friends and family who they use for their eye care needs. Once you start discussing eyes and vision with your acquaintances, you may find that you keep hearing the same name over and over again. If someone you know has a problem similar to yours, you might want to consider using the doctor who has helped them.

Table 2-1 Who Should You See?

Problem/Need	Eye Care Professional
glasses prescription	optometrist, ophthalmologist
contact lens prescription	optometrist, ophthalmologist
contact lens fitting	optometrist, ophthalmologist, optician
glasses lenses	optometrist, optician
frames	optometrist, optician
low vision aids	inquire: optometrist, retinal or general ophthalmologist, optician
routine eye exam	optometrist, general ophthalmologist
minor injury	optometrist, ophthalmologist
severe injury	ophthalmologist, emergency room
infections	ophthalmologist (optometrist may treat in some states)
cataract observation	optometrist, ophthalmologist
cataract surgery	ophthalmologist
glaucoma	general or glaucoma ophthalmologist (optometrist may treat in some states)
prosthesis	Ocularist (also some optometrists, opticians, and ophthalmologists)
eyelid surgery	ophthalmologist, plastic surgeon
macular degeneration	general or retinal ophthalmologist
corneal dystrophy	general or corneal ophthalmologist
diabetic observation	optometrist, ophthalmologist
diabetic laser	general or retinal opthalmologist

An excellent source for references is your family doctor. He or she is familiar with your general health, and can advise you about what type of eye doctor you should see, as well as give you names. In addition, some hospitals have a referral service that you can call for information. Another way to find an eye physician is to watch for advertisements. The easiest way would be to check the yellow pages of the phone book. (To find an optometrist, look under "Optometrists." To locate an ophthalmologist, look under "Physicians and Surgeons, Ophthalmology.") But you might also be alert to any ads in newspapers, newsletters, radio, and television. An office might advertise about a certain procedure or condition that you are interested in.

The location of a doctor's office might be important to you. If you have a limited driving range, you might feel you have to use someone close to home. But don't rule out a certain physician just because transportation is a problem. Many offices have a transport system and will be glad to send someone to pick you up. Call the office and ask.

Before you commit to an appointment with a new doctor, call the office and talk to the secretary. These are some sample questions you may want to ask:

- Where did the doctor receive his/her training?
- How long has he/she been practicing?
- Where does he/she do surgery? (if an ophthalmologist)
- To whom does he/she refer surgical cases? (if an optometrist)
- Do you have evening hours? Weekend hours?
- Does the doctor take emergencies?
- Do you accept my insurance?
- Do you file insurance?
- Do you provide transportation?
- When is your next available appointment?
- Does the doctor's schedule usually run behind?
- Does the doctor use this new treatment I'm interested in?
- What does a full eye exam include?
- What is the charge for an eye exam?
- Do you sell glasses there? Contact lenses?

While we don't think you should decide to use a particular doctor only because he/she will accept your insurance, we realize that this may be a major influence for you. The same applies to some of the other items. For example, if you have heard that a doctor is particularly good, you will probably have to wait several weeks before you can get an appointment. You'll have to decide which items are the most important to you, and make your decision accordingly.

Using the phone book, watching ads, or staying in your own neighborhood will not insure that you get a good doctor. Ask a few folks how they're treated by the doctor you're considering. If you don't know anyone who goes to that doctor, ask the office's secretary for a few names you can contact as references.

Making An Appointment

You've chosen a doctor and you're ready to take the first step and set a date for your exam. This is best done by phone. There are several important things to keep in mind when you call. (Many of these items apply whether this is your first visit to the doctor or not.)

1. Tell the receptionist if you have seen the doctor before, or if this will be your first visit. This helps them know if there will be a record on you or not. If you've seen the doctor before, tell them when.

2. If you have seen a physician who recommended that you see this particular eye doctor, tell the secretary. (There is a difference between a doctor recommending you be seen and a referral. If the doctor makes a recommendation, it is a suggestion. You are on your own to make the appointment. However, in the case of a referral, the doctor usually calls and makes the appointment for you.)

3. Be sure to mention what type of problem you are having, if any. Be specific. **This makes a big difference, and may affect how soon you are able to get an appointment**. Examples could include:
   —"It's time for my annual exam."
   —"My regular doctor thought he saw cataracts in my eyes."
   —"I'm seeing a curtain over my vision that seems to float down from the top."
   —"I was working in my wood shop and got something in my eye."
   — "I broke my reading glasses."
   —"I've noticed a problem seeing road signs lately."

Some of the above descriptions are emergencies that will need to be seen on the day you call. Some of them indicate a minor problem that can wait a few weeks for a regular opening. The receptionist will probably ask you a few more questions about your eye condition. Sometimes the nurse or assistant may talk to you. This is to help clarify whether or not an emergency exists. But the receptionist won't know what you need unless you tell her what's going on.

4. Be specific about what you want done. For example, if you have a growth on your eyelid, you may want the doctor to check that and nothing else. There's a big difference between looking at a growth versus a full check-up to update glasses and check on overall eye health.

5. If there is a particular day of the week or time of day that you **cannot** come in for an appointment, tell the receptionist right away. This will save a lot of time.

6. Some other things you may want to ask:
   —How long will the exam take?
   —Should I come a few minutes early to fill out paper work?
   —Will my pupils be dilated? Will I need someone to drive me home?
   —What should I bring?
   —Can you get records from my last doctor?
   —Do I need to leave my contacts out?
   —Where is your office located?

Who's Who in the Office

When you choose a doctor or clinic, you aren't just choosing the doctor. You are choosing the practice. That includes a staff of dedicated people who are there to help you. Each has a special function. We discussed medical personnel above. There are also clerical employees such as receptionist, phone operator, appointment clerk, file clerk, medical records, insurance clerk, cashier, payment clerk, etc. In small offices, one person might wear many of these hats. (In fact, it is not unusual for medical personnel to double up and help out, too.) It is not necessary to talk to the doctor for every request. The following suggests who you might contact for what:

• I need my medicine prescription refilled.
   Whoever answers the phone should take your request. Your

chart and the order may be passed along to an assistant or nurse to call in. (Some state laws may require the physician to call it in.)

- I need a copy of my lens prescription.

    Again, the person answering the phone should make a note and give it to the proper authority. An assistant can call the information in to your optician. Or, a written prescription can be mailed or picked up.

- I need information about my medication.

    If your question is about dosage, anyone who can read the chart can give you the information. Usually this will be an assistant or nurse, but it may be one of the clerical staff. If you are experiencing side effects or have questions about the drug itself, an assistant or nurse will help you. If they can't answer your questions, they will ask the physician and call you back.

- I didn't understand what the doctor said about my problem.

    A clerical person may be able to help with this if he/she knows how to read the chart. An assistant or nurse will probably be able to explain the diagnosis in more detail.

- I don't remember (or don't understand) what the doctor told me to do.

    Once again, you need someone who can read the chart. A clerical person may be able to fill you in. An assistant or nurse can probably help you with the specifics.

- I need to schedule an appointment.

    The appointment secretary or receptionist is a specialist in this area.

- I can't remember when the doctor told me to come back.

    Clerical personnel (who will pull your chart or look on the computer record) can help with this.

- I don't understand my bill.

    This is a question for the people who handle the finances: cashier, secretary, insurance clerk, or payments clerk. Many medical employees won't know about billing procedures. (They will, however, probably know which procedures are billed separately from the exam fee.)

- I have questions about my insurance.

    Insurance clerks to the rescue! This is a very specialized function, so you should talk directly to whoever files claims.

- I need to make arrangements to make periodic payments.

The cashier or payment clerk can help with this. In some offices, the office manager may make such decisions.
- I need a copy of my records.

    Whoever answers the phone should be able to take your request. A file clerk may make photocopies, or a member of the medical team may dictate a letter. (Before your records can be released, however, the office will require your signature.)
- I have a new eye problem. Can you tell me what's wrong?

    No one in the office can diagnose a new problem over the phone. An assistant or nurse may be able to tell you what a problem MIGHT be, based on your description. They can also help decide whether or not your condition is an emergency. If they have any doubts, they will consult the doctor. But there is no way to know for sure (or begin treatment) without being seen.
- I had a recent exam, and I'm ready to schedule surgery.

    The secretary will probably turn your chart over to someone in the surgical department (an assistant or nurse).
- My new glasses aren't right.

    You will probably talk to an assistant or nurse. Once you have described the problem, they will advise you or ask the doctor what to do.

Staff Problems

Personnel in doctors' offices are hired to be courteous and helpful. But we're all human. If you have a recurrent problem with an employee, consider discussing it with the office manager. Management may be unaware of how an employee interacts with patients. Perhaps the employee does not even realize that he/she seems gruff or rude.

An over-booked-and-running-behind schedule is not usually the staff's fault. The schedule is set up by management or the physician based on how long it takes for the average exam and various procedures, the number of assistants, the number of exam rooms, etc. They also try to take emergencies into account. But getting a schedule to run perfectly all the time is impossible. An exam may take longer than usual. A patient may need extra attention. A procedure may take longer than first expected. More emergencies than usual may crop up that day. If you find, over a period of time, that the waiting time continues to be extensive, discuss it with the doctor him/herself. The doctor is the one with ultimate control to change things.

Phone Savvy

We covered a lot of phone know-how above by suggesting who you can ask about certain problems. A few more hints will make your phone relations with the doctor and office a breeze.

• Give your name as it appears on your record.

  This may seem obvious. But record keeping (and finding) can be a complex job! The same patient may be listed as: Margaret J. Shepherd, Peggy J. Shepherd, M. Joan Shepherd, M. J. Shepherd, Mrs. Carl Shepherd. Be sure and tell the clerk if you've had a name change, and what name appears on the record.

• Give other identifying information such as social security number or date of birth.

• If you are calling to refill a medication prescription, have the following available: name of medication, prescription number, name and phone number of pharmacy, and pharmacy hours.

  If you have run out of a medication and do not have any for the next dose, tell the secretary.

• If you are calling for a copy of your lens prescription:

  It is helpful if you can give the date of your last exam. Tell the secretary if you want the prescription mailed to you, called in, or prepared for you to pick up. If you are picking it up, ask when is a good time to drop by. If it is to be called in, give name and phone number of optician or optometrist. (You will still need to talk to the optician or optometrist yourself about frames, tints, etc.)

• Be patient.

  If the secretary takes a message, you might ask him/her when you can expect the return call. Sometimes the staff have a certain time scheduled for making phone calls. If you feel you have an emergency and have not been called in a reasonable amount of time, call back. Be sure the secretary understands your situation. If there is no emergency, you will generally be called sometime that same day.

  Many doctors do not handle phone calls personally. Office hours are busy, often with little time for lunch or other breaks. They have trained their staff to answer common questions and requests. Thus if you call and ask to speak to the doctor, you will probably be asked to talk to an assistant or nurse first. If the staff member cannot help you, he/she will usually ask the doctor, then call you back with the physician's reply.

If your call is of such a personal nature that you wish to discuss it only with the doctor, you are within your rights to refuse to talk to anyone else. In this case there are a few things you can do to help the doctor and office fill your request. First, tell the secretary if this is a medical matter. Then your chart will be made ready for the doctor when he/she calls you back. Next, ask when the doctor usually returns calls. If you call during patient hours, it is probably unrealistic to expect the doctor to call you within an hour. If you call on a surgery day, the doctor may not even come to the office for messages. When the doctor does call you, get right to the point. Have a note pad nearby to record instructions, and be sure to say "Thanks!"

• Be there.

If you are expecting a return call and have to be away from your phone, tell the secretary. Knowing when to call you (or when not to call you!) can save a lot of frustration on both ends. Give home and work phone numbers, if appropriate, and the times you can be reached at these lines.

Changing Doctors

There may be several reasons why you decide to change doctors. The most obvious is moving to another town. Or, it may have be closer to home. Other, less pleasant, reasons may include a personality conflict or a question of the doctor's integrity.

What should you do if you've decided to find a new doctor? If you are moving, ask your current doctor for a referral. He/she may have a colleague in your new town. Or he/she may at least be able to provide you with a list of doctors in that area.

If your problem is a personality conflict, consider discussing this with your physician before making a change. Maybe you can work out the misunderstanding. If you have questions about the doctor's ability, then it may be best for you to find someone else to care for you. In either of these situations, you may not feel comfortable asking for a referral, and may search for a new physician on your own.

Once you are definitely leaving the practice, there are several things you may want to ask for. One is your medical records, which we'll talk about in the next section. Other things you need are: a copy of your current glasses prescription, a prescription for enough medication to last at least one month, and copies of any special tests that have been performed. Be sure to check with the cashier to clear up any charges due before you leave. Give a forwarding address (if applicable) so any refunds due you can be forwarded.

Whose Records are They?

The legal world says that your medical records belong to you. But that does not mean that you can walk into a doctor's office, ask for your records, and carry them out the door. What do you do to get your medical files?

There are several ways to get your records. You can ask that they be released to you personally. This gives you a copy for your private files or to hand-carry to another doctor. Or you can have the office mail them directly to your new doctor. Finally, you can ask your new doctor to make the request.

Each of these methods has a common factor. They all require your signature. Without your hand-written signature or mark, the records cannot be released. You cannot get records with a phone call. This is done for your protection, to prevent unauthorized parties from obtaining your private medical information.

Many offices have a pre-printed form for you to sign. Some may be willing to mail the form to you. Others may require a witness to the signature. You can write the letter yourself, as long as you sign it. A sample appears on page 45.

It's a very simple letter. Notice that Mrs. Taylor included her social security number and date of birth. This helps the office find the correct record. If appropriate, you could state in the letter that you are moving or whatever, and thank the doctor for his/her care in the past.

The next question is, once you've requested the records, what will you get? Many offices simply make a photocopy of the entire chart (they always retain the original). In other offices, the doctor may dictate a summary of your care. In either case, photocopies of important tests (such as visual fields) are included. Some offices may charge you for each page copied or for the letter. This is perfectly legal. In addition, an office cannot refuse to release your records because you owe them money. But they can include your

---

Faye P. Taylor
123 Any Street
Any Town, USA 12345
May 25, 1995

Dr. William J. Collins
777 Heavenly St.
Somewhere, USA 54321

Dear Dr. Collins,
Please forward my records to:
Dr. Marcus Adelbert
321 First St.
Someplace, USA 98765

Sincerely,
Faye P. Taylor
SS# 123-45-6789
Birthday 10-24-57

---

financial record with your medical information.

In a busy medical practice, record copies are not usually available "on demand." It is best to allow several weeks for an office to process your request for medical files.

Getting a Second Opinion

Choosing a doctor for a second opinion should be done as carefully as selecting your original physician. What are some instances where you might benefit from a second opinion?

Some insurance companies require a second opinion before they will approve payment for surgery or treatment. This means that you must see the second doctor before the procedure is done. Your regular eye doctor should be able to recommend someone for you to see. If you call to make the second opinion appointment yourself, be sure to tell the secretary why you need to be seen.

Another case where you may want a second opinion is to get the advice of a specialist. Again, your original doctor should be able to recommend someone. If you have heard or read about special tests or treatments that your doctor does not offer, ask where you might go to have them done.

On the other hand, if a doctor recommends an unusual or "new" treatment, you may want to seek a second opinion on your own. The same holds true if you have been given a serious diagnosis such as impending blindness or life-threatening malignancy. Cer-

Paul L. James
123 Main Street
Some Town, USA 54321
May 25, 1995

Dr. Joshua F. Tam
456 First St.
Danville, USA 54321

Dear Dr. Tam,

I was in your office for an eye exam on 2/20/94. On that date I learned that I have cataracts. You and I discussed the matter, and you suggested I have cataract surgery. I wanted to think about it and talk to my family before scheduling.

About a month ago I was visiting my sister in another state. She convinced me to see her ophthalmologist. Dr. Faux agreed that I had cataracts, but said that they were not ready to be removed.

You can understand my confusion! Please write or call me with your suggestions of what I should do next. Is there some type of test that might tell me, on paper, if the cataracts are ready to come out yet?

I appreciate your kind attention to this matter.

Sincerely,
Paul James
SS# 987-65-4321
Birthday: 06/11/28

tainly in these cases you will want an additional opinion.

When Opinions Differ

In its most basic sense, medical care involves hiring a doctor to give you an opinion. What do you do when one doctor says one thing, and another doctor says another?

First, no one is perfect, and no one can know everything. Medicine itself is not perfect, and there are never any guarantees. Without any evidence to the contrary, it is best to assume that each doctor is acting out of his/her knowledge and experience.

But what can you do? How far you go in trying to find the answers depends on how important finding those answers are to you.

1. One option is to get a third opinion. Be up front and honest with the third doctor. Let him/her know about the other two opinions. You don't have to say who the other doctors were if you don't want to.
2. If you have been seeing "general" eye care physicians, consider seeing someone who specializes in your condition.

3. Talk to one or both of the doctors. Remember that we are all human. Try to choose words that are non-threatening and don't blame anyone. If you decide to discuss the problem on the phone, be considerate. You may feel more comfortable writing a letter. See sample letter on the previous page.

Notice that the letter does not accuse anyone. There are no strong words and no threats. It is a letter that a physician can feel comfortable about answering. (Once again the patient has included information to make finding his chart easier: social security number and date of birth.)

Now that you know who's who and where you're going, we'll take a look at what to expect from a "routine" eye exam . . . in the next chapter.

CHAPTER 3

Your Eye Exam

HOW prevalent are vision and eye problems? Approximately one third of the 80 million Americans with eye disease wait to seek help until it is too late to prevent vision loss. An annual eye exam can help you be sure that your vision is up to par and detect any disease or other problems.

What To Take To Your Eye Exam

1. Your glasses. Take the glasses that you *usually wear,* even if they're only reading glasses from the dime-store. There is no need to take all the glasses you've ever owned. (Why don't you consider donating those old frames to a charitable organization like the Lion's Club?)

   There are instances when taking other glasses may be helpful: Rebecca Hess had her eyes examined two years ago. She got a prescription for new glasses at that time. When she got the new glasses, however, she couldn't seem to get used to them. So she went back to her old glasses. She should bring *both pairs* of glasses to her next eye exam: the pair she usually wears (the old ones) and the pair that didn't work (the new ones).

2. Your contact lenses. If you've been instructed not to wear them, take your lenses along. The doctor may want to look at the lenses under magnification, or he/she may ask you to put them on briefly. Be sure to take your case and solutions.

3. Medications. Put *all* the medications you take in a bag and take them with you. Don't forget vitamins and any over-the-counter medications you use regularly (for example aspirin taken daily as a blood thinner). Remember your birth control pills and hormones, ladies. Don't forget any patches, liquids, and injections. If you get injections or treatments at another doctor's office, write it down to tell your eye doctor. (Examples

are allergy shots, hormone injections, radiation treatment, and chemotherapy.) Above all, don't forget any eye drops that you use. If you have been treating an eye problem, take along any over-the-counter or prescription treatments that you've tried.

4. A list of medications that have caused allergic reactions or side effects. Give the name and the specific reaction (such as rash or shortness of breath).

5. Your insurance cards. Also, be sure to take any Medicare, Medicaid, and supplemental insurance cards that you may have. You don't need the policies, just the cards. Most offices will make a copy of your cards to keep in your record. Some offices file for visits and some don't, but no one can file unless they have your company and policy number.

6. Any records from previous doctors. If you have records from seeing another doctor, be sure and take them along. It is usually best to have your records mailed directly to your new doctor. But if you happen to have a personal copy, take it along. (It's a good idea to have an extra copy made: one for your new record and one for you to keep in your files.)

7. A list of questions you want to ask. This is a great way to be sure that you get all the answers you need. It will also save phone calls later.

8. A record of your problem. If you have read about your symptoms in Chapter 4, your answers to "What your doctor needs to know" provide important information.

9. Measurements of work distances. If you need a special pair of glasses for a specific activity, or if you work at an unusual distance, the doctor needs to know. Examples could include the distance to: speedometer, podium, sewing machine, desk, computer screen, typewriter, saw, drafting table, shelf, cash register.

10. An old photograph of yourself. If you are seeing the doctor because you believe something about your appearance has changed (such as a lid droop or head tilt), an old photo can be invaluable.

11. A book, magazine, puzzle book, handwork, stationary, or something else to occupy your waiting time (in case you don't care for the office magazines).

12. A friend or family member. This will give you someone to chat with while you wait. Also, if you are nervous about your exam, taking someone who cares can ease your mind. Most offices

are glad to let your friend accompany you into the exam room if you wish. While most people can drive with dilated pupils, you may feel more secure having a driver along.

13. A pair of sunglasses. Even if you are not driving, you will be more comfortable wearing sunglasses outside after your pupils are dilated.

When You Arrive

When you get to the doctor's office, you will need to let someone know you're there. Some offices have a sign-in sheet. At others, you report to the receptionist. If this is your first visit, remind the receptionist. She will probably need you to fill out a patient form for your medical record. Be sure to fill it out completely. This will help the office get to know you and help them serve you better. Once you have finished the form, take it back to the receptionist along with your insurance cards. Some offices also like to make a copy of your driver's license for identification purposes. At this point, you may want to ask the receptionist if the doctor is running behind. That way you'll have some idea of how soon you'll be called. (Waiting isn't as bad if you know you're going to have to do it!) If you have some type of special circumstance (such as caring for an invalid spouse, or you are a diabetic who must eat at certain times, etc.) be sure to let the receptionist know. She may be able to help reduce your wait, or she may suggest that you return on another day that is more convenient.

The next thing you should to do is relax! Find a comfortable chair. If 45 minutes go by, you might want to politely check with the receptionist again about when you'll be called. If the doctor has had an emergency or is running behind, she should tell you. Plus, it is always impossible to tell just how much time any one exam will take. Be as patient as possible. However, if the waiting time exceeds your ability to wait, you may want to consider rescheduling your appointment for another day.

The History

Often an assistant will call you back to an exam room. Sometimes the doctor does. If you have brought a family member or friend with you, feel free to ask that they accompany you into the exam room. This gives you an extra pair of ears to hear what the doctor says. This is especially important if you have a hearing problem or need an interpreter (in the case of deafness or foreign language).

The exam usually begins with introductions. Then the assistant will begin asking you questions. This is called "taking the history." These are among the things you will be asked:

- the type of eye problem that brings you in
- your past eye problems (including trauma, surgery, etc.)
- family history of eye problems (such as cataracts and glaucoma)
- your general health
- medications you take
- allergies

To the assistant, the history is like being a detective and following a trail. Certain responses on your part indicate further questions that need to be asked. If a question seems too personal, you might want to ask, "Why do you need to know that?" The assistant shouldn't mind explaining why a certain piece of information is needed. If you feel more comfortable discussing certain topics with the doctor only, politely tell the assistant. In general the questions asked during an eye exam aren't that intimate. However, the information that you give during the history is strictly confidential.

Once the history is taken, the testing generally begins. This is often done by an assistant, but may be done by the physician. Follow directions as best you can. Ask questions if you don't understand what you're being asked to do. The following sections describe the most common screening tests done in the average office or clinic.

Visual Acuity

This is merely "reading the eye chart." It is generally done at distance and near, with and without glasses. One eye is covered while the vision in the other eye is tested. For the patient who cannot read, a chart with numbers or pictures can be used. You are simply asked to read the smallest line that you can see well enough to recognize. The distant chart in many offices may be a poster on the wall. Other offices use projectors or have viewers that you look into. Checking near vision may be done with a hand-held card or a viewer. It is alright to guess when reading the eye chart if you think you can make a reasonable stab at it. Even an incorrect answer can be helpful. (For example if you call an F a P, the assistant knows you can *almost* see it. Calling a V an O is a different story.)

Patients often want to know what their vision is. What does 20/20 mean, anyway? The first "20" refers to the actual distance from the chart. This is standardized at twenty feet. (Not all exam rooms are 20 feet long, of course. These offices have adjusted their projectors to simulate 20 feet.) The second number refers to the size of letters that a person can read. For example, 20/40 means that this patient read from 20 feet away what someone with normal vision could see from 40 feet away. 20/200 means that the patient read from 20 feet away what a person with normal vision could see from 200 feet. "20/20 vision" is considered normal because the patient saw from 20 feet away what a person with normal vision can see at 20 feet. Thus the higher the second number is, the weaker the vision is.

Eye Muscle Movement Testing

Medically, this test is known as the "range of motion" evaluation. Six muscles are attached to each eye. Watching the way the eyes move gives valuable information on both the muscles and the nerves that control the eyes' motion. You will be asked to keep both eyes open and follow a light or other object as the assistant moves it.

Eye Muscle Balance Testing

This is a test that evaluates how well the eyes move and work as a team. There are a variety of ways that this can be tested . . . too many to describe here. The simplest way, though, is to have the patient look at an object (maybe a single letter on the eye chart) while the assistant covers one eye, then the other. The assistant watches to see if the eyes shift as the cover is moved.

Muscle balance can also be tested using prisms, a viewer, a red and/or white light, and other methods. Any of these tests is painless and takes a minute or less. If you're really curious, ask the assistant how your muscle balance will be tested, and he/she can explain the test that the office uses.

Pupils

Examination of the pupils gives an indication of how the optic nerve is functioning. The assistant uses a small flashlight to look at your pupils in a darkened room. He/she will note the size and shape of the pupils, as well as how they react to light. This takes less than half a minute.

Confrontation Visual Fields

A screening of your side, or peripheral vision, takes only a minute. One eye is covered, and you are asked to look at the assistant's nose. The assistant then brings his/her hand in from the side (or top, or bottom) and asks you when you can first see the hand. Or he/she may ask you to count how many fingers are being held up. All this is done without looking at the assistant's hand: you are looking straight at the assistant's face, and using your side vision to see the hand. This test can be surprisingly accurate, but it is only a rough test. For more sophisticated measurement, a perimeter will be used (described in Chapter 18)

Reading Lens Prescriptions

The assistant will put your glasses on a machine (called a lensometer) that reads the prescription of your lenses. This gives a starting place to use when testing to see if the glasses need changing. It is also used to see if glasses are filled according to the prescription. If you brought a pair of glasses that you "couldn't get used to," these are read to let the doctor know what doesn't work. This can help prevent repeated problems.

Refraction

"Refraction" refers to the test that determines what glasses prescription you need. There are several instruments the assistant or physician can use in this important part of your exam:

Auto-refractor: The auto-refractor is a computerized instrument with a viewer that you look into. It evaluates your eye using a light, and gives a readout of the prescription you need. The doctor does not prescribe this reading, but uses it as a starting point. You will still be checked using lenses. Not all offices have an auto-refractor. They're nice, but you're not missing too much if your doctor doesn't use one.

Retinoscope: This is a special hand-held light that the assistant or physician uses to evaluate your eyes for glasses. You are usually asked to look at an object in the distance while the assistant looks at each eye with the light. Often lenses will be added as the assistant moves the light up and down, back and forth. Like the auto-refractor, the retinoscope gives a starting point. You will still be checked using regular lenses.

Trial frames: The trial frames are a special pair of glasses that have rims for holding lenses. Lenses are inserted and removed by hand. Although most offices will use a refractor (below), trial frames are still needed in some cases. Most every office will have a set.

Refractor: The refractor is an instrument with rotating lenses inside it. Most offices have one because it is much more convenient to use than trial frames. Also, it does not sit directly on the patient's face like the trial frames.

The refraction itself is simple and takes only five or ten minutes. The assistant asks you to look at the letters as he/she changes the lens. The lenses are often referred to by number, and the assistant may say, "Which lens makes the letters seem clearer? Number One . . . or Number Two?" All you have to do is identify which lens seems the sharpest. Tell the examiner if:

1. you don't understand what he/she is asking you to do.
2. the letters look the same with either lens (actually, this is good news).
3. the lenses are changed too quickly for you to tell the difference.
4. you would like the assistant to show you the two lenses again before you decide.

You may be wondering why it's good news if the lenses look the same. It would seem that this would make things more complicated. Actually most of what we are doing when we change lenses during a measurement is *straddling* a specific setting. If one lens is better, that means we need to change the lenses in a certain direction. If the lenses look the same, then we know we are straddling the correct setting.

Be sure to blink during the test. If you stare, your eye may dry out and blur your vision. Don't press too tightly against the refractor, as this may fog the lens. If your eye starts to water and your vision blurs, ask for a tissue. If you are uncomfortable and would like the refractor moved to a different position, tell the assistant.

A few people really hate this test and are nervous about it. They worry that they will give the "wrong" answer, and their prescription won't be accurate. Try to relax! The only "wrong" thing you can do is to *lie* about which lens is best! An experienced assistant or physician is accustomed to interpreting responses and reactions. If they have any doubts about a reply, they will double check. One little "click" one way or the other *usually* doesn't make that much difference anyway. So just do the best you can without undue strain.

Microscope Evaluation

The microscope used to evaluate the eye is called a slit lamp microscope. It is actually an ordinary microscope that has been fitted with special light controls and filters for examining the eye. You simply lean up to the instrument and place your chin and forehead in the headrest. The assistant or physician then carefully observes each eye. He/she will survey the skin, lashes, eyelids, conjunctiva, sclera, cornea, iris, pupil, and lens (see Chapter 1 for a description of each of these structures). Contact lenses are also evaluated with the slit lamp. An additional attachment to the microscope, called a Hruby lens (pronounced "ruby"), allows a view of the vitreous and retina.

Although the light may be bright, it is not an X-ray or laser. The assistant or physician may spend several minutes looking at your eyes in various lights and magnifications. Virtually every eye physician's office will have a slit lamp, and it is generally used on every patient during every exam.

Tonometry

Tonometry is a test which measures the pressure inside the eye. Aqueous (the watery fluid inside the eye) is constantly being formed and then drained out of the eye. This creates a normal pressure inside the eye. However, if the fluid does not drain out properly, the fluid can build up and cause the pressure to rise. If the pressure rises high enough or stays high over a period of time, the optic nerve can be damaged. (This condition is known as glaucoma, Chapter 14). Tonometry is a quick, painless test that should be part of every full eye exam. People whose family members have glaucoma, plus those over 40, should have their pressure checked every year.

The instrument used to measure pressure is called a tonometer. The most common and accurate type, called a Goldmann tonometer, is attached to the slit lamp microscope. First a drop of yellow numbing drops is placed in each eye. Then you lean up to the slit lamp. The assistant will ask you to keep both eyes open and look straight ahead (perhaps at a small light). Often he or she will hold your eyelids open for you. The tip of the tonometer is brought forward to contact the eye. Because of the drops, this is not uncomfortable. If you can keep from blinking, you should not feel anything at all. If you blink, you may feel the tonometer tip against your lids. Even though this is not painful, it may make you blink even more. Try to keep both eyes open. The measurement itself takes five or ten seconds. Most offices will have this type of tonometer.

There are other types of tonometers, but they are generally not as accurate. Most of these are held in the assistant's hand. Some instruments can be used while you are sitting up; for others you must lie back. After a numbing drop, the assistant gently applies the tip of the tonometer. Try to keep both eyes open and look straight ahead (or up).

In the past, you may have had your pressure checked using an air-puff tonometer. This instrument does not touch the eye, so no drops are needed. After aligning the instrument with your eye, it releases a puff of air. The air puff may startle you, but it does not hurt. The measurement is automatically printed out. This type of tonometer is often used for public screening, such as a health fair. Some industries also use them as a part of the company physical. The air-puff is useful for evaluating large numbers of people quickly, but it can miss some cases of high pressure. It is also useful in children or patients who cannot tolerate the Goldmann (usually because they can't stop blinking). Some eye physicians use the air puff to screen their patients. Other offices don't have this type of tonometer.

What is a normal pressure? Medical opinions vary. Usually if the pressure is 20 or below, it is considered normal. But there are individual exceptions to the rule. Whether or not a pressure is normal depends on whether or not the optic nerve is being damaged. For example, Amanda Rice's pressure is 24. Normally that would be considered high. But her optic nerve is healthy. Her physician considers this "high" pressure to be normal for her, although he cautions her to have her pressure checked every six months. Then there's Shelly DuMont. His pressure is 16, but his optic nerves show signs of damage. He has been diagnosed as having glaucoma and placed on eye drops to lower his "normal" looking pressure even more.

The pressure is checked in each eye. The pressure in one eye may be a point or two higher that the other eye. It is also possible to have normal pressure in one eye and glaucoma in the other. See Chapter 14 for more on glaucoma.

Dilation and Fundus Exam

Dilating the pupils is a very important part of your eye exam. The eye drops cause the pupils to open wide, and hold this position for several hours. There are different types of drops that can be used for this purpose. Some are stronger, open the pupils wider, and take longer to wear off. Some are weaker and wear off quicker. The strongest type can last for over a week. The weaker type, the kind usually used for exam purposes, wear off in several hours. In most cases, the drops blur only your close-up (reading) vision. Your driving vision is not usually altered (but there are exceptions). Since the pupils cannot constrict (become smaller) for a while, you may be light sensitive. Take a pair of sunglasses to wear when you drive home after your exam, to cut down on the glare. Most offices provide sunglasses for their patients who have been dilated. You don't have to wear the sunglasses if you don't want to: your eyes will not be damaged if you choose not to wear them. But you will probably be a lot more comfortable if you do!

Dilation is important because it allows the doctor to get a good look at the vitreous, retina, optic nerve, blood vessels, and other parts of the eye's interior. The special light that the physician uses to see the retina is rather bright. The pupil would normally get smaller in response to the light. Then the doctor would be able to see less. Dilation holds the pupils open so he/she can get a good look.

Dilation should be done annually. People with diabetes and high blood pressure should take special care to be dilated once a year, because those conditions can damage the retina and blood vessels. Patients with retinal problems may be dilated more often.

To examine the fundus ("fundus" is the general term for everything the doctor can see in the back of the eye), the physician uses

an instrument called an ophthalmoscope. One type of ophthalmoscope is held in the doctor's hand. He/she looks through the
instrument into your eye from an inch or so away. The light may
be bright, but the instrument does not touch the eye . . . so there
is no pain. Another type of ophthalmoscope has two parts. One
is worn on the doctor's head. Then a hand-held lens is positioned
several inches from your eye. Again, nothing touches the eye. You
may be lying back or sitting during this exam. Finally, a special
lens on the slit lamp microscope, the Hruby lens, may be used to
view the eye's interior. In this case, you sit up to the microscope
with your chin and forehead in the head rest. The lens gets close
to the eye, but does not touch it.

For any type of fundus exam, it is best if you can keep both eyes
open. It is alright if you must blink, but try to keep from closing
or fluttering your eyelids. The physician will tell you where to look.
He/she will generally have you look straight ahead, up, down, right,
and left. This allows him/her to look at different parts of the retina.

Diagnosis and Treatment

Once the assistant has completed the screening tests and the
physician has examined you, the doctor will go over his/her findings
with you. He/she should explain your condition in words that you
can understand. Often the physician first tells about the condition
of your eyes, then gives the reason(s) for that condition. Finally,
you will be told what needs to be done, and what to expect. Several
examples follow:

1. "Mrs. Andrews, our tests show that you are having some trouble
   seeing up close. This is just a normal progression of your presbyopia. Presbyopia is the loss of reading vision that generally
   starts around age 40 and continues to worsen until about age
   60. I'm writing you a prescription to strengthen your bifocals.
   Otherwise your eyes are healthy, and I'll see you back in one
   year."
2. "Mr. Phillips, your distant vision has fallen off a lot. When I
   examined you with the microscope, I could see cataracts. Cataracts are a clouding of the eye's natural lens, behind the pupil.
   This cloudiness has caused your vision to get worse. Our testing
   shows that changing glasses won't help. It's gotten bad enough

that I suggest we do surgery to remove the cataract. The back of your eye looks pretty good, and your pressure is fine. My nurse will set up a date that's convenient for you to have the surgery. Do you have any questions?"

3. "Mr. Roberts, I could see the floaters you had noticed when I looked inside your eye. The flashes of light that you mentioned are caused by the jelly inside your eye being pulled away from the retina. It's not unusual for this to happen to someone over forty, like yourself. Now, I want you to understand that this is *not* a retinal detachment. I checked your retina and saw no holes or tears. Only the jelly, called the vitreous, has pulled away. It's nothing to worry about. Very rarely, a person will develop a retinal detachment later after the vitreous detaches. So I want you to help me out. As long as the floaters and flashes stay the same or get no worse, you're fine. But if you get a shower of more floaters, you notice a curtain or veil over part of your vision, or your vision blacks out, I want you to call me right away. I don't expect that to happen, but we do want to keep tabs on it. Here is a brochure explaining your condition. Look it over at home. Then let me know if anything comes up. Otherwise I'll see you in six months."

Before You Leave

Before you leave your physician's office, you should:

1. be sure that you have any prescriptions for glasses or medications (including refills).
2. be sure that you understand what you've been told about your condition and treatment.
3. know when you need to return for another exam (and to whom, if you are being referred to another doctor).
4. have any written instructions needed (such as how to instill eye drops or how often to use medications).
5. have any brochures or written material about your condition, if they are available (Some offices have audio tapes and/or video tapes that you can have, borrow, or use in the office. Be sure to ask!).

Types of Examinations

A regularly scheduled eye exam is one of the most important

keys to maintaining visual health. An annual, complete, or routine eye exam will generally include all of the tests we've discussed here.

There is more than one type of eye exam, however. A follow up exam may be scheduled to check on a specific on-going problem, such as glaucoma. In this case, the testing will be limited to the problem itself. If you need such follow up exams, there may be a charge for every visit. If you have had surgery, the surgery fee may include the follow up appointments. Check with your doctor or cashier to find out.

Testing is often limited in an exam for an emergency problem. For example, if you call the office about a red watery eye, you will probably not be scheduled for a complete exam including dilation and refraction. You will be given a shorter appointment slot that will allow the doctor to address the problem causing you distress. If you also need a full exam, you can schedule that at a later date, once your problem has been taken care of.

Other procedures may be too time-consuming for the staff to perform on the spot, so they set aside certain days for them. These specialty appointments might include a photography session, being measured for surgery, surgery counseling, contact lens fitting, a visual field test, or other specific tests.

Now that you are familiar with the routine workings of an eye exam, you can see why each test is important to your annual check-up. But what are some of the unexpected symptoms that might drive you to the eye doctor between yearly visits? We'll take a look at them in the next chapter.

CHAPTER 4

Symptoms of Eye Trouble

L IKE most of us, Marion Marcella took her vision for granted until something went wrong. She began to notice halos around lights at night. She called her eye doctor. The receptionist began firing questions at her: Was it one eye, or both? (She hadn't tried covering one eye to find out.) Is either eye red? (She hadn't noticed.) Marion hung up the phone wishing she had been more observant. The tone of the receptionist indicated that this could be a serious problem. *But just exactly what was she fishing for with her questions?*, Marion wondered.

This chapter lists various symptoms that may indicate eye problems. The information is divided into two sections. Section One (starts on this page) discusses symptoms of a visual nature. Section Two (page 71) lists physical symptoms. Symptoms are listed alphabetically. If you don't find a particular item, try wording it a different way. (For example, "flashing lights" is listed as "light flashes.")

Following each symptom is a list of questions that your doctor will need answered. After the questions is a list of possible causes of each symptom. This list is included to help you understand what may be happening and why. (Please check the Index or Contents to find more information on these conditions.)

But remember: ONLY YOUR EYE CARE PHYSICIAN CAN DIAGNOSE ANY PROBLEMS! Don't decide for yourself what's wrong based on these lists. Our goal is to inform you, not tell you how to diagnose yourself. Only your eye doctor is trained to do that.

Section One: Visual Symptoms

Blurry Vision

What your doctor needs to know:
- When did the blurred vision start?

- Did it begin gradually and get worse slowly, or was it sudden?
- Is it blurred only in the distance? Only close up? Or both?
- Does the blurring come and go?
- Is it in one eye or both?
- Is it a general blurring, or just in a certain spot (like a cloud or a curtain)?

Possible causes: change in glasses prescription, cataract, blood sugar fluctuations, diabetes, poor blood pressure control, drug reaction, angle closure glaucoma, retinal detachment, inflammation inside the eye, fatigue, hunger, vitamin deficiency, hormonal disorders, fainting, heart failure, arteriosclerosis, large floater

Color Vision, Change In

What your doctor needs to know:
- When did you first notice the change?
- Have both eyes changed? Or just one?
- What colors seem to be most affected? Greens? Blues and Purples?
- Have you been told that you have cataracts?
- Are you taking Placquinil™ (hydroxychloroquine)?

Possible causes: cataracts, drug reaction, diabetes, glaucoma

Curtain Over the Vision

What your doctor needs to know:
- When did you first notice the curtain?
- Which eye is affected?
- Can you see through the curtain, or is it solid?
- Where does the curtain seem to be coming from: the top, bottom?
- Have you had a blow to the eye?
- Have you had any type of eye surgery?
- Have you seen any light flashes?
- Does the curtain swish around when you move your eye?

Possible causes: retinal detachment, posterior vitreous detachment, hemorrhage

Distorted Vision

What your doctor needs to know:
- When did you first notice this?
- Is the distortion in one eye or both?

- Is it constant, or does it come and go?
- Describe the distortion. (Parts of words missing or crooked, round objects appear oblong, straight lines appear wavy, etc.)

    Possible causes: macular degeneration, astigmatism, inflammation inside the eye, retinal detachment or hole

Double Vision

What your doctor needs to know:
- When did the double vision start?
- Is your vision double all the time or just some of the time?
- Is your vision doubled when you look into the distance, up close, or both?
- Is the second image above, to the side, or at an angle from the first image?
- Does the double image go away if you cover one eye?
- Does the double image go away or get worse if you tilt or turn your head a certain way?
- Is your vision doubled with your glasses, without, or both?
- Could your glasses be out of line, or have you just gotten new glasses?
- Have you been told that you have a cataract?
- Have you had a head injury?
- Are you diabetic?
- Do you take Vitamin A? How much?

    Possible causes: Paralysis of one or more of the muscles that move the eye, misaligned glasses, cataract, dislocation of intraocular lens implant, head trauma, dislocation of the lens, fluid behind the eye, fracture of the bones around the eye, large difference in glasses correction between the eyes, stroke, multiple sclerosis, thyroid trouble, diabetes, vitamin toxicity

Fluctuating Vision

What your doctor needs to know:
- How long has this been going on?
- Does this occur in one eye or both?
- Does the vision just get blurry, or does it black out?
- Do you have diabetes?
- When did you last have your blood sugar checked?
- Is there a history of diabetes in the family?

- Have you been told that you have cataracts?
- Have you had any type of eye surgery?
- Do you use any type of eye drops or ointment?
- Do you have any type of discharge from the eyes?
- When does the blurring occur? For example: Just in the mornings? Or mostly when reading?

    Possible causes: diabetic blood sugar fluctuations, cataracts, ointment or matter in the eye, dry eyes, blood vessel disease

Glare

What your doctor needs to know:
- How long has this been bothering you?
- Does your vision worsen in bright sunlight?
- Are you having a problem with headlights from oncoming cars at night?
- Have you been told that you have cataracts?
- Have you had cataract surgery?

    Possible causes: cataract, corneal scar or dystrophy, capsule opacity after cataract surgery, drug reaction

Halos Around Lights at Night

What your doctor needs to know:
- How long have you noticed this?
- Is it happening in one eye or both?
- Have you been told that you have cataracts?
- Is the eye ever painful?
- Are you having headaches?
- Is the eye ever red?
- Do you notice this all the time, or just now and then?

    Possible causes: glaucoma, cataracts, mucus on the cornea, corneal scar, drug reaction, exposure to intense light, dislocated intraocular lens implant, water-logged cornea (corneal edema)

Improvement of Near Vision

(OR noticing you don't need your reading glasses anymore, when you used to HAVE to have them.)

What your doctor needs to know:
- When did you first notice this?
- Has it been a gradual change?

- Is it in one eye or both?
- Have you been told that you have cataracts?
- Have you had cataract surgery?
  Possible cause: cataracts, cloudy capsule after cataract surgery

Light Flashes

What your doctor needs to know:
- When did this start?
- How often do you see the flashes?
- How long does it last? A second? Thirty minutes?
- Is it constant, or does it come and go?
- Which eye is affected?
- Have you also had any floaters (specks), spots, or curtains?
- Do you see the lights even with your eyes closed?
- Have you had a blow to the eye?
- Have you had eye surgery?
- Has your vision been affected?
- Do you have a headache after the lights disappear?
  Possible causes: posterior vitreous detachment, retinal detachment or tear, migraine headache, ocular migraine (without headache), brain concussion, glaucoma

Loss of Central Vision

What your doctor needs to know:
- When did you first notice this?
- Did your vision fade out gradually or go out suddenly?
- Does this come and go, or is it constant?
- Is your center vision totally blacked out or just foggy?
- Did you have a headache after this occurred?
  Possible causes: stroke, macular degeneration, retinal tear or hole, migraine, drug reaction, nutritional deficiency

Loss of Depth Perception

What your doctor needs to know:
- When did you first notice this?
- Have you recently lost vision in one eye?
- Is your vision good in one eye and poor in the other?
- Have you been told that you have cataracts?

- Possible causes: cataract, difference in vision between the two eyes, loss of vision in one eye

     Possible causes: cataract, difference in vision between the two eyes, loss of vision in one eye

Loss of Near Vision

What your doctor needs to know:
- When did you first notice this?
- Has it changed gradually, or suddenly?
- Is it in one eye or both?
- Is it with your glasses on? Off? Or both?
- Is it constant, or does it come and go?
- What exactly have you noticed that you are unable to see? The newspaper or phone book? Threading a needle? The speedometer? Something on a grocery shelf?
- Are you using any type of eye drop with a red top?

     Possible causes: age, need for glasses change, cataract, drug reaction

Loss of Side Vision

What your doctor needs to know:
- When did you first notice this?
- Is it in both eyes or just one?
- Does it come and go, or is it constant?
- Have you noticed any flashes of light?
- Have you had a blow to the eye?
- Have you been told that you have glaucoma?

     Possible causes: retinal detachment, glaucoma, pituitary tumor, stroke

Loss of Upper Vision

What your doctor needs to know:
- When did you first notice this?
- Is it in one eye or both?
- Does it come and go, or is it constant?
- Have you noticed any flashes of light?
- Have you had a blow to the eye?
- Is extra skin from your upper lids hanging down into your eyes?

     Possible causes: drooping eyelids, retinal detachment

Loss of Vision (Gradual)

What your doctor needs to know:
- When did you first notice the decrease?
- Is the decrease in one eye or both?
- Is the decrease constant, or does it come and go?
- Do you notice this more close up (for reading) or at a distance?
- When did you last have your glasses changed?
- Do you take Vitamin B? How much?

   Possible causes: need to change glasses, cataracts, diabetes, vitamin toxicity, drug reaction

Loss of Vision (Sudden)

What your doctor needs to know:
- When did you first notice this?
- Which eye is affected?
- Is your vision totally blacked out in that eye, or can you see light? Movement?
- Do you have hardening of the arteries?
- Is the eye painful?
- Is the eye red?
- Have you had injury or surgery to the eye?

   Possible causes: angle closure glaucoma, stroke, brain injury, retinal detachment, temporal arteritis, hemorrhage inside the eye, drug reaction, optic nerve disease, blockage of vein or artery inside eye, psychological

Poor Night Vision

What your doctor needs to know:
- When did this start?
- Is there a history of night blindness in the family?
- Are you mainly bothered by glare from oncoming headlights at night?

   Possible causes: cataracts, retinitis pigmentosa, malnutrition (Vitamin A deficiency), advanced glaucoma

Specks Before The Eyes (Floaters)

What your doctor needs to know:
- When did you first notice the floaters?

- Which eye, or both?
- When do you see them?
- Describe the shape: spider-web, hair, specks/bugs, a circle or half-moon, a curtain, a spot?
- Have you had a blow to the eye?
- Have you had eye surgery?
- Do they scoot around when you move your eye? Or stay in the same place?
- Has your vision decreased?
- Have the floaters increased in number or size since you first noticed them?
- Have you seen any light flashes?

    Possible causes: retinal detachment, retinal hemorrhage, posterior vitreous detachment, high nearsightedness (myopia)

Star-Bursts From Headlights

What your doctor needs to know:
- When did this start?
- Have you been told that you have cataracts?
- Have you had cataract surgery?
- Have you had corneal surgery?
- Do you have astigmatism?
- Have you had a corneal injury?
- Does this occur with your glasses on? Off? Or both?

    Possible causes: cataracts, uncorrected astigmatism, capsule opacity, displaced intraocular lens, corneal scar

Uncomfortable Vision

What your doctor needs to know:
- When did this start?
- Is it in one eye or both?
- Is the discomfort constant, or does it come and go? Does it occur during a certain part of the day?
- Describe the discomfort. (Examples: tired feeling, drawing, "just not right")
- How long has it been since you had your glasses changed?
- Have you recently had your glasses changed?

    Possible causes: eye strain, need glasses changed, incorrect prescription, eye muscle imbalance, glasses need adjusting

Section Two: Physical Symptoms

Burning

What your doctor needs to know:
- How long has this been bothering you?
- Does this happen especially during a certain part of the day?
- Does this happen when you are doing a certain activity? (Such as reading or watching TV?)
- Do your eyes also water?
- Have you tried any kind of eye drops to clear this up? Did it help?
- Are you taking any kind of antihistamines, sinus, cold, or allergy medication?

Possible causes: dry eyes, staring (forgetting to blink while reading or watching TV), allergy, drug reaction

Crusting Lids

What your doctor needs to know:
- When did this start?
- Is it in one eye, or both?
- Are your eyes matted shut in the morning?
- Are the crusts on your lashes? Or just in the corners of your eyes?
- Is there any redness, watering, itching, burning, or pain?
- Have you tried treating this yourself? How? Did it help?

Possible causes: low-grade lid infection (blepharitis), infection

Difference in Pupil Size

What your doctor needs to know:
- When did you first notice this?
- Do you use a green-top drop in one eye?
- Do you use a red-top drop in one eye?
- Have you had an injury?
- Have you had any type of eye surgery?
- Is the vision in either eye blurred?
- Is the eye with the smaller pupil sensitive to light? Red?
- Is the eye with the larger pupil sensitive to light? Red? Painful? Blurred vision?

Possible causes: congenital (born with it), angle closure glaucoma, surgery, trauma, inflammation inside the eye, drug reaction, optic nerve damage

Growths

What your doctor needs to know:
* When did you first notice the growth?
* Has it changed? Grown? Changed color?
* Does the growth ever bleed? Ooze or weep? Crust over?
* Have you tried to treat it yourself?
* Is the growth tender and sore?
* Have you ever had any type of skin cancer?
   Possible causes: mole, allergic reaction, cholesterol deposit, stye, chalazion, cancer, wart, cyst

Headaches

What your doctor needs to know:
* How long has this been bothering you?
* What part of your head hurts?
* How long does the headache last?
* How often do you have a headache?
* Have you taken any medication to relieve it? Did that help?
* What activities make the headache better? Worse?
* Is the headache centered around one eye? If so, does the eye turn red and the vision decrease when it hurts?
* Does it hurt worse when you bend over?
* Do you have high blood pressure?
* Is there a rash on your forehead?
* Are you using any type of eye drops?
* Have you just started any new medication?
   Possible causes: angle closure glaucoma, migraine, sinus, eye muscle imbalance, drug reaction, shingles, high blood pressure

Itching

What your doctor needs to know:
* When did this start? Is it in one eye, or both?
* Where does it itch? (Example: lids, edge of lids, corners of eye)
   Possible causes: allergies (hay fever), drug reaction, contact allergy (to makeup, lotions, etc.)

Jumping Eyelid

What your doctor needs to know:
- How long has this been bothering you?
- Do you consume a lot of caffeine (coffee, tea, colas, chocolate)?
- Have you been having trouble sleeping?
- Are you under more stress than usual?
- Have you had injury or surgery to the eye?

Possible causes: too much caffeine, fatigue, stress, drug reaction, Parkinson's disease, response to eye injury/pain

Lid Droop

What your doctor needs to know:
- When did you first notice this? Has it been this way all your life?
- Is this in one eye or both?
- Are the upper lids drooping or the lower lids? Both?
- Is the lid swollen?
- Have you had cataract surgery on the drooping side?
- Have you had an eye injury?
- Does there seem to be a lump or growth in the lid?
- Do you have any type of muscular disorder?

Possible causes: birth defect, loss of muscle tone, redundant skin of upper lids, growth, injury that has damaged lid muscles, nerve paralysis, muscular dystrophy, myasthenia gravis

Light Sensitivity

What your doctor needs to know:
- When did this start?
- Is it in one eye or both?
- Do you also have eye pain? Redness? Discharge?
- Have you had any type of eye surgery?
- Have you had an injury to your eye (even years ago)?
- Are you using any type of eye drop with a red top?
- Has your vision also decreased?

Possible causes: inflammation inside the eye, dilated pupil, drug reaction, migraine

Matter/Discharge

What your doctor needs to know:
- When did this start?
- Are both eyes affected, or just one?
- Are your eyes uncomfortable? Itch? Burn? Hurt? Red? Have you used any eye drops or done anything else to try to clear this up? Did it help?
- Have you been exposed to someone with an eye infection?
    Possible causes: infection, allergy

Pain

What your doctor needs to know:
- How long has this been bothering you?
- Is it in one eye, or both?
- Is the pain constant, or does it come and go?
- Does it bother you more during a certain part of the day?
- How long does the pain last?
- Does it hurt so bad that you also feel sick to your stomach?
- Do you also have a headache?
- Has your vision changed?
- Does your vision decrease when the eye is hurting?
- Describe the pain: throb, shooting, ache, gritty/sandy.
- Does your eye turn red when it is hurting?
- Do you use any type of eye drop? Or have you just begun using some sort of eye drop?
- Have you had eye surgery?
- Have you ever had an eye injury (even years ago)?
- Do your eyes close all the way when you sleep?
- Have you been exposed to a sun lamp, strong sun, or reflected sun (water or snow)?
- Have you been welding without eye protection?
    Possible causes: dry eyes, foreign body, angle closure glaucoma, drug reaction, corneal abrasion, inflammation inside the eye, eye infection, recurrent erosion syndrome, ultraviolet burn

Pressure Sensation Behind the Eyes

What your doctor needs to know:
- When did this start?

- Is it in one eye, or both?
- Do you have sinus problems?
- Have you recently had your glasses changed?
     Possible causes: sinus, misaligned glasses

Protrusion of the Eye(s)

What your doctor needs to know:
- How long have you noticed this?
- Does only one eye seem to be pushing out, or both?
- Do you have thyroid problems?
- Do you take steroids?
- Do you take Vitamin A, B, and/or D? How much?
- Is there any pain?
- Do you have sinus problems?
     Possible causes: thyroid (Graves' disease), drooping lid (lid droop of one eye can make it look as if the other eye is protruding), growth behind the eye, drug or vitamin toxicity, inflammation or infection behind the eye (as in sinus)

Pulling Sensation

What your doctor needs to know:
- When did this start?
- Do both eyes seem to pull, or just one?
- Does this occur with glasses on? Off? Either way?
- Do you have double vision?
- Is it constant, or does the sensation come and go?
- Have you recently had your glasses changed?
     Possible causes: misaligned glasses, incorrect glasses prescription

Rash

What your doctor needs to know:
- When did this start?
- Have you started some new medication?
- Have you been out in the woods, or doing yard work?
- Have you changed brands of eye makeup?
- Are just the lids affected? Or the eyes, too?
- Do you have a rash on any other part of your body?
- Describe the rash. Tiny red bumps? Blisters?

- Is there any pain?

    Possible causes: allergic reaction to drugs or chemicals, poison (ivy, oak, etc.), shingles (Herpes zoster)

Redness

What your doctor needs to know:
- When did this start?
- Is it one eye, or both?
- Is there any tearing or other discharge?
- Is there any pain or discomfort?
- Has the vision decreased?
- Is the eye sensitive to light?
- Is the eye red all over? Or is there a single blood-red patch?

    If there is a blood-red patch (burst blood vessel):
- Do you have high blood pressure?
- Have you had a blow to the eye?
- Have you been straining (hard coughing or sneezing vomiting or retching, constipation, heavy lifting, etc.)
- Do you take blood thinners or aspirin?

    Possible causes: angle closure glaucoma, inflammation inside the eye, eye infection, allergic reaction, dryness, hay fever and asthma. Burst blood vessel: high blood pressure, injury, blood disorder, Vitamin C deficiency

Swelling

What your doctor needs to know:
- When did this start?
- Is it in one eye, or both?
- Might you have been bitten by a bug of some sort?
- Are both the upper and lower lid affected?
- Is the lid tender?
- Is the lid red and angry looking? Fevered?
- Do you feel ill?
- Is the whole lid swollen, or just one area?
- Have you been using any type of eye wash, drops, or ointment?
- Have you been doing any yard work and perhaps rubbed your eyes?

    Possible causes: fluid retention, stye, chalazion, cellulitis, injury, allergic reaction (hay fever), contact allergy (make-up, lotions, etc.) drug reaction, malnutrition

Watery Eyes

What your doctor needs to know:
- How long has this been bothering you?
- Do the tears actually stream down your cheeks?
- Are the tears clear? Or sticky?
- Do your eyes feel scratchy and gritty, and/or itchy?
- Do your eyes tear during any particular time of day?
- Have you been using any type of eye medication to try to clear this up? Does it help?
- Are you taking any type of antihistamine or sinus/cold/ allergy medication?

Possible causes: dry eyes, allergy, drug reaction, infection, blocked tear duct

A few of the symptoms we've discussed can be caused by a need to change your glasses. The next chapter will explore nearsightedness (myopia), farsightedness (hyperopia), lazy eye (amblyopia), and other vision problems.

CHAPTER 5

Everything But Hindsight
(Vision Problems)

MARCIA Fern proudly displayed her new glasses to her friends in the women's circle.

"Oh, those are such lovely frames!" gushed Mary Ricks. "Are you nearsighted or farsighted?"

Suddenly the conversation erupted. Are you nearsighted if you can see far away? Or up close? Or is that what happens when you need bifocals?

Refractive Errors

Ideally, every eye should focus light onto the retina (see Figure 5-A). But most bodies are not "ideal." An image may come to focus in front or behind the retina (or even both). The result is blurred vision. When light coming into the eye is not focused properly, this is called a refractive error. A refractive error can be corrected with glasses, contact lenses, and surgery (see Chapter 6)

Astigmatism

Do you have astigmatism? Try answering the following questions:

- Before age forty, did you have blurry vision at distance *and* near?
- Do you have problems adjusting your focus from distance to

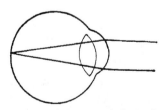

Figure 5-A Incoming light properly focused on the retina.

near and back again?
- Do you find yourself constantly tilting your head one way or the other to see?
- If you hold your glasses about eight inches from a printed page and turn them, does the print distort and stretch? (This won't work with progressive power trifocals.)
- Look at the astigmatism card in the back of this book (Appendix G). Are some of the lines darker, blacker, sharper than the others?

Light coming into the eye must be focused. The cornea (clear window over the front of the eye) bends light even more than the lens does. Light coming through the cornea is bent inward, condensing the image.

The ideal cornea has the same amount of curve in every direction, like a basketball. In this perfect condition, incoming light is bent equally in all directions. Many corneas are not "ideal," however. In this case, the cornea is curved *more* in one direction and *less* in another, like the back of a spoon. This condition is called astigmatism.

In astigmatism, light is not bent equally in every direction. This breaks up the image, sort of stretching it out (see Figure 5-B). Thus, part of the image may focus on the retina and part of it may focus in front of the retina. Or both ends of the stretched-out image may be in front of or behind the retina. You could even have one end in front and the other end behind. There are several possible combinations. These mixtures result from the fact that an eye with astigmatism may ALSO be myopic (nearsighted) or hyperopic (farsighted).

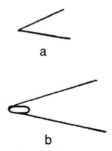

Figure 5-B (a) Light focused to a point and (b) stretched-out image of astigmatism.

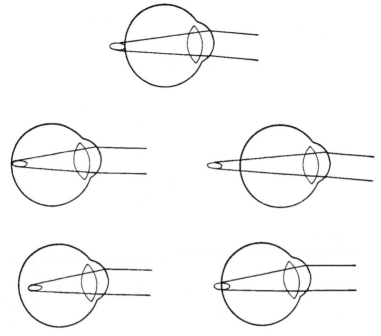

Figure 5-C Combination possibilities in astigmatism.

What this all amounts to is blurry vision, often for both close up and far away (see Figure 5-C).

Some people talk about their astigmatism as if it is a disease. It's not. It is merely a special kind of refractive error that can usually be corrected with glasses. Contact lenses can be used in some cases.

Contacts and glasses both use a special type of lens called a *cylinder* for correcting astigmatism. The cylinder must be measured for two items: its power and its direction. This is done during the examination for glasses. It is possible that, although you never had astigmatism before, it could be found now during a routine eye exam.

It may take some adjustment on your part to get used to a change or addition in cylinder power. Sometimes round objects will appear oval or a straight line will appear bowed. Give yourself at least two weeks (without going back to your old glasses) to adjust. Going back to your old glasses interferes with the adjustment process. You may also notice a change in cylinder position. Some people observe a slight drawing or pulling sensation. If this doesn't improve after two weeks, contact your eye care physician. In spite of the above discomforts, the vision should be as good as, or better than, your old glasses.

Astigmatism may be measured by retinoscope, refractor, auto-refractor, keratometer, or corneal topography. Astigmatism can also be evaluated by Placido's disk or keratoscopy.

Astigmatism is an important factor when considering cataract surgery. The placement of the incision (through which the cataract is removed) can sometimes improve or worsen the astigmatism. These procedures are discussed in Chapters 6 and 11.

Hyperopia

* other names: farsighted
Are you hyperopic? Answer these questions:

- Did you have trouble seeing to read without glasses BEFORE age forty?
- Before age 40, did you have trouble seeing BOTH at distance and near without glasses?
- Are the lenses of your glasses thicker in the middle and thinner at the edges?
- If you hold your glasses about 8 inches from a printed page, does the TOP portion make the print look larger?
- Do you have to have your glasses to read?

Hyperopia occurs when an image is focused behind the retina instead of on it (see Figure 5-D). If the farsightedness is mild, you can focus at a distance but not up close. In high amounts of hyperopia, distant vision may be blurred as well.

Hyperopia is corrected with "plus" power lenses. The correct power is measured with the retinoscope or auto-refractor, then

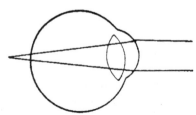

Figure 5-D Hyperopia (farsightedness); image is focused behind the retina.

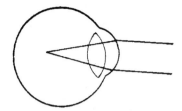

Figure 5-E Myopia (nearsightedness); image is focused in front of the retina.

refined with the refractor (each of these instruments is discussed in Chapter 3). Or it can be measured with the refractor alone.

A change in your lenses may take some getting used to. If the power was increased, you may notice that flat things seem slanted. Or you may feel like you are "stepping down." Objects may seem to be larger. Even so, your vision should be as good as or better than your old glasses. Wear your new glasses (without switching back to the old) for two weeks. Then, if the problems have not cleared up, notify your eye care practitioner.

Myopia (Nearsightedness)

Do you have myopic eyes? Please ask yourself:

- Do you have trouble seeing at a distance without glasses?
- Can you see to read without glasses?
- Are the lenses of your glasses thicker at the edge and thinner in the middle?
- If you hold your glasses about 8 inches above a printed page, does the TOP portion make the print look smaller?

In nearsightedness, the image is focused in front of the retina (see Figure 5-E). A nearsighted person has blurred distance vision but clear near vision without glasses. In high myopia, an object may have to be brought up to several inches from the face before it can be seen clearly.

Myopia is corrected with a "minus" lens. The power of the lens can be measured with a retinoscope or auto-refractor, then refined with a refractor (each of these instruments is discussed in Chapter 3). Or it can be measured with the refractor alone.

If you have an increase in your minus power, it may take a little getting used to. You might notice that objects appear smaller. Even so, your vision should be as good as if not better than your previous glasses. Try wearing the new lenses for two weeks (without going back to your old ones). Then if you still have problems, contact your eye doctor.

Presbyopia

Are you presbyopic? You need only answer one question to find out: Are you over age forty?

We see it in eye doctors' offices every day. It's inevitable. Sooner or later everyone succumbs to it. It's inconvenient, frustrating, and misunderstood.

The symptoms are usually classic. The phone book, the newspaper, threading a needle . . . it all starts getting a bit fuzzy. Then you discover that things are a bit clearer if you just hold them away from you a little. A bit farther, a bit farther...you suddenly realize the problem. Your arms are too short!

This vision problem is known as presbyopia. The first symptoms usually appear around age forty, although it can occur earlier or later. It is a gradual decrease in the eye's ability to focus up close, which steadily continues until around age 60.

Here's how it happens. The crystalline lens is the focusing mechanism of the eye, and lies behind the pupil (Fig. 11-A). It is attached to a washer-like muscle (the ciliary muscle) by tiny ligaments (called zonules). The ciliary muscle controls the shape of the lens, enabling it to change and focus. It takes more focusing power to look at something up close, so the ciliary muscle makes the lens fatter (thicker) when you read. This is known as *accommodation*. It takes less focusing power to look in the distance, so the ciliary muscle pulls the lens taut making it thinner when you look into the distance.

In the newborn eye the lens is soft, and its ability to change shape (and thus to focus) is tremendous. As a person grows, the lens lays down more layers from the outside. The original inside layers become compacted and less elastic. (It's somewhat like a tree laying down rings over the years.) Eventually the harder central core gets hard enough to reduce the stretchiness of the lens as a whole. Then the lens can't thicken for extra reading power as it used to. That's when you begin noticing a problem with close work.

If you've never worn glasses, it may be just a matter of getting reading glasses. This replaces the power your crystalline lens has lost. Reading glasses are only good for up close, however, and if you look into the distance when wearing them, anything much farther away than your book will be blurry. You may also choose bifocals that are clear at the top.

Those already in glasses when presbyopia begins are another story. One who wears glasses for farsightedness (already cannot see up close) will need to add a bifocal segment to get the extra boost needed for seeing up close. A person wearing correction for nearsightedness (can't see well at a distance) may have two choices. First, he might be able to take his glasses off to read. (His glasses have negative power, so taking them off actually adds that necessary close-up boost.) Others with nearsightedness will want a bifocal segment like their far-sighted counterparts.

A bifocal has the advantage of providing distance and near vision in one frame (top part for distance and lower segment for reading), eliminating the need to put glasses on and off. Thus someone who's never worn glasses might also choose a bifocal with essentially plain glass on top and extra "reading power" in the bifocal.

A glasses lens is obviously not flexible, and there is a certain range where it focuses best. Usually the reading segment is focused at about 14 to 16 inches. Correction for distance is focused at 20 feet and beyond. Thus, there is a "no man's land" between 16 inches and 20 feet that causes a problem for some folks. For example, a person may read music from a stand that is 24 inches away. Or you may prefer holding reading material in your lap instead of closer at the "normal" 16 inches. Your eye care specialist needs to know these distances to make the necessary adjustment to your prescription. A trifocal may be the answer, since the middle segment will focus around three feet. This is a good solution for someone doing desk work, typing, or computer work. Trifocals are available in the attractive and popular no-line or progressive style. Or you can get them with three separate segments. (See Table 6-1 on page 98 for notes on choosing various types of bi- and tri-focal lenses.)

As an alternative to bifocals or trifocals, you may want a separate pair of glasses for a special activity such as painting, reading music, etc. These lenses are focused at one specific distance (the easel or music stand, for instance), and will be blurred at any other distance.

When presbyopia arrives, a lot of people decide now is the time for contacts. They think, "I'll just put them in and be able to see everything like I could before." But it's not that simple. A contact, like a glasses lens, has no ability to adjust its power. It is focused at one particular distance just as glasses are. So contact lens wearers (whether new or current) must make some adjustments. We'll discuss the options in presbyopia here, but please refer to Chapter 6 for general information on contacts.

A person already wearing glasses or contacts may choose to have contacts that focus both eyes at a distance, and then get a pair of reading glasses to wear over them for the extra power needed for close-up. Another option is bifocal contacts with the extra reading power at the bottom of the lens. Yet another choice with growing popularity is known as the *monovision* technique. One eye wears a contact to give distance vision, and the other eye wears a contact for close vision. It takes some co-ordination at first to get used to it, but if one has the drive to succeed, it is a good option. Of course, you need an evaluation by an eye doctor to determine if you are a good candidate for contact lenses and the choices mentioned here.

Other Visual Conditions

Amblyopia (Lazy Eye)

Do you have amblyopia? Here are some questions to ask yourself:

- Has the vision in one eye been weaker since childhood?
- Has one of your eyes turned in or out since childhood?
- Did you have a childhood eye injury?
- Is one of your eyes very nearsighted or farsighted, and the other eye normal?
- Is there a history of amblyopia in your family?
- Have you had a cataract in one eye since birth or childhood?
- As a child, was one of your eyes treated by patching it?
- Has the upper lid of one eye drooped down over your pupil since childhood?

- Did you have a cataract removed from one eye as a child, without an implant or contact lens?

If you answered yes to any of the above questions, you may have amblyopia. Amblyopia, commonly called "lazy eye," occurs when one eye does not see as well as the other from childhood. This happens when a child does not use one eye as much as the other. There can be many reasons why one eye would not be used. The vision in that eye might be covered by a cataract, eyelid, or scar from some injury. Or, the lazy eye might need glasses while the other eye doesn't. An eye that had a cataract removed, but no intraocular lens (IOL) or contact lens was used, would not develop visually. Finally, if the same eye turns in or out all the time, it doesn't get used and becomes amblyopic.

Treatment for lazy eye usually works only in childhood. After a child reaches age ten or so, the vision in that eye generally cannot be improved. In treating a young child, the strong eye is patched and the lazy eye is forced to work. (If there are other problems involved, such as a cataract, needing glasses, or scarring, those problems would need to be fixed before patching would help.) If you remember wearing an eye patch as a child, it may have been to treat amblyopia.

Because the common term for amblyopia is "lazy eye," some people may misunderstand what it is. Amblyopia is *not* an eye with a droopy lid, or an eye that crosses (although either of these conditions can cause amblyopia).

How does a doctor determine if an adult is amblyopic? The first clue is when the vision in one eye is worse than the other, but there is no disease causing the poor vision. The doctor will also do tests to determine if your eye crosses, or if the eyes are very different from each other. These conditions, if present, have probably been there since birth, and suggest amblyopia.

It is true that there are many reasons why an eye may not see well. Poor vision in one eye may indicate a need to change the glasses, the presence of a cataract, or some other condition. If the poor vision can be explained and there is no childhood history of lazy eye, the eye is not usually considered to be amblyopic.

If amblyopia can't be treated as an adult, what does it matter if an eye is lazy or not? From a medical point of view, vision that is below normal must be explained. If the physician finds the vision in one eye to be poor, he/she must attempt to find the cause of the poor vision.

This brings up an important point. Some folk like to go to a new doctor and not give any information about previous eye exams. "I want to see what *this* doctor finds, without knowing what other doctors have said," they may say. This attitude can backfire. In attempting to find the "cause" of poor vision in an amblyopic eye, the physician may order extra tests . . . tests that would not be necessary if the patient had explained that the eye has been weak since childhood.

It is also important to know that an eye is lazy when predicting post-operative vision before cataract or other eye surgery is done. If a normal-looking eye has undetected amblyopia, the doctor and patient may expect post-operative vision to be better than it actually turns out to be. Even with perfect surgery and a healthy eye, a lazy eye is simply not capable of 20/20 vision.

One way to estimate what vision will be after cataract surgery is to do a potential acuity meter test. This test works even on a lazy eye. A cataract *can* be removed from a lazy eye, but the doctor will consider how much improvement is expected before agreeing to perform surgery.

There are two ways that amblyopia may affect your every day life. First, if the lazy eye is extremely poor, you will want to wear glasses at all times in order to protect your good eye. Second, you may have trouble every time you renew your driver's license if the lazy eye does not meet the vision standards of your state. As long as your good eye has driving vision, all that is required is a note or form from your eye doctor.

Aphakia

Aphakia means that the lens of the eye has been removed (see Figure 5-F). This could happen from trauma that causes the lens to dislocate or detach. But the most common case is when a cataract (cloudy lens) has been removed and *no* intraocular lens (IOL) is placed inside the eye. (See Chapter 11 for a full discussion of cataracts and implants.)

Without correction, the vision of an aphakic eye is very poor. The natural lens of the eye does a lot of focusing for the eye. When the

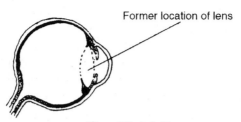

Figure 5-F Aphakia.

lens is removed, so is all of that focusing power. That power must be replaced if the vision is to improve. If there is no eye disease, most people with aphakia see clearly with correction (see Figure 5-G).

Glasses can be used to correct the vision in aphakia. This may seem like the easiest solution. Unfortunately, there are many drawbacks:

1. The lenses are very thick. This creates problems such as magnification, distortion (lines seem to bow out), poor side vision, and "jack-

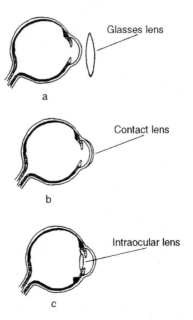

Figure 5-G Correction of aphakia by: (a) Glasses, (b) contact lens and (c) intraocular lens (IOL).

in-the-box" sight (objects seem to "jump" suddenly into view). Also, the glasses have to be fit just right. Too much error in aligning the glasses up or down, in or out, will decrease the effectiveness of the glasses. The prescription must be very accurate as well.

2. The thick lens won't work for just one eye (that is, if one eye is normal and the other is aphakic). The brain can't handle such a large difference between the eyes.

Aphakia can also be corrected with a contact lens. This eliminates the problems created by the glasses. There is no distortion, little magnification, and good side vision. Even if one eye is normal, you can wear a contact on the aphakic eye and the brain will accept it. Chapter 6 covers contact lenses in more detail.

But contact lenses have problems of their own:

1. A contact lens has to be removed and cleaned. Even if you wear extended wear lenses (the kind you can sleep in and leave in for several weeks at a time), they must be removed and cleaned periodically. This is a problem for anyone with stiff joints or shaking hands.
2. Contact lenses increase your risk of getting an eye infection. Soft lenses especially may harbor bacteria, fungus, even viruses.
3. The cost involved in cleaning solutions and replacing lenses may be a problem for someone on a fixed income.
4. You can develop an allergy to the solutions, or even the plastic in the lens itself.
5. Dry eyes, common as we age, make contact lens wear more difficult and maybe impossible.

Not really a disadvantage, but perhaps a consideration, is that you will most likely need to wear reading glasses along with the contact.

A third option is to have an intraocular lens (IOL) placed in your eye. The IOL eliminates all of the problems associated with the thick glasses or contact lenses. The implant can be inserted into the eye in a 20 minute out-patient surgery under local anesthesia. An IOL is considered permanent. (See Chapter 11 for more details.) You might still need regular glasses after IOL surgery, but they are not the thick kind used in aphakia.

Evaluation For An Implant

First, you'd need to be examined by an ophthalmologist and have a full eye exam (Chapter 3). The doctor will determine if you're a good candidate for an IOL. An IOL might not be recommended if you have:

1. recurrent episodes of inflammation inside the eye
2. corneal damage
3. eye disease such that an implant will not improve vision.

If an IOL is right for you, the physician will determine which placement is best: behind or in front of the iris (colored part of the eye). Measurements and tests will be done including refraction, keratometry, and A-scan. These readings are used to calculate the power of implant to be placed in your eye.

Implant surgery is similar to cataract surgery, except that there is no cataract to be removed. Please refer to Chapter 11 for general information about cataract and implant surgery.

Had you realized there were more vision problems than just being nearsighted and farsighted? Now that you understand refractive errors, the next chapter will discuss how they are corrected.

CHAPTER 6

Glasses, Contact Lenses, and Refractive Surgery

IT is estimated that 100 million Americans require glasses. It is also calculated that in 1987 18 million people in the U.S. (many of whom were 40 or older) wore contact lenses.

Glasses

Glasses are the simplest way to correct refractive errors. These days glasses are expected to do more than hold lenses in front of the eyes. They must also enhance our looks and provide protection. There are so many styles of frames and options on lenses, that we can only cover general information here. For all the choices available to you, find an eye care professional you trust, then follow his/her advice.

Frames

The frame is required to be durable and fashionable (see Figure 6-A). Each frame has the same basic parts. The eyepiece surrounds the lenses and holds them in place. The nosepiece bears the weight

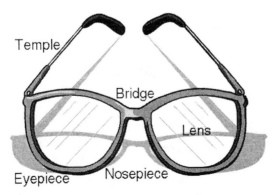

Figure 6-A Parts of a glasses frame.

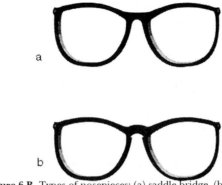

Figure 6-B Types of nosepieces: (a) saddle bridge, (b) keyhole bridge.

of the frame on the front. The two basic nosepiece styles are the saddle and keyhole (see Figure 6-B). The frame may have mounted eye pads that "float" and are easy to adjust. The temples run from the eyepieces along the side of the face and over the ears. There are several types (see Figure 6-C). The cable temple (also known as the riding bow or curl side) have a flexible portion that goes around the ear. This keeps the glasses from sliding when you look down. The straight temple (also called the library or loafer temple) is straight, and does not curve around the ear at all. These are great for those who take the glasses on and off constantly. They

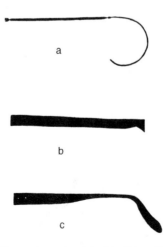

Figure 6-C Types of temples: (a) cable, (b) straight, (c) paddle.

are also good if you must wear something on your head or around your face (such as a nurses' cap, habit, scarf, etc.). Finally, the paddle temple (other names are the skull or hockey end temple) is the most common type and good for all-purpose use.

Frame selection can be a complicated (and frustrating) task. Someone trained in helping others choose frames can be a real blessing. We will cover a few basics here.

A frame can be used as an optical illusion to "change" facial features. First, consider the shape of your face. For a long face, use a broad frame. "Shorten" a long nose with a low bridge-bar and dark color frame. "Lengthen" a short nose with a narrow bridge-bar set high. Separate closely set eyes by frame that is wider at sides than at center. Bring in wide-set eyes by a frame that is wider at center than sides, or a frame with darker color at sides than at center. A large frame makes the face look smaller and daintier. A small face can be "enlarged" by using a small frame. Bright colors are good for fair complexions, dark colors for dark complexions. Heavy temples "shorten" the profile, and thin temples "elongate" it.

Basically, there are two materials available for frames: metal and plastic. Metal looks good and goes with everything. Metal is not "noticed" as much as plastic, so is a good choice if you are trying to down-play the glasses. Those who work with electricity or around heat should choose a plastic frame, however. Metal is a conductor!

Plastic frames tend to draw attention more than metal. There are several types of plastic frames. Many consider Optyl™ to be the best. Optyl tends to return to its original shape after being distorted. Another advantage to Optyl is that it does not cause allergies. (Certain other types of plastics can cause an allergic rash.) The range of colors available is practically unlimited. Choose a color that blends well with your hair, eyes, and complexion.

Rimless glasses don't really have a frame. The nose piece and temples are attached directly to the lenses. This style offers a wider field of vision without the interference of the frame edge. They are also light-weight. On the down side, this style is more fragile. If you take your glasses off a lot during the day, you should choose a sturdier frame. Also, if you are highly farsighted, the edges of the lens may be too thin and weak to work well in a rimless style.

The size of the eyepiece is often a matter of fashion. A strong prescription works better in a smaller sized eyepiece. There is usually an adjustment period when you change from one size of eyepiece to another. If your prescription is moderately strong, you may notice some distortion at the lens edges when you switch to a larger eyepiece. If you are going from a large to a smaller size, you may have to learn to ignore the visible edge of the frame.

A saddle bridge nosepiece "shortens" a long nose. Keyhole styles or mounted pads are good when the nose is short and round. If the lenses are heavy, you may want over-sized pads.

Frames can be special ordered or modified for certain needs. Side shields may be necessary for a person with dry eyes. These slip on over the temples. If the dryness is severe, moisture chambers can be added to the frame. These chambers are soft plastic cups, rather like goggles, that completely enclose the eyes and prevent evaporation. Another example of a special accessory is the ptosis crutch. (Ptosis is a drooped lid). The crutch is a small wire attached to the frame and holds the lid up. While the crutch does not solve the problem, it might be useful if eye lid surgery is not possible. Another frame adaptation is used when the frames cannot rest on the nose. These off-the-face frames hold the glasses on by pressure on the temples. Ask your eye care physician for recommendations on frame modifications if you have a special need.

Lenses

Bifocal, Trifocal, Etc.

Single vision lenses give you vision at a single level (called the focal distance). The optician can adjust the prescription to suit your working distance. Distant glasses, used for driving, are measured to give clear vision at about 20 feet and beyond. If you try to read with them on, the vision will be blurry. Reading glasses are set at about 14 inches. Objects that are farther away will not be clear. Various professionals and hobbyists request single vision glasses at other levels so that they can see their notes on a podium, the music on the piano, or the canvas on the easel. A single vision lens will give sharp vision at the level it is made for, but any other distance will not be as sharp.

Since most everyone over age 40 is presbyopic, multifocal lenses are extremely useful. A multifocal lens is a single lens that provides more than one focal distance. A bifocal has two distances: distant (20 feet) and near (14 inches). The trifocal has an additional third level for mid-range (28 inches). The progressive power lens has a gradual power change that gives many intermediate distances between 20 feet and 14 inches. With any multifocal lens, you avoid the hassle of putting your glasses on and off constantly as you change your focus from one distance to another.

Bifocals and trifocals are made in a variety of styles to fit various needs. The flat-top has the familiar half-circle segment, and the round top looks like a circle. (The round top is available in an "invisible" bifocal variety that has blended edges.) The executive style has a line all the way across. There is even an occupational lens that has segments at the bottom *and* top, for those who do close work over their heads (like mechanics). Your eye physician or optician can advise you on which style will best suit your needs. Table 6-1, page 98 will give you some idea of your options.

When you get your first pair of multifocal lenses, there will probably be a period of adjustment. You will have to experiment a little to know where to hold close-up material. Look through the bifocal (or the bottom of the trifocal) and pull your book closer, then further back. The point where the print is clearest is where you need to hold your reading from now on. If that point is too close or too far away for comfort, tell your eye doctor. The lenses can be remade to adjust the power and change the reading distance.

You will have to learn to raise and lower your head in order to look through the correct segment. For example, if you are shopping and want to read a price on an overhead shelf you will have to raise your chin to see the self through your reading segment. When you walk you will have to tuck your chin to see the ground through the top distant portion of the lenses. These changes may be a hassle at first, but rest assured, you will adjust and soon use the correct segment without even thinking about it.

The adjustments for no-line trifocals are the same, whether you start out with them or switch after using regular bi- or tri-focals for years. Please read about them on pages 104-105.

Lens Materials and Treatments

Options for lens materials, styles, and types are even greater

Table 6-1 Choosing a Bifocal or Trifocal.

Is a BIFOCAL best for you? Ask yourself:
• Is your near work mainly at a single level (that is, no typing or computer)? • Are you already wearing and comfortable with a bifocal? **Which type of bifocal style might be best for you?** *Flat top (other names: straight top, D segment)* • Must you look frequently from distant to near? • Is your close work in a narrow area? • Do you have a moderate or high prescription? Advantages: light weight, economical, comfortable for the eyes *Round top (other names: curved top (or "CT"), Kryptok; blended variety is sometimes called "invisible" or "no line blended")* Brand names: Ultex A; blended: Younger, Flexite Advantages: Economical, least noticeable of all segment types, light weight, comfortable for the eyes Disadvantages: You must look further down the segment to properly focus at near *Executive (other names: president, desk bifocals)* Do you work mainly up close? Does your near work cover a wide field (such as left to right across a desk or table)? Advantages: gives a broad field of vision, good with the low and moderate prescriptions Disadvantages: Thicker and heavier, harder to clean because ledge runs all the way across the lens, thick edge may cause "rainbow" colors at edge of lens, eyes may "pull" when reading

Table 6-1 (continued).

Is a TRIFOCAL best for you? Answer these questions:
• Do you do a lot of desk work at varying distances (typing, computer, etc.)?
• Do you do a lot of shopping or filing?
• Do you frequently operate vehicles with control panels that are about 2–3 feet away (professional driver, airplane pilot, etc.)?
Which type of trifocal style might be best for you? The flat top, round top, and executive bifocal styles discussed above are all available as trifocals.
No-line (other names: progressive, invisible, gradient, multifocal)
Brand names: Varilux, Varilux 2, Multilux, Ultravue, Omnifocal, Progressive R, Truvision
Advantages: cosmetically great all levels of vision present
Disadvantages: may be difficult to adjust to, must learn to move head instead of eyes when looking to the side, narrow field of vision

than frame choices. Glass lenses are durable but heavy, and inappropriate for safety glasses. Welders should avoid glass, because the "spatter" sticks to it. Plastic lenses are strong enough to be considered safety lenses, and are much lighter than glass. Even though a plastic lens must be thicker than a glass lens, the decrease in weight makes plastic great for high powered lenses. The main drawback is that plastic tends to scratch easily. You may also notice rainbows at the lens edges. There may be an adjustment period if you switch from one type of lens material to the other.

A modern option for a glass lens is high index glass. Lenses made with high index glass are thinner than conventional glass. They are also a little heavier. But since there is less bulk, it's a good trade-off. High index glass is a good choice for stronger prescriptions.

Regular plastic lenses are so tough that they are rated as safety lenses without additional treatment. Glass must be treated to make it impact-resistant. One way to do this is heat treating (known as "hardening" the lens). The only way to tell if a glass lens has been heat-treated is to take it to the optical shop and have them look at it under a special light. Unfortunately, a deep scratch in a hardened lens can weaken it to the point where it no longer qualifies as a safety lens.

A "toughened" glass lens is *not* the same as a hardened safety lens. True, it has been heat treated and is tougher than untreated glass, but it has not been treated to the point of qualifying as a safety lens. Be sure you know what you are buying.

Glass can also be chemically treated, which gives the best type of glass safety lens. Another, less used, option is laminated (plastic sandwiched between glass).

The world of lens tints and colors is a big one. Tints may be used for sunglasses, glare protection, or looks. Glass can be made with the tint incorporated in it, or applied later as a coating. Plastic lenses can be dyed or coated.

The amount of tint ranges from ten to 90 percent. Anything less than 50% is not very effective in reducing glare.

Colors for sunglasses include green, brown, and gray (blue and yellow aren't usually recommended). Tint used just for looks is lighter, and you can pretty much get any color you want. (There are some limitations with tinting glass lenses, though.) An advantage of dyed plastic lenses is that the tint can later be darkened or lightened if desired.

Another lens option is UV dye. In this process, lenses are treated so they filter out harmful ultraviolet, or UV, light (from fluorescent lamps as well as the sun). UV light is suspected of playing a role in corneal and retinal disease as well as cataracts. The UV dye does not actually color or tint the lenses, so it is virtually impossible to look at the lenses and tell if they've been dyed. Your optician can detect UV dye by putting the lenses under a special light. Many eye care physicians request this filtering dye for all lenses they prescribe.

A special kind of tinted lens has been developed that filters out blue and ultraviolet light. These lenses, made in shades of yellows and reds, get darker outside and lighter indoors. They decrease glare and sharpen vision. They may be useful in a person developing cataracts, before surgery becomes necessary. Other patients who might benefit are those with extreme light sensitivity. Your eye care professional may have a set of these lenses for you to evaluate. Ask!

Other lens coatings besides tints are also available. Since these are applied to the finished lens, they can be removed if desired. One popular coating is used to make plastic more scratch resistant, although some professionals question its effectiveness. Anti-reflective coating can also be applied. This makes the lens itself look clearer, so the eyes appear less "glassy." It also reduces glare from lights and computer screens. Be sure to ask your optician how to clean these lenses. Improper care can cause the coating to peel. Another type of glare-reducing lens is the polarized lens. This is a specially-processed lens, not a coating, and is rather expensive.

A one-way mirror coating is useful if there is facial disfigurement. The observer can't see the eyes, but the wearer can see through.

Some people don't like having a separate pair of sunglasses. Photosensitive lenses turn dark in bright light and clear in normal light. It takes the lenses about 60 seconds to change from light to dark. A little more time is required for them to lighten. The crystals in "photo gray" lenses respond to the amount of invisible ultraviolet light present. Thus, they will turn dark even on a cloudy day, because UV light passes through the clouds. These crystals never wear out, but may "slow down" in their reaction time. If they do, your optician can easily "renew" them. "Photo brown" lenses react to visible light, and thus do not darken on a cloudy day.

Prisms

Prism in lenses is used to treat double vision. Prism can be ground into the lens when it is made. Another option is to "de-center" the optical center of the lens. The optical center of a lens is the strongest point of the lens. Ideally, it is placed in front of the pupil so that you look through it. In cases where prism is needed, however, an easy technique is to move the optical center slightly. This creates prism without having to grind it into the lens.

A third type of prism is called a press-on prism. This prism comes as a plastic sheet. The sheet is cut to match the lens, then pressed on. It is generally intended for temporary use, for example in a patient gradually recovering from a palsy. The press-on prism is thin and can be removed easily.

If the prescription between the two eyes is very different, it may result in double vision for reading. This can be eliminated by a technique called slab-off. Slab-off grinding changes the way light enters the eye through the segment, bringing the images together. There is a faint line all the way across the lens at the top of the bifocal or trifocal.

Caring for Lenses and Frames

A hard case protects glasses best. A soft case subjects the frames to a lot of pressure: being crammed into a purse or crushed in a back pocket. Frames treated roughly like this will need readjustment frequently. Use two hands when removing glasses, rather than tearing them off with one hand. Your car (especially the glove box) is like an oven in hot weather, and can warp frames.

For general cleaning, soak your glasses once a week in mild detergent, then clean with a soft brush. Don't wipe a dry lens: use water or cleaner. Do not use paper towels with designs. The painted-on decoration can scratch the lenses.

To de-fog your lenses, smear dry soap on them then wipe gently. This soap coating will last several days. Defogger is also available at most stores.

Moving parts (hinges and floating nose pieces) can loosen up with wear. Loose screws can be "tightened" with a drop of clear nail polish. Moving parts can also "freeze" from corrosion due to perspiration. (Another reason to keep them clean!) Corrosion spots on metal frames can be kept from spreading by applying clear nail polish.

Glasses Problems

Getting new lenses and/or frames is exciting. Adjusting to them may require a little patience. This process is rather like breaking in a new pair of shoes. Your brain is used to seeing in one way, now it must get used to another. We generally recommend wearing the new glasses for two weeks without going back to the old ones. If, at the end of that time, you are still having problems, contact your eye care specialist. *Please* don't just throw the new glasses in a drawer and forget the whole thing! Nor should you wait several months before seeking help. Give your eye professional a chance to make things right. We are going to list some common problems here, but you should trust and work with the doctor or optician who knows your case.

Common problems include:

- inadequate distant vision- new lenses not as clear as old
- inadequate near vision- unclear, has to hold too close, has to hold too far back

- discomfort- "swimmy-headed," eyes feel drawn, can't walk in bifocals, headache, vague discomfort
- distortion- slant, "stepping down," straight lines are bowed, "standing in a hole," "standing on a hill"

The above difficulties usually subside during the two-week adjustment period. If not, the cause needs to be identified and fixed (if possible). These difficulties may have several different causes. Frame adjustment, alteration of the prescription, or remaking the lenses may be all that is needed to correct them.

- double vision- at distance, near, or both. This may be a matter of getting used to the glasses. If the doubling is only for close-up, you may want to go ahead and work with it for the two weeks. But doubled distant vision can create hazards when driving. Check it out promptly.

Some folks are distressed when they notice that the edge of one bifocal or trifocal segment is higher than the other. The real test, however, is where the lines are when the glasses are worn. One eye may actually be a little higher than the other.

Another item of dissatisfaction may be when the edge of the bifocal or trifocal is ridged. The stronger the segment, the more noticeable the ridge may be. Even without a change in lens power, there may be a ridge in the new glasses if you have changed to frames with a different size eye piece. In addition, this ridge can vary among manufacturers...just as tire tread varies among the different companies.

Mr. Crumb tossed his glasses on the counter at our office with a snort. "They're not even!" he says. He bounces one temple, and sure enough, the frames rock. But Mr. Crumb is like me (Jan): one ear is slightly higher than the other. When the glasses are on his face, they are straight. ("The table's not going to wear them," Dr. Gayton quips.)

The new lenses may be thicker than you'd like. Actually, the Food and Drug Administration has issued safety standards governing lens thickness (at both center and edges). If your new prescription is stronger, or if you have changed materials (for example, gone from plastic to glass), then the new lenses may be thicker than your last pair.

Those who have been using reading glasses, bifocals, or trifocals for several years have already made the initial adjustments for coping with presbyopia. But you may still have to undergo some adjustments when the power of your reading correction is changed, or if you switch from one type of lens to another.

First, when your bifocal (or trifocal) power is increased, you may notice that you need to hold reading material closer than before. This doesn't mean that the lens is incorrect. However, if you are uncomfortable with the new distance, let your eye doctor know. This can be altered to make you more comfortable, usually by remaking the lens. If you have to tip your chin way up to see through the bifocal, the segment may be too low. If you see the line of the segment when you are looking straight ahead, the segment may be too high. (The general rule of thumb is that the top edge of the segment should be even with the lower lid.) Both of these problems can be fixed, perhaps by a simple frame adjustment or by remaking the lenses. Those in certain professions, however, may want the segments set a little higher or lower on purpose. A barber or beautician, for example, may want a higher segment to avoid having to tip the chin back in order to use the segment.

If you have trouble walking in your bi- or trifocals, remember: the ground is farther away than the 14 inch distance that the bottom segment is created for. Be sure to tuck your chin down when looking where to step, thus using the top (distant) portion of your glasses.

If you switch to a no-line trifocal at this stage, there will definitely be a period of adjustment. But most people agree that it is worth the effort! The power of a no-line lens changes gradually as you move down the lens. The top is still for distance and the bottom is still for about 14 inches. The great thing is that every intermediate distance is there, too, somewhere in between the top and the bottom. The trick is that you have to learn where all these places are. This comes with patience and working with the glasses. To find the right spot for any distance, slowly tip your head up and down until the object is in focus. After a while you won't have to search for the right place...you'll use it automatically.

Another thing to be aware of in adjusting to no-line lenses is that there is a "garbage area" out to either side. Objects viewed through these areas are wavy and distorted. You must learn to look through the center part of the lens. Instead of cutting your eyes to the side, you need to turn your head. This, too, eventually becomes second nature.

No matter how careful the measurements, no matter how careful the fit, there are some things that glasses cannot cure. Glasses cannot relieve migraines or eye symptoms such as watering, itching, or burning.

Let's take a quick look at how lenses are made. First, you have an eye exam. The doctor or assistant measures you carefully with a refractor. The numbers on the machine are copied by hand into the chart. The doctor decides on a prescription. He copies numbers from the chart onto a prescription form. You take the prescription to the optician. The optician performs a mathematical formula on the prescription, and writes this down. Then he/she may call a lab and give them the numbers over the phone. Someone at the lab handwrites the numbers. Or the optician may grind the lenses himself. ("Grinding" refers to the process of putting the prescription onto a blank lens.) Next the optician "edges" the lens, cutting it to the shape and size that fits your frame. When not being worked on, the lenses are placed in a plastic tray labeled with your name or other identification.

The point of going through all this is to let you see that there are a lot of places where a mistake can occur. If you have difficulty with your lenses, it's unfair to assume that the person who measured you didn't know what they were doing, or that the person who made them did poor work. Every one who plays a part in generating your lenses wants to help you see better. Don't hesitate to ask for help!

Contact Lenses

Contact lenses aren't just for teenagers! If your eye care practitioner agrees and you are determined to succeed, contact lenses may be a viable choice at any age.

If you already have an eye doctor, contact the office to see if he/she fits contact lenses. (Some ophthalmologists do not.) Here are some questions you may want to ask:

- Can I be fit during my routine exam, or do I have to make a separate appointment?

- If I had a recent full eye exam, must I have another to be evaluated for contacts?
- Can I buy the lenses through your office?
- Can I get a prescription for contacts and then buy or order them elsewhere?
- What is the fee?
- What does the fee include? (This will vary according to the type of lenses you get.) Does it include:
  — eye exam?
  — evaluation for contacts?
  — the lenses?
  — a kit of cleaning solutions?
  — instructions on handling and care?
  — follow up exams? How many or for how long?
- How much of the fee is refundable if I cannot wear contacts after getting them?
- Is there a time limit on returning the lenses?
- Do you offer contact lens insurance?

It is important to have realistic expectations when deciding to try contacts. Contact lenses will not restore the focusing ability you had before age forty. You may need to wear reading glasses over them or have one contact for distance and one for near. (Please read about contact lens options and presbyopia in Chapter 5.) If there is a problem with the eye, such as a cataract, contacts will not help you see any better than glasses.

It is also important to understand that wearing contacts lenses carries some risk. A contact lens is a foreign body placed in the eye. The risk of getting an eye infection is increased with contact lens wear, especially with the soft lenses.

Fitting

Fitting contact lenses is not very complicated in most cases. A full eye exam which includes a refraction is the first step. The refraction gives the prescription portion of the contact. In addition, keratometry readings are needed to measure the curvature of the cornea. (Keratometry is not usually a part of a routine eye exam, and will probably not be done unless you have requested to be evaluated for contact lenses.) If dryness is suspected, a tear test may be done as well.

Not every one is a good candidate for contact lenses (See Table 6-2). However, many of the objections listed can be overcome if there is a good reason to do so. For example, a dentist might wear goggles while working. Or a care-giver may be taught how to insert, remove, and clean lenses.

In a moment we will discuss different types of contacts. The fitting procedure is similar in most cases, regardless of the type of lenses you wear. Once the measurements are taken, you will try the lenses on. (An exception is if the lenses must be ordered, or if fittings are scheduled separately from exams.) This gives you a chance to see what it feels like to have a lens on your eye. Your vision will be recorded. You will probably look through the refractor again for a refinement of the prescription. Then you will be checked with the slit lamp microscope. The examiner is evaluating how the lens rests on the eye and how it moves. You will be asked to blink and move your eye around. This may feel odd with a lens in your eye, but it should not be painful.

If the practitioner is satisfied with the way the lenses look and move, you're all set! If the lenses are part of the office stock, you may be allowed to get them the same day. If not, they will have to

Table 6-2.

You may not be a good candidate for contact lenses if:
• you have dry eyes   • you have conditions that predispose you to dry eyes (thyroid, arthritis, etc.)   • you take medications that end to cause dry eyes   • your occupation or hobbies involve lots of contact with soil or dirt (farming, gardening, pottery, etc.)   • your occupation or hobbies involve using tools that generate high-speed particles (grinding, sanding, dentistry, etc.)   • you have very high astigmatism   • you have a condition that affects your ability to use your fingers and/or hands (arthritis, Parkinsons's, etc.)   • you have frequent eye or eyelid infections   • you have difficulty caring for yourself

be ordered. In this case, it may take several days or a week before they come in. Some offices make a separate appointment for dispensing contacts, even if they are in stock.

General Lens Care

Regardless of when you get the lenses, you will need to be instructed on how to insert, remove, and clean them before taking them home. This instruction may be one-on-one or as part of a class. You will be told, shown, then assisted in handling the lenses. You may be given written instructions as well. (For more detailed handling information, read about your specific type of lens.)

Many offices give a kit containing a case and cleaning solutions to get you started. Unless you have problems with a particular brand, it is best to stick with the solutions your eye care professional recommends. Don't just buy whatever is on sale. The chemicals of some brands are not compatible with others.

Be sure and follow your schedule for wearing time. You have to start slowly and build up your time, especially with rigid lenses.

No matter what type of contact lenses you choose, there are several important pointers to remember:

1. Wash your hands before handling.
2. Establish the habit of removing the right lens first, then the left lens.
3. Never exceed your recommended wearing time.
4. Never, never, never put your lenses in your mouth to wet them.
5. Do not wear a painful lens. Remove it. If the eye is still uncomfortable one hour after taking the lens out, call your eye doctor.

Follow-Up and Replacement Lenses

Your doctor will want to see you again after you've been wearing the lenses for about a week, and several times thereafter. Don't skip these appointments! It is possible for corneal damage to occur even though the vision is clear and the lens feels fine.

In fact, this brings up an important point. If you get a prescription for contacts from one doctor, then buy the lenses somewhere else, who is going to examine you? Someone has to be sure that the lenses fit and your eyes are not being harmed. For this reason (that is, that SOMEONE has to be responsible), some doctors will not release a contact lens prescription to allow you to buy lenses elsewhere. An exception might be if you have worn contacts for a long time and are doing well. Or that whomever you buy your contacts from agrees to do the follow up.

This may sound like a hassle, but you can understand the physician's concern. Suppose you have never worn lenses before and take your prescription to the drug store. (Yes, some drug stores sell contacts!) Who is going to teach you how to handle and clean them? Not the drug store! Who is going to be sure that enough oxygen is getting to the cornea? That the lenses are not too tight or too loose?

While the lenses may be cheaper through mail order or other sources, remember that the price of follow-up exams is often included in the practitioner's charge. (Such a package deal is usually cheaper than a per-visit-fee to the same practitioner.) Be sure you understand the policies of your particular office from the outset.

Changes made in the contact lens during the initial trial period (often six to eight weeks) usually don't carry an additional charge. An example is if the power is too strong and you need a weaker lens.

Lost or damaged lenses, however, are your responsibility. That is why contact lens insurance is a good idea. The cost of such a policy is modest, and you can choose the period of coverage (usually 12 or 24 months). Then if you lose a lens, you pay a small deductible and the office's handling fee. The total of those two charges is still considerably less than the cost of the lens without insurance.

Types of Contacts (see Figure 6-D)

Hard Contacts

To the public, the term "hard contacts" has come to mean any rigid contact that is not of the soft variety. To professionals, however, there is a difference. In optical circles, a "hard" contact is made of rigid plastic from a material called PMMA. PMMA does not allow much oxygen to pass through. Since the cornea needs to "breathe", the hard lens is small and must float on the tears of the cornea. Every blink moves the lens and pumps fresh tears under it. This way the cornea gets some oxygen.

Hard contacts aren't being fit that much these days. They can be uncomfortable while you are first learning to wear them. They need periodic professional polishing to remove scratches. Yet the

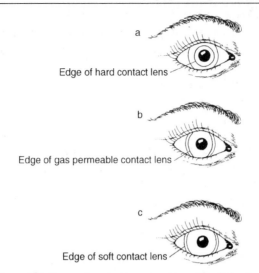

Figure 6-D Types of contact lenses and how they fit on the eye.

fact remains that conventional hard lenses are durable, easy to handle and care for, give sharp vision, and are reasonably priced. Unfortunately it is also true that they can slip off center or pop out, cause vision with glasses to be less clear, and can cause corneal warping. If you wear a hard lens now and need to change to another type of contact, you will need to leave the lenses out for several weeks before you can be refit. This is required to allow the cornea to return to its normal state.

Gas Permeable Contacts

Like the hard lens, the gas permeable (GP) lens is made of rigid plastic. A GP lens also floats on the layer of tears covering the cornea. Like the hard lens, a GP lens moves with every blink. But the material used in the GP lens allows oxygen to pass through it, nor does it warp the cornea.

The GP lens is larger than the traditional hard lens. It is also easy to handle and clean. GP's are durable, resistant to deposit build-up, and provide sharp vision. Many eye care professionals consider the gas permeable contact to be the "lens of the hour," and would prefer to fit everyone possible with this type of lens.

Disadvantages include several of the same downfalls of the hard lens: discomfort when first learning to wear them, popping out, slipping off center. These three items generally decrease and are not a problem after the initial adjustment period. Gas permeable lenses are the most expensive type of lens (with the exception of some specialty lenses). Since they last much longer than a soft lens, however, the cost may even out. GP's may get scratched and need periodic polishing by your practitioner.

Care and Handling of Rigid (Hard or Gas Permeable) Lenses

Since you need to rely on your eye care practitioner, we will only mention several points.

First, a hard lens is generally placed on the eye with a (clean) fingertip. It can be removed by using a suction cup or pulling on the eyelid and blinking it out. If using a suction cup, wetting the cup before touching it to the lens can help the lens stick. It is very important that you know where the lens is before you touch the suction cup to your eye. Never use the suction cup to "fish around" in your eye for a "lost" lens.

If the lens slips off the front of the cornea, it is easy to move it back into place.

1. Look AWAY from the place where the lens has slipped to.
2. Close your eye.
3. Gently put your finger over the lens to hold it still.
4. Roll your CLOSED eye toward the lens. This should get the lens back into place.

If you can see the lens (and ONLY if you can see it), you may use a suction cup to remove it.

Cleaning usually includes at least two solutions, although some companies make a solution that does everything. First, the lenses need to be cleaned every night when you remove them. Place the lens in the palm of your hand, apply the cleaner, and rub gently. Follow the manufacturer's instructions about rinsing them. (Some brands require you to rinse the cleaner off with tap water. Others don't.) It is best to store the lenses wet in some type of conditioner/soaker. The lenses should never be dry when inserted. Use a wetting solution recommended by your eye care professional. Do not use tap water and NEVER put the lenses in your mouth to wet them.

Some offices advise their patients to use an enzyme cleaner on rigid lenses. This is an extra cleaning step done once a week.

Soft Contacts

The soft contact lens is made of flexible plastic. Oxygen passes through a soft lens, some types allowing more oxygen to pass through than others. The lens is large, covering the entire cornea and extending onto the sclera. Blinking moves the lens a little, but not as much as a rigid lens. This, plus its flexibility, makes the soft contact lens the most comfortable even from the first time they are inserted. Soft lenses are inexpensive (except for some specialty lenses) and rarely slip out of place or pop out.

Soft lenses are not as durable as rigid lenses, however. They can be torn, discolored, and tend to form deposits on them. Patients with glaucoma may not be able to wear a soft lens because of the eye drops they use. Cleaning soft lenses is a constant battle to keep the deposits from forming. Another concern is that the soft plastic can harbor bacteria. Because of this, the lenses must also be disinfected as well as cleaned. While soft lenses are cheaper, they must be replaced more often than a rigid lens. Vision with a soft lens may not be as clear as with glasses.

Handling may be difficult, too. A soft lens can fold over and stick to itself. It can stick to your finger when you want it in your eye, and stick to your eye when you want to get it out! (All that said, I have to tell you that *I* wear soft lenses! JRL)

You must be examined periodically to check the lenses and cornea. If your cornea is not getting enough oxygen, abnormal blood vessels may grow. The cornea is normally clear, with no vessels. If blood vessels form and expand, vision can be threatened. It is possible for this to get so severe that a corneal transplant must be done.

Daily Wear Soft Contacts

This type of soft contact is meant to be removed (and cleaned!) every day. Generally speaking, it is the most durable and easy-to-handle soft lens.

Extended Wear Soft Contacts

The main idea behind an extended wear soft contact is to enable the wearer to sleep in the lenses. This lens is generally thinner (and flimsier, and harder to handle) than a daily wear lens to allow more oxygen to pass through it, since it is rarely removed.

The opinion about extended wear varies from one extreme to another. Some companies claim that their lens needs to be removed and cleaned only once a month. Some eye physicians will not recommend sleeping in *any* lens. Follow your doctor's advice and keep your follow-up appointments religiously.

An extended wear lens is frequently used in aphakia. It is convenient for patients who cannot handle the lenses themselves, since the contacts are not removed on a daily basis. Some patients go to the eye doctor's office every two weeks or so to have the lens cleaned by a staff member. If it is not practical for a person with aphakia to wear a contact lens, an intraocular lens implant should be considered.

Disposable Soft Contacts

Disposable contacts are similar to extended wear with one important exception. Instead of being removed and cleaned every so often, disposables are removed and thrown away. A new pair is then inserted. This avoids the hassles of cleaning. Again, some physicians recommend that disposables be removed and cleaned daily. Follow your doctor's advice.

Care and Handling of Soft Contacts

Our purpose here is to give you some general information. We want you to rely on your eye care practitioner for personal instruction.

Soft lenses are inserted by a (clean) fingertip. They are removed by "pinching" them out with thumb and forefinger. It is best to use a mirror when learning.

Soft lenses tend to become coated with whatever touches them . . . cold cream, make-up, lotions, hair spray, etc. Before handling your lenses, wash your hands with plain soap that doesn't contain any "extras." Close your eyes when using hair spray.

Cleaning usually involves two or more solutions. Some companies make one solution that "does it all." Follow your doctor's advice and the directions included with your solutions.

First, the lenses are cleaned when they are removed. Place the lens in your palm and apply the cleaner, then rub very gently with a finger. Follow directions about rinsing. Soft lenses are not rinsed with tap water . . . you need to use bottled sterile saline.

The lenses are soaked overnight. Never store them dry (they will shrivel up). Some solutions undergo a chemical change while they work. This type of solution will burn the eye if it hasn't had time to convert totally. Be sure to read the directions.

Most practitioners recommend using a weekly enzyme cleaner. This is designed to remove deposits and lengthen the life of the lens.

Other Uses of Contact Lenses

Up to this point, we have been discussing the use of contact lenses to improve vision. There are several instances in which a contact might be worn for other reasons.

Bandage Lens

A soft contact lens can be used temporarily as a sort of "bandage" for the cornea. A disposable or extended wear lens is generally used, so the patient does not have to handle or clean the lens. This treatment might be used in cases of corneal abrasion, recurrent corneal erosion, or corneal ulceration.

Prosthetic Lens

A prosthetic soft contact is used to hide or mask a disfigured eyeball. For example, if an eye has a distorted pupil, a contact with a "pupil" on it can make the eye look more normal. A prosthetic lens needs to be removed and cleaned . . . follow your doctor's advice.

Refractive Surgery

A few years ago, the only way to correct vision was with glasses or contact lenses. It is now possible to correct some refractive errors with surgery. The goal of refractive surgery is to alter the cornea so that incoming images focus directly on the retina. In addition to correcting existing refractive errors, refractive surgery can be done during or after cataract surgery in order to reduce astigmatism.

It is important to understand that refractive surgery will not restore the eye's ability to focus. Presbyopia is permanent and irreversible. However, some methods make it possible to have a distance-vision eye and a reading-vision eye (a technique known as monovision), eliminating the need for glasses.

If you are considering having refractive surgery, the first thing you will need is an ophthalmologist who does this type of surgery. You will be required to have a full eye exam to check the health of the entire eye. This examination will include a refraction, slit lamp microscope evaluation, keratometry, and pachymetry. All of these tests are quick and painless (and explained in detail in Chapters 3 and 18). If the equipment is available, your physician may also request a corneal topography study.

Radial Keratotomy

There are several types of refractive surgery. Radial keratotomy (RK) has received the most publicity. RK is used to correct nearsightedness (or myopia) and/or astigmatism.

In RK, small incisions are made in the cornea. These incisions do not go all the way through the tissue, just far enough to change the shape of the cornea.

The results of RK used to be rather inexact. Although no surgical outcome can ever be guaranteed, RK has become more predictable and controllable over the past several years. The information from each of the preoperative tests is used to decide where the incisions should be placed, how long they should be, how deep they should be, and how many there should be. There is now a computer program available that makes the calculations regarding the incisions. (Okay, we'll brag. Dr. Gayton designed the program!)

Regardless of preparation and careful measurements, it is impossible to predict how any one eye will respond. Sometimes a touch-up surgery is required to get the desired results. In this case, repeat measurements are needed to calculate the second procedure. (The above-mentioned computer program is also equipped to handle such repeat surgical information.)

RK is done on an out-patient basis. Often no pre-operative lab or physical is required. As in any surgery, leave valuables at home, wear comfortable clothing, and arrange for someone to drive you home.

Only topical anesthetic (numbing eye drops) is used. You may be given a mild tranquilizer if you need help relaxing. In most cases you will not have to wear a hospital gown. Before entering the operating room your hair will be covered with a paper "shower cap". Once in the operating room, you will be given some eye drops, and your eye will be cleansed. (The cleaning solution will probably feel cold and drippy.) A plastic drape is placed over your face. (This may be taped up out of the way so your mouth and nose aren't covered.) A small instrument is placed between the eyelids to keep the eye open. This may feel strange, but it should not be uncomfortable.

You will not be able to "see" the doctor working on your eye. You will be able to see the overhead operating light or the light from the operating microscope. Depending on the number of incisions, the surgery may take ten to forty minutes. A touch-up is usually shorter.

When the procedure is over, the eye is patched. You will be given instructions about using medications and told when to return for a follow-up exam. Once you get home, just take it easy.

Like any surgery, RK has risks. The most common are over-or-under-correction. Fluctuating vision and glare have also been reported. Since there are actual incisions, there is a risk of infection.

Arcuate Keratotomy

Arcuate keratotomy (AK), like RK, involves making partial incisions in the cornea. Instead of the straight incisions of RK, however, AK uses arc-shaped incisions at the edge of the cornea. AK is used to correct astigmatism. AK and RK may be used together if a person has both myopia and astigmatism. AK may be used during cataract surgery to correct astigmatism the patient already has, or after cataract surgery if astigmatism has worsened.

Excimer Laser

The excimer laser is used to treat myopia (nearsightedness). Using laser to perform refractive surgery has recently gained FDA approval in the United States. According to the most recent reports, there are rarely any complications.

Excimer laser is done in the office using numbing drops. First, the outer tissue layer of the cornea is removed, then the laser itself is performed with the patient lying down. After the laser, the eye is patched or a contact lens is put in as a bandage. Your eye is examined daily until the cornea is healed (usually 2-4 days). At that point the patch or contact lens is discontinued. Eye drops are used on a decreasing basis for about 4 months. It takes 18-24 months for vision to stabilize.

Keratomileusis and Epikeratophakia

Up to now, we have been discussing procedures that correct nearsightedness and astigmatism. Keratomileusis and epikerato-phakia can also be used to treat those, as well as farsightedness (including aphakia, the condition of having no natural lens in the eye).

Both procedures involve lathing (or "grinding") corneal tissue to a specific prescription. In keratomileusis, your own cornea is removed, ground, and sewn back into place. Donor tissue is used in epikeratophakia.

The cornea of the recipient is prepared by removing the top tissue layer, then the corneal tissue is sewn in. Some have referred to this arrangement as a "living contact lens." A donor "button" can be removed later if necessary. The procedures are done using local anesthetic drops, and can take as little as 10 minutes.

Your vision affects your life. But your life can also affect your vision. To find out how, move on to Chapter 7.

CHAPTER 7

Your Body and Your Eyes

S TEVEN Allan limped into his eye doctor's office.
"Looks like you're in the wrong place!" the receptionist teased.
"You need to see a foot doctor."

Mr. Allan grinned at her. "Yeah, I know. My gout is acting up lately. But I'm here about my eye."

Later, in the exam room, Mr. Allan talked with Dr. Christopher. "My right eye is red, watery, and sensitive to light. It sort of aches when I look around,too," he finished.

After the doctor had examined him, she said, "Mr. Allan, you have a condition called episcleritis."

Mr. Allan knotted his eye brows and leaned forward. "Where in the world did I catch that?"

Dr. Christopher shook her head. "It's not an infection or disease. In fact, it's probably related to your gout."

Mr. Allan sat back in the exam chair, surprised. "Gout affects my eyes?" he asked.

This chapter deals with various diseases and conditions, and how they affect the eyes. Each topic has a list of various symptoms that may occur as signals of trouble. Symptoms should also be a "signal" that you need to contact your eye doctor.

Never ignore a symptom simply because you think it is "normal" for someone with your condition. Many people with these various diseases never experience the eye problems listed. And, of course, any single symptom may have more than one cause. Your best defense is to stay in touch with your regular doctor and your eye care physician. If you call your eye doctor to report symptoms, be sure to tell the secretary about any condition or disease you have. This will influence the decision as to whether or not you have an emergency or can wait several days or weeks to be seen.

Acquired Immune Deficiency Syndrome (AIDS)

1. Problem: decreased immunities
   Symptoms: tendency to develop recurrent infections such as corneal ulcers, Herpes simplex, and shingles
2. Problem: dry eye
   Symptoms: excessive tearing, light sensitivity, pain (sandy/gritty sensation), itching, burning, redness
3. Problem: development of tumors (Kaposi's sarcoma)
   Symptoms: painless tumors may be flat patches or raised nodules appearing on the lids (external or inner), or conjunctiva (membrane lining over the white of the eye)
4. Problem: viral inflammation of the retina (retinitis)
   Symptoms: light flashes, floaters, blurred vision, loss of side vision, loss of central vision
5. Problem: areas of decreased blood flow in retina
   Symptoms: no immediate symptoms, but a gradual loss of vision
6. Problem: spread of pneumonia infection to the choroid (lining of blood vessels under the retina)
   Symptoms: maybe none, or can include floaters and loss of side vision
7. Problem: inflammation of optic nerve (optic neuritis)
   Symptoms: sudden vision loss, vision loss that comes and goes, decreased depth perception, change in color vision, pain, loss of central vision
8. Problem: nerve palsies
   Symptoms: double vision
9. Problem: involvement of the orbit (bony structure containing the eyeball)
   Symptoms: protrusion of the eye, double vision

Recommendations: Report to your eye physician if symptoms of infection, tumors, retinitis, neuritis, double vision, or orbital involvement occur. Use artificial tears for comfort of dry eyes, see eye care physician if not relieved. Keep appointments as recommended by your doctor.

Alcoholism

1. Problem: nerve palsies

Symptoms: double vision, blurred vision from shaking eyes, lid droop, paralyzed pupil (does not adjust to light)
2. Problem: inflammation of the optic nerve (optic neuritis)
Symptoms: sudden vision loss, vision loss that comes and goes, decreased depth perception, change in color vision, pain, loss of central vision
3. Problem: deterioration of the optic nerve (optic atrophy)
Symptoms: sudden vision loss
4. Problem: development of lazy eye (alcohol amblyopia)
Symptoms: gradual loss of vision in one eye
5. Problem: loss of areas of vision
Symptoms: blind spots, black-out of an area of vision

Recommendations: Find a program to help you quit. Get adequate nutrition. Report the above symptoms to your eye doctor. Have annual check-ups.

Allergies/Sinus Problems/Hay Fever

1. Problem: allergic reaction
Symptoms: redness, excessive tearing, glare, light sensitivity, headache, matter/discharge
2. Problem: reaction to drying properties of medication
Symptoms: excessive tearing, light sensitivity, pain (sandy/gritty sensation), itching, burning, redness
3. Problem: inflammation inside the eye (iritis)
Symptoms: redness, pain, light sensitivity, decreased vision

Recommendations: Use artificial tears for lubrication. See your ophthalmologist for allergy eye drops. Report symptoms of iritis at once.

Anemia

1. Problem: burst conjunctival blood vessel
Symptoms: bright red spot on white of eye
2. Problem: hemorrhage inside the eye
Symptoms: spots or floaters or blacked-out areas of vision, fog or veil over vision, sudden loss of vision
3. Problem: areas of decreased blood flow in the retina
Symptoms: no immediate symptoms, but a gradual loss of vision

Recommendations: See your medical doctor for recommendations about diet and iron supplements. Report symptoms of hemorrhage to your ophthalmologist at once.

Ankylosing Spondylitis

1. Problem: inflammation inside the eye (iritis)
   Symptoms: redness, pain, light sensitivity, tearing, blurred vision
2. Problem: glaucoma caused by iritis
   Symptoms: none

Recommendations: Report symptoms of iritis to your ophthalmologist at once. Have an annual eye exam that includes a pressure check for glaucoma.

Arteriosclerosis

1. Problem: external changes
   Symptoms: creamy colored ring around the colored part of the eye (this is a benign condition)
2. Problem: hemorrhage inside the eye
   Symptoms: spots or floaters or blacked-out areas of vision, fog or veil over vision, sudden loss of vision
3. Problem: swelling of retina (retinal edema)
   Symptoms: decreased vision
4. Problem: macular degeneration
   Symptoms: loss of central vision
5. Problem: weakening of blood vessels
   Symptoms: no immediate symptoms, but makes vessels more likely to bleed
6. Problem: leakage of fat-filled cells out of the blood vessels and into the retina
   Symptoms: no immediate symptoms, but a gradual loss of vision

Recommendations: See your regular physician as directed. Take any medications as directed. Report symptoms of hemorrhage to your ophthalmologist at once. Some physicians recommend taking Beta Carotene, Vitamin C, and Vitamin A.

Asthma

1. Problem: inflammation of conjunctiva (conjunctivitis)
   Symptoms: redness, excessive tearing, light sensitivity
2. Problem: cataracts secondary to steroid treatment

Symptoms: gradually decreased vision, new ability to read without reading glasses, change in color vision, change in depth perception, halos around lights at night, glare from lights at night, double vision, light sensitivity
3. Problem: glaucoma secondary to steroid treatment
Symptoms: none

Recommendations: Maintain close contact with medical doctor. Take steroids only as directed. Be aware of symptoms of cataracts. If on steroid therapy, see eye doctor annually. This yearly exam should include a pressure check for glaucoma. See eye care physician for symptoms of conjunctivitis.

Cancer

1. Problem: spread of cancer to eye
Symptoms: blurred vision, loss of vision, loss of peripheral vision, visible mass, pain, redness, protrusion of the eye, double vision

Recommendations: Report any of the above symptoms to ophthalmologist immediately.

Carotid Artery Disease

1. Problem: inflammation inside the eye (iritis)
Symptoms: redness, pain, light sensitivity, decreased vision
2. Problem: dilation (enlargement/swelling) of blood vessels in conjunctiva
Symptoms: redness
3. Problem: hemorrhage inside the eye
Symptoms: spots or floaters or blacked-out areas of vision, fog or veil over vision, sudden loss of vision
4. Problem: areas of decreased blood flow in the retina
Symptoms: no immediate symptoms, but a gradual loss of vision

Recommendations: Follow your medical doctor's advice regarding exams and medications. Report symptoms of iritis or hemorrhage to your ophthalmologist at once. If redness is a problem, see eye care physician about medication to help.

Diabetes (see Figure 7-A)

1. Problem: sugar fluctuations
   Symptoms: blurred vision that comes and goes (this is reversible and does not damage the eye)
2. Problem: nerve palsies
   Symptoms: double vision
3. Problem: external changes
   Symptoms: yellowish growth above upper lid or below lower lid (xanthelasma; this is a benign condition)
4. Problem: cataracts
   Symptoms: gradually decreased vision, new ability to read without reading glasses, change in color vision, change in depth perception, halos around lights at night, glare from lights at night, double vision, light sensitivity
5. Problem: hemorrhage inside the eye
   Symptoms: floaters (may be large), blurred vision, loss of central vision (all may be sudden)
6. Problem: leakage of fat-filled cells out of the blood vessels and into the retina
   Symptoms: no immediate symptoms, but a gradual loss of vision
7. Problem: areas of decreased blood flow in retina
   Symptoms: no immediate symptoms, but a gradual loss of vision
8. Problem: growth of new, abnormal blood vessels

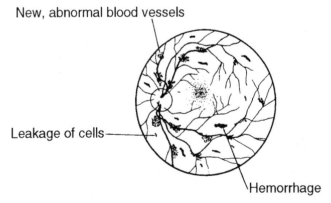

Figure 7-A Diabetic retinopathy.

Symptoms: no immediate symptoms, but a gradual loss of vision
9. Problem: inflammation of optic nerve (optic neuritis)
Symptoms: sudden vision loss, vision loss that comes and goes, decreased depth perception, change in color vision, pain, loss of central vision
10. Problem: deterioration of the optic nerve (optic atrophy)
Symptoms: sudden vision loss
11. Problem: retinal vein occlusion
Symptoms: blurry area or blurred vision (may be sudden)

Recommendations: See your medical doctor as scheduled. Have your blood pressure checked frequently. Be conscientious about medications: sugar control (including weight control and exercise) helps minimize damage to the retina. See your ophthalmologist as scheduled (in the absence of problems, once a year for a dilated exam). Report symptoms of hemorrhage, optic neuritis, or optic atrophy immediately. Be aware of symptoms of cataracts.

Emphysema

1. Problem: cataracts due to steroid treatment
Symptoms: gradually decreased vision, new ability to read without reading glasses, change in color vision, change in depth perception, halos around lights at night, glare from lights at night, double vision, light sensitivity
2. Problem: glaucoma due to steroid treatment
Symptoms: none

Recommendations: Keep scheduled appointments with medical doctor. Be aware of symptoms of cataract. If using steroids, see eye doctor annually for an exam that includes checking pressure for glaucoma.

Endocarditis

1. Problem: hemorrhage of tiny vessels in conjunctiva
Symptoms: tiny red spots on white of eye
2. Problem: hemorrhage inside the eye
Symptoms: spots or floaters or blacked-out areas of vision, fog or veil over vision, sudden loss of vision
3. Problem: nerve palsies

Symptoms: double vision, blurred vision (from eyes shaking), pupils not the same size

4. Problem: inflammation inside the eye (iritis)
   Symptoms: redness, pain, light sensitivity, tearing, blurred vision
5. Problem: inflammation of optic nerve head (papillitis)
   Symptoms: decreased vision, decreased peripheral vision
6. Problem: areas of decreased blood flow in retina
   Symptoms: no immediate symptoms, but a gradual loss of vision
7. Problem: infection that spreads to the eye (metastatic endophthalmitis)
   Symptoms: sudden (over a period of 1–2 days) appearance of pain, redness, lid swelling, lid twitching, loss of vision

Recommendations: Keep scheduled appointments with medical doctor. Take medications as ordered. Report double vision and symptoms of iritis, hemorrhage, papillitis, or endophthalmitis at once.

Gout

1. Problem: inflammation of tissue layer between conjunctiva and sclera (episcleritis)
   Symptoms: redness, pain (usually when the eye is moved), tearing, sensitivity to light
2. Problem: inflammation of white of eye (scleritis)
   Symptoms: redness, pain (may be severe, may be a deep boring ache), light sensitivity, tearing, decreased vision
3. Problem: crystals in cornea
   Symptoms: scattered light-burst effect, halos, light sensitivity
4. Problem: inflammation inside the eye (iritis)
   Symptoms: redness, pain, light sensitivity, tearing, blurred vision
5. Problem: glaucoma secondary to iritis
   Symptoms: none

Recommendations: See your regular doctor and take medications as directed. Report any pain and/or symptoms of iritis, episcleritis, or scleritis to your ophthalmologist at once. An annual eye exam should include a pressure check for glaucoma.

High Blood Pressure (Hypertension)

1. Problem: external changes
   Symptoms: creamy colored ring around the colored part of the eye (this is a benign condition)
2. Problem: hemorrhage inside the eye
   Symptoms: spots or floaters or blacked-out areas of vision, fog or veil over vision, sudden loss of vision
3. Problem: swelling of the retina (retinal edema)
   Symptoms: decreased vision
4. Problem: swelling of the optic nerve (papilledema)
   Symptoms: sudden blurred vision or vision blackouts that come and go (lasts less than one minute) with normal vision in between attacks, double vision, loss of side vision, headache (worse in morning, worse when straining)
5. Problem: leakage of fat-filled cells from the blood vessels into the retina
   Symptoms: no immediate symptoms, but a gradual loss of vision

Recommendations: See your medical doctor and take medications as directed. Monitor and control blood pressure. Report symptoms of hemorrhage or retinal edema to your ophthalmologist at once. Papilledema is an emergency and should be reported immediately. In the absence of other problems, have an annual dilated eye exam.

Leukemia

1. Problem: leukemia cells in area around eye
   Symptoms: protrusion of the eye(s)
2. Problem: hemorrhage in the back of the eye
   Symptoms: spots or floaters or blacked-out areas of vision, fog or veil over vision, sudden loss of vision
3. Problem: leukemia cells in aqueous
   Symptoms: may have no symptoms or may see floaters
4. Problem: glaucoma due to leukemia cells in aqueous
   Symptoms: none
5. Problem: leukemia cells clogging optic nerve
   Symptoms: sudden loss of vision (may occur over a period of several hours)

6. Problem: swelling of retina (retinal edema)
   Symptoms: decreased vision
7. Problem: inflammation of optic nerve head (papillitis)
   Symptoms: decreased vision, decreased peripheral vision
8. Problem: areas of decreased blood flow in retina (cotton wool spots)
   Symptoms: no immediate symptoms, but a gradual loss of vision
9. Problem: infection that spreads to the eye (metastatic endophthalmitis) due to chemotherapy
   Symptoms: sudden (over a period of 1–2 days) appearance of pain, redness, lid swelling, lid twitching, loss of vision

Recommendations: Follow your medical doctor's instructions about visits and medications. Report ANY of the above symptoms to your ophthalmologist at once. In absence of problems, have annual eye exam that includes a pressure check for glaucoma.

Lupus

1. Problem: hemorrhage inside the eye
   Symptoms: spots or floaters or blacked-out areas of vision, fog or veil over vision, sudden loss of vision
2. Problem: retinal swelling (retinal edema)
   Symptoms: decreased vision
3. Problem: areas of decreased blood flow in the retina
   Symptoms: no immediate symptoms, but a gradual loss of vision
4. Problem: external changes
   Symptoms: round marks on skin of lids, redness
5. Problem: inflammation of cornea (keratitis)
   Symptoms: pain, light sensitivity, decreased vision, tearing
6. Problem: inflammation inside the eye (iritis)
   Symptoms: redness, pain, light sensitivity, decreased vision
7. Problem: glaucoma due to iritis
   Symptoms: none

Recommendations: See your medical doctor and take any medications as directed. Report symptoms of hemorrhage, iritis, keratitis, or retinal swelling to your ophthalmologist at once. An annual exam should include a pressure check for glaucoma.

Malnutrition

1. Problem: external changes
   Symptoms: lid swelling, sensation of "fullness" in the eyes
2. Problem: dry eyes
   Symptoms: excessive tearing, light sensitivity, pain (sandy/gritty sensation), itching, burning, redness
3. Problem: decreased functioning of retinal cells
   Symptoms: night blindness

Recommendations: Consult with medical doctor regarding diet and vitamins. Try artificial tears for relief of dry eyes; see eye doctor if not relieved. Do not drive at night if night vision is affected.

Menopause

1. Problem: dry eye
   Symptoms: excessive tearing, light sensitivity, pain (sandy/gritty sensation), itching, burning, redness
2. Problem: loss of skin and muscle tone
   Symptoms: increased wrinkles, dry eye, ectropion, entropion, baggy eyelids, drooped eyelids
3. Problem: sudden development of migraine headaches (see next section, Migraine Headaches)

Recommendations: See your doctor for advice on hormone replacement therapy. Use artificial tears for comfort of dry eyes, see eye care physician if not relieved. Have evaluation by oculoplastic surgeon if eyelid position problems occur. In the absence of other problems, have an annual eye exam.

Migraine Headaches

1. Problem: spasms of blood vessels
   Symptoms: "blind spots" in the vision (these are missing areas of vision, different from floaters or specks)
2. Problems: spasms of blood vessels
   Symptoms: loss of side vision, closing in of side vision
3. Problem: spasms of blood vessels
   Symptoms: jagged lights around the vision

Recommendations: See your regular physician for therapy that might help. If directed to do so, take medication immediately when visual symptoms occur, as this may ward off the headache. Consult your physician whether calcium and magnesium supplements may help. Have an annual eye exam. Above symptoms may occur singly or together, usually before the headache starts. Visual symptoms may occur with no headache afterwards. Headache may occur without visual symptoms.

Multiple Sclerosis

1. Problem: inflammation of optic nerve (optic neuritis)
   Symptoms: blurred vision, periods of decreased vision, pain, blind spot(s) in vision
2. Problem: nystagmus ("dancing eyes")
   Symptoms: jerking movements of eyes, blurred vision, objects seem to move
3. Problem: weakness of eye muscles
   Symptoms: double vision
4. Problem: palsy of nerves to eye muscles
   Symptoms: drooped upper lid, double vision, difference in pupil size

Recommendations: Report symptoms of optic neuritis at once. Be aware of symptoms of eye muscle disturbances, contact ophthalmologist or neurologist if these occur. In absence of problems, have eye exam annually.

Muscular Dystrophy

1. Problem: muscle deterioration
   Symptoms: double vision, lid droop
2. Problem: dry eyes
   Symptoms: excessive tearing, light sensitivity, pain (sandy/gritty sensation), itching, burning, redness
3. Problem: cataracts
   Symptoms: gradually decreased vision, new ability to read without reading glasses, change in color vision, change in depth perception, halos around lights at night, glare from lights at night, double vision, light sensitivity

Recommendations: Follow your medical doctor's advice regarding exams and medications. Try artificial tears for relief of dry eyes; see eye doctor if not relieved. Be aware of symptoms of cataract.

Report double vision to your eye doctor. In absence of problems, have annual eye exam.

Myasthenia Gravis

1. Problem: nerve palsies
   Symptoms: double vision, lid droop, abnormal pupil size

Recommendations: See your medical doctor and take any medications as directed. Report double vision to eye doctor. In absence of problems, have annual eye exam.

Neurofibromatosis (von Recklinghausen's Disease)

1. Problem: external changes
   Symptoms: protruding eye, lid droop, thickened lids, fibroma growth on lids
2. Problem: internal changes
   Symptoms: vision loss, loss of peripheral vision
3. Problem: glaucoma
   Symptoms: none

Recommendations: See medical doctor as directed. Report lid droop if it cuts off vision. Report symptoms of internal changes. In absence of problems, have annual eye exam that includes a pressure check for glaucoma.

Occlusive Vascular Disease (Sudden)

1. Problem: clots moving through blood vessels inside eye
   Symptoms: vision goes out then comes back
2. Problem: blockage of blood vessels inside eye
   Symptoms: sudden loss of vision

Recommendations: Follow medical doctor's directions regarding exams and medications. Take medications as directed. Report symptoms of clots or blockages to ophthalmologist immediately. Have a dilated eye exam every year. If scheduled for eye surgery, be sure to tell the eye surgeon if you are taking blood thinners.

Parathyroid (Overactive)

1. Problem: breakdown of outer surface of cornea
   Symptoms: pain, light sensitivity, blurred vision, tearing

2. Problem: calcium deposits in conjunctiva
   Symptoms: foreign body sensation/pain, scratchy feeling, tearing
3. Problem: calcium deposits in cornea (corneal opacities)
   Symptoms: scattered light-burst effect, halos, light sensitivity

Recommendations: See your medical doctor and take medications as directed. Report symptoms of corneal breakdown to your eye doctor at once. In absence of problems, have annual eye exam.

Parathyroid (Underactive)

1. Problem: inflammation of conjunctiva (conjunctivitis)
   Symptoms: redness, excessive tearing, light sensitivity
2. Problem: inflammation of cornea (keratitis)
   Symptoms: pain, light sensitivity, decreased vision, tearing
3. Problem: cataracts
   Symptoms: gradually decreased vision, new ability to read without reading glasses, change in color vision, change in depth perception, halos around lights at night, glare from lights at night, double vision, light sensitivity
4. Problem: swelling of optic nerve head (papilledema)
   Symptoms: sudden blurred vision or vision blackouts that come and go (lasts less than one minute) with normal vision in between attacks, double vision, loss of side vision, headache (worse in morning, worse when straining)
   Other miscellaneous symptoms: lid twitching, light sensitivity

Recommendations: Keep scheduled appointments with medical doctor, take any medication as directed. Report symptoms of keratitis to your ophthalmologist. Papilledema is an emergency, and should be reported immediately. Be aware of symptoms of cataract. Have annual eye exam if no other problems arise.

Psoriasis

1. Problem: inflammation of conjunctiva (conjunctivitis)
   Symptoms: redness, excessive tearing
2. Problem: chronic low-grade lid infection (blepharitis)
   Symptoms: itching, swollen lids, crusting
3. Problem: corneal involvement

Symptoms: pain, foreign body sensation, blurred vision, light sensitivity, tearing

Recommendations: See medical doctor as directed. Seek non-emergency treatment for conjunctivitis and blepharitis. Report symptoms of corneal involvement to eye doctor at once. Have annual eye exam.

Rheumatoid Arthritis

1. Problem: dry eyes (Sjögren's Syndrome)
   Symptoms: excessive tearing, light sensitivity, pain (sandy/gritty sensation), itching, burning, redness
2. Problem: inflammation of conjunctiva (conjunctivitis)
   Symptoms: redness, blurred or fluctuating vision, excessive tearing, matter/discharge, light sensitivity
3. Problem: inflammation of tissue layer between conjunctiva and sclera (episcleritis)
   Symptoms: redness, pain (usually when the eye is moved), tearing, sensitivity to light
4. Problem: inflammation of white of eye (scleritis)
   Symptoms: redness, pain (may be severe, may be a deep boring ache), light sensitivity, tearing, decreased vision
5. Problem: inflammation inside the eye (iritis)
   Symptoms: redness, pain, light sensitivity, tearing, blurred vision
6. Problem: cataracts secondary to steroid treatment
   Symptoms: gradually decreased vision, new ability to read without reading glasses, change in color vision, change in depth perception, halos around lights at night, glare from lights at night, double vision, light sensitivity
7. Problem: glaucoma secondary to steroid treatment
   Symptoms: none

Recommendations: Maintain contact with your medical doctor and take medications as directed. Use artificial tears for comfort of dry eyes, see eye care physician if not relieved. Report symptoms of iritis, episcleritis, or scleritis to ophthalmologist at once. If on steroids, have eye pressure checked annually (more often if pressure goes up). In absence of problems, have an annual eye exam.

Sarcoidosis

1. Problem: inflammation of iris (iritis)
   Symptoms: redness, pain, light sensitivity, tearing, blurred vision
2. Problem: inflammation inside the eye (uveitis)
   Symptoms: pain, redness, light sensitivity, blurred vision
3. Problem: inflammation inside the back of the eye (chorioretinitis)
   Symptoms: mild pain, mild light sensitivity, mild blurred vision

Recommendations: See your medical doctor and take medications as directed. Report symptoms of iritis, uveitis, or chorioretinitis to your ophthalmologist at once. In the absence of problems, see you eye care physician yearly for an exam.

Shingles (Herpes zoster)

1. Problem: blister-like lesions on skin
   Symptoms: pain, lid droop, lid swelling, lid redness
2. Problem: lid paralysis (lid does not close completely)
   Symptoms: excessive tearing, light sensitivity, pain (sandy/gritty sensation), itching, burning, redness
3. Problem: nerve palsies
   Symptoms: double vision
4. Problem: inflammation of white of eye (scleritis)
   Symptoms: redness, pain (may be severe, may be a deep boring ache), light sensitivity, tearing, decreased vision
5. Problem: inflammation of cornea (keratitis)
   Symptoms: pain, light sensitivity, decreased vision, tearing
6. Problem: swelling of the cornea (corneal edema)
   Symptoms: blurred vision, halos around lights, light sensitivity
7. Problem: inflammation inside eye (iritis)
   Symptoms: redness, pain, light sensitivity, decreased vision
8. Problem: inflammation of the optic nerve (optic neuritis)
   Symptoms: sudden vision loss, vision loss that comes and goes, decreased depth perception, change in color vision, pain, loss of central vision
9. Problem: secondary glaucoma due to inflammation in the drainage network
   Symptoms: none

Recommendations: See your medical doctor, who may treat blisters on lids. Contact your ophthalmologist for any of the other above symptoms.

Smoking

1. Problem: deterioration of the optic nerve (optic atrophy)
   Symptoms: sudden vision loss
2. Problem: development of lazy eye (tobacco amblyopia)
   Symptoms: gradual loss of vision in one eye
3. Problem: cataract formation
   Symptoms: gradually decreased vision, new ability to read without reading glasses, change in color vision, change in depth perception, halos around lights at night, glare from lights at night, double vision, light sensitivity
4. Problem: increased risk of diabetic retinal disease
   Symptoms: see page 124
5. Problem: increased incidence of macular degeneration
   Symptoms: loss of central vision
6. Problem: dry eyes
   Symptoms: excessive tearing, light sensitivity, pain (sandy/gritty sensation), itching, burning, redness

Recommendations: Find a program to help you quit. Report symptoms of optic atrophy or tobacco amblyopia to ophthalmologist at once.

Temporal (Giant Cell) Arteritis

1. Problem: nerve palsies
   Symptoms: double vision, lid droop
2. Problem: inflammation inside the eye (iritis)
   Symptoms: redness, pain, light sensitivity, tearing, blurred vision
3. Problem: hemorrhage inside the eye
   Symptoms: spots or floaters or blacked-out areas of vision, fog or veil over vision, sudden loss of vision
4. Problem: blockage of retinal artery
   Symptoms: total loss of vision
5. Problem: inflammation of the optic nerve (optic neuritis)
   Symptoms: sudden vision loss, vision loss that comes and goes,

decreased depth perception, change in color vision, pain, loss of central vision

6. Problem: decreased blood supply in arteries of the optic nerve (ischemic optic neuropathy)
   Symptoms: sudden loss of vision (1–2 days) or gradual loss of vision (3–12 weeks), vision loss that comes and goes (blurred vision or "gray cloud" lasts 2–3 minutes, sometimes 30 minutes), loss of peripheral vision, unreactive pupil

7. Problem: fluid leaking from the blood vessels of the retina
   Symptoms: no immediate symptoms, but a gradual loss of vision

Recommendations: See your medical doctor as instructed, use medications as directed. Report symptoms of iritis, hemorrhage, and optic neuritis to your ophthalmologist. Report symptoms of artery blockage or ischemic optic neuropathy AT ONCE. In absence of problems, have yearly eye exam.

Thyroid (Overactive)

1. Problem: external changes
   Symptoms: protrusion of eye(s), puffiness around eyes, lids don't close all the way

2. Problem: exposure of eye (from lids not closing)
   Symptoms: excessive tearing, light sensitivity, pain (sandy/gritty sensation), itching, burning, redness

3. Problem: deterioration of the optic nerve (optic atrophy)
   Symptoms: sudden vision loss

4. Problem: swelling of optic nerve head (papilledema)
   Symptoms: sudden blurred vision or vision blackouts that come and go (lasts less than one minute) with normal vision in between attacks, double vision, loss of side vision, headache (worse in morning, worse when straining)

Recommendations: See your medical doctor and use medications as directed. Be aware of symptoms of external changes. Report lack of lid closure and symptoms of optic atrophy or papilledema to your ophthalmologist. Have an annual eye exam.

Thyroid (Underactive)

1. Problem: external changes
   Symptoms: swelling around eyes, eyelid swelling, loss of outer third of eyebrows
2. Problem: cataracts
   Symptoms: gradually decreased vision, new ability to read without reading glasses, change in color vision, change in depth perception, halos around lights at night, glare from lights at night, double vision, light sensitivity
3. Problem: inflammation of the optic nerve (optic neuritis)
   Symptoms: sudden vision loss, vision loss that comes and goes, decreased depth perception, change in color vision, pain, loss of central vision
4. Problem: deterioration of the optic nerve (optic atrophy)
   Symptoms: sudden vision loss

Recommendations: Take medications and keep medical appointments as directed. Be aware of symptoms of external changes and cataracts. Report symptoms of optic neuritis and optic atrophy to your ophthalmologist at once.

Tuberculosis

1. Problem: inflammation of sclera (scleritis)
   Symptoms: redness, pain (may be severe, may be a deep boring ache), light sensitivity, tearing, decreased vision
2. Problem: hemorrhage inside the eye
   Symptoms: spots or floaters or blacked-out areas of vision, fog or veil over vision, sudden loss of vision
3. Problem: inflammation of optic nerve (optic neuritis)
   Symptoms: sudden vision loss, vision loss that comes and goes, decreased depth perception, change in color vision, pain, loss of central vision
4. Problem: inflammation inside the eye (uveitis)
   Symptoms: pain, redness, light sensitivity, blurred vision

Recommendations: Maintain close contact with your medical doctor, take medications as directed. Report any of the above symptoms to your ophthalmologist. In absence of problems, see eye care physician for annual check-up.

The body is a collection of united parts. Beginning with the next chapter, we'll look at each section of the eye and the problems associated with it. Did you know that the skin is an organ of the body? (It's also the largest!) That's where we'll start, in Chapter 8.

CHAPTER 8

Eyelids and Skin

CYNTHIA VanDusen was concerned. About a week ago, she had noticed a new growth on her lower lid. Mrs. VanDusen was a nurse, so she pulled out one of her medical books. "Non-malignant growths of the lids are common, and more likely to occur as one ages," she read. That sounded good. But the next section discussed skin cancer. That didn't sound so good. Even with her medical experience, she knew she couldn't tell one from the other. She called her eye doctor for an appointment.

Oculoplastic surgery is plastic surgery of the eyelids, eyebrows, tear system, or eye socket (see Figure 8-A). The surgery may be performed in order to improve function, comfort, or appearance, or to remove a mass. Most oculoplastic surgery can be done in an office under local anesthesia. Chapter 15 contains information common to many ocular procedures. Scanning that chapter will be helpful for anyone who is considering facial surgery.

Blepharitis (Granulated Lids)

Blepharitis Survey

Risk factors:

- Do you have dry eyes?
- Do you have dandruff, eczema, psoriasis, or seborrhea?

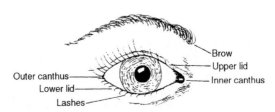

Figure 8-A The external eye.

Symptoms:

- Do your lids itch?
- Are the edges of your lids red?
- Are your eyelashes falling out?
- Do you have crusts on your lashes?

"Granulated lids" is the old-fashioned name for blepharitis. In basic terms, blepharitis is a low-grade lid infection caused by bacteria.

Blepharitis is often associated with dry eyes. Tears have a natural cleansing action, washing away germs and debris from the eyes and lids. Without enough tears to do this job, bacteria remain and cause an infection. Itching, redness, and crusting are common. In more severe cases the corner of the lids may crack, ooze, and become sore (angular blepharitis). Eyelashes may fall out.

The infection may spread from the lids and into the eye, causing pink eye (conjunctivitis) or corneal ulcers. Severe cases may scar the eyelid.

Treatment

Blepharitis can be an aggravating problem. In general, you don't get rid of it. The goal is to control it. Maintenance treatment must be continued indefinitely or the symptoms will come back.

If the problem is due to dry eyes, the dryness must be treated (outlined in Chapter 9). The lids themselves are usually treated with cleansing and antibiotics.

Cleaning the lids, or lid scrubs, can be done with no-tears baby shampoo. Mix a capful of shampoo with a capful of warm water (a paper cup is handy for this). Use a cotton-tip applicator. Dunk the applicator in the shampoo water, then carefully scrub the lids. Rub along the base of the lashes. Be careful not to poke your eye! Do NOT pull your eyelid down and scrub the inside of the lid. The idea is to cleanse the lash line. Instead of baby shampoo, you may want to use an over-the-counter cleanser made especially for cleaning the lids.

Lid scrubs are done twice daily at first. When the symptoms begin to clear up, you may scrub once a day. If you stop altogether, the symptoms will probably come back. Warm compresses are good for both comfort and healing.

If there is scalp dandruff, use a good shampoo on your head and eyebrows (brows, *not* lashes). Your doctor may also ask you to massage your lids. This is to empty the oil glands that harbor bacteria.

Antibiotic drops or ointment will probably be prescribed as well. Follow your doctor's instructions. Ointment should be applied to the lash line rather than in the eye. After the problem is under control, you may be told to use the drops or ointment at regular intervals (for example, twice a day for one week out of every month). If you do not follow instructions, the symptoms will probably come back.

Most cases of blepharitis will respond to the above treatment. If you are following your doctor's instructions and the symptoms don't clear up, let your doctor know. He may want to do a culture to determine what kind of bacteria is causing the infection. Once the doctor knows what type of bacteria is causing the problem, he can choose a medication that is especially effective. In addition to drops or ointment, you may be given an oral antibiotic. Be sure to take ALL of them; don't stop taking them because the symptoms are gone.

Brow Ptosis (Drooped Eyebrows)

As the muscles of the forehead lose their strength with age, the brows may droop so low that they interfere with vision. When this occurs, the brows must be raised high all the time in order to see. (You might even feel like holding your brows up with tape!) This can cause fatigue and headaches.

Brow ptosis can be corrected by a procedure called a brow lift. In this surgery, an incision is made just above the brow, in the forehead, or in the scalp. Skin and muscle tissue is removed so that the brow is lifted to a more normal position. The scar is camouflaged among the natural lines in the forehead, or is hidden in the scalp. If the lids are also baggy, a blepharoplasty might be done at the same time.

Preparation, surgery, and post-operative care are very similar to any eye surgery. (See Chapter 15 for more details.)

Cancer

Cancer of The Lids and Skin Survey
Risk factors:

• Has someone in your family had skin cancer?

- Did you have one or more severe sunburns during childhood or adolescence?
- Did you or do you work in a job with a lot of exposure to the sun? (Examples: farming, construction work)
- Are you fair-skinned and tend to sunburn easily?

Symptoms:

- Asymmetry—Compare one side of the mole to the other. Are the halves un-matched?
- Border irregularity—Are the edges of the mole irregular, notched, or blurred?
- Color—Is the mole more than one color, with different shades of tan, brown, black, or patches of red, white, or blue?
- Diameter—Is the mole larger than 1/4 inch (the top of a pencil eraser)?
- Does the growth bleed, scab over, then bleed again without completely healing?
- Does the growth have a "dimple" in the center?
- Has the growth changed in size or color?

Please remember that these are guidelines meant to lead you to your doctor. Any lesion around the eyelids should be checked out by your eye care physician or dermatologist. We are including skin cancer in this book because the eyelids are common sites of skin cancer. This is because the face is exposed to the sun. (Other types of growths are discussed starting on page 154.)

In general, there are three types of skin cancer.

1. Basal cell carcinoma—This is the most common type of skin cancer. It usually starts as a small bump that may have a shiny or pearly appearance. If not removed, it may bleed, crust over, then bleed again. Basal cell cancer is slow growing. It is rarely life-threatening because it does not spread to other parts of the body (metastasize). But it should be removed because it can destroy the tissues around and underneath it.

2. Squamous cell carcinoma—This type of skin cancer may begin as nodules or red patches with obvious borders. The face is the most common place for squamous cell cancer. Like basal cell carcinoma, squamous cell causes damage to the tissues around it. But squamous cancer can also spread to other parts of the body.

3. Malignant melanoma—This is the least common of the three types, but the most serious. Melanoma arises from cells that contain skin pigment (color), so the most common starting-point is in or near a mole. Any sign of change in a mole should send you immediately to the doctor: a change in color (may be different shades of brown, tan, or black; may have red or blue parts), or a mole that has jagged or uneven edges. Early detection is vital. Melanoma tends to grow rapidly, and can spread throughout the body. If discovered and removed early enough, melanoma can be cured. But if not treated promptly, it can be life-threatening. Of the new cases of melanoma diagnosed each year, 75% are in patients over age 40.

Diagnosis and Treatment

Detection is the first line of defense in the fight against skin cancer. If you have a growth on your eyelids or around your eyes, ask your ophthalmologist to check it. (Growths on other parts of the body should be checked, too—probably by your regular physician or dermatologist.)

If your doctor feels that the growth might be cancer, he will probably do a biopsy. A biopsy may be done by totally removing the growth, along with a tiny border of the healthy tissue right around it. Or, if the growth is large, a small piece may be removed and sent to the lab. The area is numbed before the procedure. Stitches may be used if the excision area is large. Follow your doctor's instructions about bandages, ointment, and follow-up visits.

Once a growth has been confirmed to be cancer (either by biopsy or appearance), it needs to be removed totally. There are four types of cancer surgery: cutting the growth out (excision), burning, freezing, and using radiation.

Surgical Excision

Please refer to Chapter 15 for general information on eye surgery. Basically, you should report for surgery on time, wear a button-front shirt, and not wear make-up. If the procedure will be long, you may have an IV. The area to be treated will be numbed with an injection of anesthetic. Ask your doctor if you will need someone to drive you home, and what your restrictions are. Apply ointment to stitches as directed, and be sure to keep your follow-up appointments.

If the growth is small and has been detected early, only the growth itself (plus a small border) may be cut out. (This is basically the same procedure as the biopsy we talked about before.) Later, if the lab report shows that the clear-looking borders were also cancerous, you may need to have another surgery to remove more tissue.

If the growth is large and has been there a while, the doctor may suspect that the cancer has grown down into the deeper tissues. In this case a more extensive procedure may be planned.

Frozen Sections

This procedure gives the surgeon a better idea of what tissue to remove while the patient is still in the operating room. Tissue is removed, taken to the lab, and quick-frozen. The pathologist looks at the sample and reports to the surgeon. If the frozen sample is clear, the surgery is over. If the pathologist finds that the sample contains cancer cells, the surgeon removes more tissue, which is again sent to the lab. The process continues until the pathologist gives the all-clear signal. The disadvantage to this technique is the time required for freezing the tissue.

Mohs Surgery

In Mohs surgery, the physician also learns how much tissue he must remove as he is operating. The obvious cancer and a tiny border of normal-looking tissue around it are removed first. This fresh tissue is immediately examined under a microscope. This eliminates the time-consuming task of freezing. The surgeon makes a map of the tissue, showing malignant and non-malignant areas. A thin layer of tissue is removed from any area that still shows malignancy. Then *this* tissue is looked at under the microscope and mapped. The process continues until all the cancer is removed.

The main advantage of Mohs surgery is that a minimum of normal tissue is removed. The surgeon uses the microscope as his eyes to "see" normal tissue that need not be removed. He is also aware of small tumor nests that might otherwise be missed, lowering the recurrence rate.

The three areas where a cancer is most likely to recur are the nose, eye lids, and ears. The low recurrence rate after Mohs makes it ideal for facial cancers, as does the fact that less tissue is removed. But there is another aspect of Mohs that is appealing when the face is involved. In traditional cancer removal methods the wound had to heal over before a repair could be done. That takes time. But with Mohs surgery, the restoration can be done the same or next day.

Burning (Cautery) and Freezing (Cryotherapy)

Burning or freezing a growth destroys it, leaving nothing to send to the lab. This means that there is no way to get a lab report confirming whether a growth was cancer or not. So freezing or burning is usually used on growths that have first had a biopsy or in cases where the doctor is already sure what the growth is. There is also no way to tell if all of the growth was destroyed, except by what the doctor can actually see. If the physician thinks that a growth may have penetrated into deeper tissues, he will usually use a method other than cautery or cryo.

In either case, the growth is numbed with an injection. The freezing or burning tip is touched to the growth until it is gone. Your doctor will tell you about bandages, ointments, and return visits. Be sure to follow directions.

Radiation

Radiation is beams of a special kind of energy. At low levels, radiation is used for X-rays. At high levels, radiation is used to treat cancer. The rays are aimed at the cancer, and the radiation is absorbed by the tissue. This causes chemical changes in the cells. The purpose of treating skin cancer with radiation is to either kill the cancer cells or to prevent them from reproducing.

Radiation may be used alone, or together with surgical removal. The combination technique is used to treat any unseen cancer cells that might be left after a growth is surgically removed. Each treatment takes anywhere from 30 minutes to 2 hours. Sometimes more than one treatment is required (often over a 2–7 week period), depending on the size and type of the growth.

Reconstruction

Any type of cancer surgery can leave a defect or scar. Plastic surgery may be needed to restore a more normal appearance, and is discussed beginning on page 157. Chapter 15 explains details of general eye surgery.

Pre-cancerous growths

A biopsy may show that a growth is not cancer, but is a type of lesion that may develop into cancer. Such a growth, sometimes called a sun spot, is removed before it can cause trouble. Surgical removal, cryotherapy, or cautery, all described above, can be used to remove a pre-cancer. In addition, such spots may be chemically treated. (Cancer itself is not usually treated chemically because most surgeons prefer methods that show whether all the cancer has been removed.)

Chemical treatment uses the same procedure as endodermology, used to remove facial wrinkles and age spots (described in detail beginning on page 161). When treating pre-cancer, however, the chemical peel is applied only to the lesions, instead of the entire face.

Some patients notice tingling or tenderness in the treated area. It is recommended that you avoid steam, and use a cool dryer to dry your hair. The most important precaution is to be very careful about sun exposure.

Cellulitis

other names: orbital cellulitis

Cellulitis Survey

Risk factors:

- Do you have lowered immunities?
- Have you had a recent eye injury that penetrated the skin?
- Have you had recent eyelid surgery?
- Do you have a sinus infection?

Symptoms:

- Is the lid swollen, red, feverish, and tender?

Cellulitis is an inflammation and infection of the tissues around the eye. It is most common in children, but can also occur in the elderly and those with low resistance.

Cellulitis is caused by bacteria, usually coming from the sinuses in the eye area. Thus it may occur during a sinus infection (sinusitis).

A penetrating injury could also allow the bacteria to enter the lid tissues. The symptoms include redness, swelling, fever, and tenderness in the lids and tissues around the eye. Eye movements may be restricted. There may be fever and a sense of not feeling well. In some cases, a draining abscess forms.

Diagnosis and Treatment

Cultures are often taken to identify the organism causing the infection. A blood sample may be cultured as well.

A CT scan or an MRI scan may be ordered to see how deep the inflammation is. If there is an abscess, a CT scan can show its location and severity.

Treatment is begun right away, even before the cultures are read. Because the bones surrounding the eyes and the sinuses are so close to the brain, cellulitis is treated promptly. The infection can corrode the bones, exposing deeper areas to the bacteria. Nerve damage or septic fever can result.

In most cases, oral antibiotics are prescribed. In severe cases, hospital admission and antibiotics by IV may be ordered. The good news is that antibiotic treatment is extremely effective. (If you are taking pills, be sure to take all of them, even if the symptoms go away.)

Hot packs are used to help keep the inflammation from spreading. Decongestant nose spray may be used to help drain the sinuses. If an abscess forms, it may be drained surgically once the infection has quieted down. This is done after the area is numbed with an anesthetic injection.

Contact Dermatitis (Rash)

Contact dermatitis is an allergy to something that you've applied to (or has gotten on) your eyes or eyelids. The rash may be bumpy, itchy, and swollen. There may be little blisters that weep and get crusty. The conjunctiva (membrane covering the white of the eye and lining the lids) may have an allergic response as well. If the allergy problem continues, the lids may look dry, wrinkled, red, and scaly.

The allergy may be to any number of things, such as: cosmetics, eye drops or ointments, plastic glasses frames (or other plastic), lotions (such as sunscreen, moisture lotion, or bug repellent), poison from plants (ivy, oak, etc.), clothing, jewelry, food, insect bites, and industrial chemicals. The rash may occur right after contact or a day or two later.

Treatment

Your physician will advise you about cleansing the area. A steroid ointment or cream is often prescribed. This is usually an eye ointment, you may get some in the eyes. In severe cases you may be given an antihistamine or some other oral medicine to relieve the symptoms. In the future, try to avoid whatever you're allergic to!

Dermatochalasis (Baggy Eyelids)

"I feel as if my eyelids are cutting off part of my vision, like blinders on a horse!" one patient complains. Another describes a heaviness of the lids and a tired feeling. Yet another reports headaches. One single problem can cause any or all of these symptoms: drooping eyelids.

There are actually several categories of droopy lids. First, one may be born with eyelids that don't open all the way (called "congenital ptosis"). In this instance, the problem is usually caused by a muscle that did not develop properly.

A second type, "acquired ptosis," occurs later in life, usually due to aging or trauma. The muscle that pulls the eyelid up slips out of position, and the lid sags. In both congenital and acquired ptosis, the lowered lids may reduce side vision drastically. The eyes look sleepy all the time. (That's where the expression "bed room eyes" came from.)

A third type of lid droop occurs when loose skin actually hangs down onto, and sometimes over, the eyelashes. This is commonly described as "baggy eyelids" (called "lash ptosis" or dermatochalasis). It is caused by the gradual loss of skin and muscle tone associated with getting older, plus the effects of gravity. This condition sometimes runs in families. Furthermore, weakening of the tissues may cause fat to bulge into the upper and lower lids, resulting in larger "bags." These folds of skin not only make one look older, but can also block off vision to the side. Often the patient tries to counteract the drooping by raising his eyebrows. The effort of holding the brows up constantly can result in a nasty headache.

What can be done? Aristotle Onassis' answer was to tape his

eyelids up, remember? Maybe he was too rich to care what he looked like. At any rate, most of us don't want to go around with adhesive strips on our foreheads! Fortunately, oculoplastic surgery provides a better looking and more permanent alternative.

In congenital and acquired ptosis, the corrective surgery consist of repairing the muscles involved. In lash ptosis, the extra skin and sometimes underlying fat are actually removed. (This surgery is called a blepharoplasty.) If acquired and lash ptosis occur in the same patient, surgery requires muscle repair as well as tissue removal. The upper lid scar is hidden in the lid crease. The lower lid incision is placed just below the eyelashes, or inside the lower lid where it isn't visible.

The surgery is done on an out-patient basis, often right in the doctor's office. Local anesthesia is usually all that is necessary. The procedure is generally successful in giving a much more youthful appearance to the eyelids, as well as improving the side vision.

Complications are uncommon and usually minor, but must be considered. The most common side effect of this type of surgery is a dry or scratchy eye. This might require indefinite treatment with artificial tear drops or ointment. Some other common complications include under or over correction, recurrence of the original problem, a change in skin pigmentation, a change in skin sensation, scarring, and loss of tissue.

Preliminaries

To determine if you are a good candidate for blepharoplasty, you need to schedule a consultation with a surgeon. Choose your doctor with care. Inquire through a referral service, or ask for recommendations from friends who have had successful results. The physician you select should be certified in the area of his or her specialty. Inquire at the doctor's office when you call. Blepharoplasties are currently done by a variety of board-certified physicians including ophthalmologists, general plastic surgeons, facial plastic surgeons, dermatologists, and otolaryngologists.

Because an upper lid blepharoplasty may be done to improve your vision, your insurance (including Medicare) may cover it either completely or in part. (Insurance companies aren't concerned that the surgery may make you look better. They consider only the practical side.) You, however, will gain the benefit of the cosmetic and visual nature of the surgery without the disadvantage of being responsible for the entire fee.

Before blepharoplasty, it is usually necessary to get prior approval from your insurance company. In this case, photographs are taken showing the position of the lids both from the front and the sides. Criteria differ among companies, but generally the photos must show that the extra skin is touching or hanging over the eyelashes.

To give evidence that the surgery will increase your peripheral vision, a special computerized test, called a visual field, is done that maps out your side vision. This analysis is run two times. The first test is done with your lids in their normal relaxed, drooped position. The second test is done with your eyelids taped up. (I know what you're thinking . . . "After all they said about Aristotle!") The test done with the lids held up simulates what your side vision will be *after* surgery is done. The insurance review board compares the un-taped to the taped test. If the maps show that the side vision will improve by having the surgery, chances are good that they will approve it. The visual field maps and photographs are sent from the physician, often accompanied by a letter giving other details about your case.

Since having a blepharoplasty on the lower lids will not affect your vision, it is usually considered to be cosmetic. However, if the lower lids are so lax that they do not function properly, insurance may provide coverage. You should discuss this with your surgeon. He or she may offer a reduced rate for having the lowers done at the same time as the uppers. The reasoning behind this is that the operating room and instruments are set up and used only one time, as opposed to twice if you had uppers and lowers done separately.

Once the proper paperwork has been submitted, there is a waiting period while the company considers your request. It often takes only ten to 12 weeks to get a reply. Then, when everything is in order, you will receive notification from your doctor with a go-ahead for surgery.

If you have chosen an ophthalmologist to do your eyelid surgery, you may be required to have a preliminary eye exam before the procedure. You will be asked about your health, allergies, and any medications you are taking. In addition to the normal tests of a routine eye exam, a tear test will probably be done. If your tear production is low or borderline, the surgeon may decide to be more conservative with the lid surgery. The physician will also consider the cause of the lid droop as he/she plans what surgical method is best.

The Surgery

Chapter 15 covers topics related to all types of eye surgery. If you are planning to have a blepharoplasty, please glance over this material.

The requirements before having a blepharoplasty are very simple. Surgeons may vary in their guidelines, so follow your doctor's advice. Some doctors recommend taking Vitamin C (1,000 milligrams a day) and zinc (50 milligrams a day) for one week before and one week after surgery. These vitamins have been shown to increase healing.

On the day of surgery, report at your appointed time. Do not wear any face make-up. Wear a shirt or blouse that buttons (no pull-overs). Have someone lined up to drive you home.

A blepharoplasty is an out-patient procedure. You will have an IV and local anesthesia. You may have to put on a hospital gown. Before starting, the physician will measure and mark the lids with a special pen. The procedure lasts about an hour for upper lids, and around two hours if both upper and lower lids are being repaired.

After surgery, the lids are gently cleansed, but not patched in most cases. Once you have recovered sufficiently, you will be allowed to go home.

After Surgery

Once you arrive home, consider yourself restricted to bed-rest except to use the bathroom. Do not lie flat . . . elevate your head with two pillows. Use ice packs as much as possible for the next 72 hours. You will be given a prescription for ointment to apply to the sutures. Do not get the stitches wet for one week.

There is rarely much pain. Occasionally there may be some mild discomfort or a "pulling" sensation which will disappear soon.

There is usually some swelling and bruising. Since every person is different, it is impossible to predict how much or how long either will last. The ice packs should keep the swelling to a minimum. Any residual swelling slowly disappears over 4 to 6 weeks. Bruising will gradually disappear over a period of two weeks or so. You may wear face make-up after one week and eye make-up after two weeks.

You will generally have a follow-up appointment sometime during the week following surgery. The stitches usually resorb. Any fragments are removed a week or two after the procedure. A final check-up is generally done about six weeks after the operation. If an ophthalmologist has done your surgery, this check-up may include checking to see if your glasses prescription needs changing. (Sometimes the weight of the lids can put pressure on the eyeball and change the way you see. Once the lids are lifted, you may need a different prescription.)

As mentioned before, the scar lines are carefully placed to be as inconspicuous as possible. At first the scar may be red and bumpy. This fades with time. Usually within a year all that remains is a permanent fine white line. The skin of the lids heals with less scarring than other areas. A few patients require a "touch up" procedure to adjust the lid position and remove suture bumps or redundant skin.

Ectropion (Out-Turned Eyelid)

Ectropion Survey

Risk factors:

- Have you had eye lid surgery?
- Do you have scarring on your eyelids?

Symptoms:

- Do your lower lids hang outward, exposing the pink membrane underneath?
- Do your eyes water almost constantly?
- Do you often have the sensation of having sand or grit in your eyes?
- Do your eyes itch and burn? (see Figure 8-B)

Loss of muscle tone can cause the lower lid to turn outward. This condition, known as ectropion, can also be caused by a nerve palsy or lid scarring. When the lid flips out, the conjunctiva (membrane lining the lid) is exposed to the air. This causes several things to happen. First, the conjunctiva, which is meant to be a moist

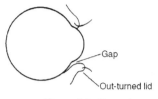

Figure 8-B Ectropion.

membrane, dries out...it may turn beefy red and the lid may thicken. Second, the punctum (tear-draining opening in the lid) is folded away from the eye. The tears cannot drain through their natural route, and so spill down the cheeks. Third, without the lower lid in proper position, the cornea (clear window over the front of the eye) is exposed. Dehydration of the cornea can cause painful dry spots and leave the eye vulnerable to infection. Finally, if the eye dries out, the tear gland may over-react by creating more moisture . . . causing further gushing of tears.

Treatment

Ectropion can be treated temporarily by putting one stitch in the lid. This tightens the lid and helps pull it back against the eye. Only a local numbing injection is needed. The stitch is not a permanent repair, however. It might be used when the patient can't tolerate having longer surgery, or as an "emergency" procedure if the cornea is severely dry.

A more lasting solution is surgery to remove a wedge of lid, then sew the edges of the wound together. This shortens the lid and pulls it up against the eyeball. This procedure is also done with a local injection to numb the area.

Entropion (In-Turned Eyelid)

Entropion Survey

Risk factors:

- Have you had eye lid surgery?
- Do you have scarring on your eyelids?

Symptoms:

- Do you often feel like there's something in your eye?

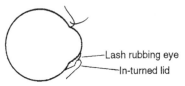

Lash rubbing eye
In-turned lid

Figure 8-C Entropion.

- Do eye drops fail to make this sensation go away?

Muscle tone tends to diminish with age. If the muscle of the lower lid degenerates, the lid may flip in (see Figure 8-C). As a result, the eyelashes rub against the cornea (clear covering over the colored part of the eye). This can be quite painful, and may even damage the cornea. Scarring from injury to the lower lid may also cause the eyelid to turn in. An in-turned lid is called an entropion.

Treatment

There are several methods of treatment. One method uses cautery (a hot probe). The lids are numbed by an injection of anesthetic (such as Xylocaine). The scar tissue from the burns tightens the lid and pulls it outward, off the eye. This treatment is usually temporary.

Another treatment that gives temporary relief is placing a suture (stitch) in the lid to hold it in place. Only a local numbing injection is needed. The stitch is used in cases where the patient cannot tolerate a longer procedure or as an "emergency" measure when it is necessary to move the lashes off the eye immediately.

A more permanent solution is surgery to tighten the lax lower lid. A horizontal wedge of the lid is removed. The wound is stitched together, which pulls the lid taut and keeps it from flipping. There are several ways to do this surgery, but all are out-patient procedures done with local anesthetic.

Growths

Growths of many kinds may appear on the eyelids. Cancerous growths are discussed above. There are so many types of growths that we will describe only the most common.

Any growth that is surgically removed is sent for biopsy. The growths listed here are all benign, but any growth may turn cancerous. It is important to have your physician check any lesion, even if it sounds exactly like the benign ones we are describing here. A change in any growth should always be drawn to your doctor's attention. Removal should be considered for any growth around the eye area that is causing a cosmetic or functional problem.

Chalazion—A chalazion is an infected oil gland in the eyelid. It is often associated with dry eyes and blepharitis. The gland gets stopped up, and bacteria grows. The gland becomes swollen, tender, and red. Hot packs and antibiotic ointment or drops are the usual treatment. Sometimes an antibiotic to take by mouth is prescribed. Once the swelling and tenderness goes down, there may be a knot in the lid. This lump may not go away unless removed by surgery. In this minor surgery procedure, the lid is numbed with an injection then the knot is cut out. Sometimes a stitch is needed in the lid. The wound is usually on the inside of the lid, so there is no visible scar. Antibiotic ointment and hot packs are used after surgery.

Moles—Like any other part of the body, moles are common on the lids and skin around the eye. They may be present at birth and enlarge or darken during adolescence. Or a mole may be colorless. A mole may be removed surgically using a local anesthetic (injection). Any mole that changes during adulthood should be examined by your physician.

Skin tags—These are little flesh-colored tags of skin. They may appear out of the blue and grow for a few weeks. They don't usually go away, and can be removed surgically.

Stye—A stye (hordeolum) is an infected hair follicle (the sac that the eyelash grows from). It is treated using hot packs and antibiotic ointment. Surgery is not usually needed.

Warts—A wart is a painless bumpy-looking growth that may appear suddenly and grow for a few weeks. It doesn't go away, and can be removed by surgery. Never use over-the-counter wart treatment on a wart near the eyes.

Xanthelasma—Xanthelasma is a flat yellowish growth on the upper or lower lids. It has been associated with high cholesterol. Small growths may be treated with cautery (burned). Large growths must be surgically removed, but may come back (see Figure 8-D).

Herpes Zoster (Shingles)

Shingles are caused by the same virus as chicken pox. It is more common among the older population and those with lowered immunities.

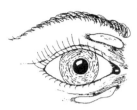

Figure 8-D Xanthelasma.

The infection can start with fever, headache, and a sick feeling. Painful, burning, itching ulcers erupt on one side of the face, sometimes including the eyelid. The cornea can also develop ulcers.

An oral anti-viral medication is often prescribed. Anti-viral cream may be applied to the ulcers. The cream is meant for the skin, and should not be used directly in the eye. Your physician will advise you about the use of pain-killers.

Lice

If the scalp is infested with lice, the eyebrows and eyelashes may need to be treated as well. The lice may live among the lashes And lay eggs (nits) at the lash line or in the brows. Waste products from lice on the lashes can cause a form of allergic conjunctivitis.

The scalp will have to be treated with lice killing shampoo. The lashes may be treated with Eserine™ (physostigmine) ointment. Apply the ointment to the lashes as directed by your physician. Eserine is an eye ointment, so it will not damage your eye if some gets in it. But try to keep the ointment on the lashes. A side effect of Eserine is to make the pupils small. It can also cause headaches. Keeping the ointment on the lashes instead of getting it in the eye will keep these side effects to a minimum.

If you also have conjunctivitis, your physician will treat that as well.

Ptosis (Drooped Eyelids)

As stated earlier, "ptosis" is the term used for a drooping eyelid. In dermatochalasis the extra skin can cause the lid to droop, creating a ptosis. Conditions other than dermatochalasis may cause ptosis. Loss of muscle tone may cause the lid to droop. Sometimes a lid may droop after eye surgery. This is probably due to the eyelid's being stretched to keep the eye open during the procedure.

A person can be born with ptosis. Look at the photos of the authors. Mrs. Ledford's left lid has been a little lower since birth. Her father and one sister have a drooping left lid as well. This hereditary condition may affect one eye or both.

Sometimes one lid will look lower not because it has drooped, but because the position of the other lid is abnormally high.

Ptosis may occur following muscle damage due to an accident. Or, damage to the nerve supply (from trauma or palsy) may cause the lid to droop. This is the case in a third nerve or seventh nerve palsy. Heavy scarring on the upper lid might also pull the lid down. So could any large tumor in the upper lid.

The first sign of myasthenia gravis is often the appearance of a new ptosis. To diagnose myasthenia, an injection of Tensilon™ is given in a vein in the arm. If the drooped lid rises, then myasthenia is probably present.

Treatment and Surgery

Treatment depends in part on the cause of the ptosis. If the lid droop is caused by dermatochalasis, then a blepharoplasty will be done to remove the extra skin and fat.

Ptosis surgery may be needed on the eyelid muscle itself. This generally involves taking a "tuck" in the muscle to make it shorter, thus raising the eyelid. These procedures are done with local anesthetic (injection) as an outpatient. (Please refer to Chapter 15 for general information on eye surgery.)

If the lid droop is due to nerve palsy, it may resolve. The physician will usually want to wait several months before attempting surgery, to see if the ptosis will clear up on its own.

Reconstructive Plastic Surgery

Plastic surgery is designed to improve appearance and function. This is especially important when the face and eyes are scarred or disfigured. Reconstructive surgery may be done at the time of the original repair (in the case of trauma) or surgery (such as in growth removal). In other cases, plastic surgery is done after the original wound has healed.

Many of the details of plastic surgery are similar to those of any eye surgery. Reading Chapter 15 will give you an idea of what will be done before, during, and after any reconstructive or ocular procedure.

For now, we will discuss the various types of techniques used in reconstructive plastic surgery.

If a wound is small, the physician may simply stitch it closed and let it heal. But in the case of a larger wound, the scar would be disfiguring. Instead of letting such a wound fill in with scar tissue, the physician would rather cover the area with skin. Or, an existing scar can be treated to improve appearance. Flaps and grafts are two ways this can be done.

Flaps

In a flap, skin next to the wound is moved over to cover the wound itself. The important thing about a flap is that it is not completely cut away, but left attached at the base. That means that the transferred skin has not lost its blood supply, so healing is more rapid. There is also less chance of rejection. The area that the flap came from is stitched closed. This creates a thin linear scar, which is better than a big hole filled with a scar.

Grafts

A graft uses tissue that is removed from one part of the body and sewn into the place that needs repairing. Usually a person's own skin is used, because the body is not as likely to reject its own tissue. This work is often done using a numbing injection at the place where the tissue is removed (which is then stitched closed) and at the place where it is to be sewn in. If the repair is going to take a long time, an IV may be used to help you relax.

Skin to repair a defect on the lids or around the eyes may be taken (or "harvested") from any of several places. If the upper lids have extra skin, they are a good source for graft tissue. Skin may also be obtained from the inner arm, behind the ear, or above the collar bone. Just the surface skin or skin with a bit of fat under it is used. This piece of skin is then placed on the repair site and sewn in.

If the area to be repaired needs a firm base, a cartilage graft may be needed. Cartilage is the tough tissue that gives shape and structure to the nose and ears. A lower lid repaired with only a skin graft would be rather "floppy." The lid needs something to help it keep its shape. So a cartilage graft is used for firmness. Then a skin graft is sewn on top of the cartilage. Cartilage grafts are usually harvested from the back side of one's own ear. Only a small amount is used, so the ear still keeps its shape.

If you pull down your eyelid, you can see that it is lined with a membrane. When an eyelid must be repaired, this membrane lining must be grafted in as well. The tissue may be taken from the conjunctiva, the tissue membrane covering the eyeball. Another place the membrane graft can come from is the inside of the cheek. The removed portion is sewn on the back-side of the cartilage graft. Repairs to areas other than the lid don't require this type of graft.

Trichiasis (In-Turned Eyelashes)

Trichiasis Survey

Risk factors:

- Have you had in-turned lashes before?
- Have you had eyelid surgery?
- Do you have scarring on your eyelids where the lashes grow?

Symptoms:

- Do you often feel like there's something in your eye?
- Do eye drops fail to make this sensation go away?
- Can you see the in-turned lashes in the mirror? (see Figure 8-E)

In-turned eye lashes are literally a pain! Instead of curving outward, the lash grows back toward the eye. This condition is known as trichiasis. The tip of the lash rubs the cornea, causing the sensation of something in the eye. Often these lashes are so fine that they can't be seen without a microscope. They can also be more brittle than ordinary lashes.

If the lash continues to rub the cornea, it can cause a scratch or raw spot on the corneal surface. That hurts even more.

What causes trichiasis? If the lid is scarred at the lash line, the

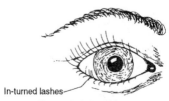

In-turned lashes

Figure 8-E Trichiasis.

lash follicles may now be pointing in a new direction. Thus when the lashes come in, they grow the wrong way. There might be just one lash that turns in, or several.

Dry eye is the most common cause of trichiasis. This is mainly because dry eye often leads to blepharitis, a low-grade lid infection. Long-term blepharitis can cause scarring and changes to the lash follicles, causing the lashes to point inward. Thus, consistent treatment of dry eye and blepharitis is a way to help prevent trichiasis from occurring in the first place.

Treatment

Usually the first method of treatment is to pull out the offending lashes. The physician or assistant does this with tweezers while looking through a microscope. (Don't try to pull them out yourself!) Unfortunately, the unruly lashes usually reappear within 6 weeks.

If the lashes recur and continue to be a problem, the doctor may suggest freezing the lashes (cryotherapy). The idea is to kill the follicle so that the lashes won't grow back. The procedure takes less than thirty minutes. The eye lid is injected with a numbing agent (such as Xylocaine). The freezing probe is small enough for the doctor to hold in his/her hand. The tip of the probe (about the size of a capital "O") is touched to the area of the lid with the ingrown lashes. The tip is cold and freezes the contact area. The probe is held to the lid for several seconds.

After the numbness wears off, the lid will probably be a little sore. The doctor will prescribe ointment to use on the area. This method is often successful in permanently eliminating the lashes, but may require more than one treatment.

Electrolysis may be used if there are only a few lashes that need treating. A wire tip applies weak electric current to the lash follicle. Only one follicle can be treated at a time. Since only a few lashes are treated, no anesthetic may be needed (although a local injection *may* be used). This treatment has a 30–50% success rate. The procedure can be repeated as long as the lid does not become scarred. Laser has been used to kill the lash follicles, but this is not a common practice.

If the in-turned lashes grow only in one small, isolated spot on the lid, that portion of the lid may be surgically removed. This is an out-patient procedure done with local anesthetic.

Severe cases may require surgery with a mucous membrane graft. (See page 158 for general information on grafts.) In this case the graft tissue may be taken from inside the mouth or nose.

Wrinkles

Skin rejuvenation, known as endodermology or chemical peeling, is a medically-approved non-surgical cosmetic facial rejuvenation procedure. Specifically, a chemical is applied to the facial skin which removes the outer layer of the skin, known as the epidermis. This stimulates the growth of new skin. The new skin is largely free of the wrinkles and spots caused by aging. As a result, it can remove five, 10, to 20 years from your appearance.

Chemical peeling is not a new procedure. It was pioneered by European dermatologists during the turn of the century. For at least the past thirty years the treatment has been available to the rich and famous, who wanted to keep the secret of their youthful appearance to themselves. During that time the procedure has been modified and improved greatly. Now chemical peeling has become a state-of-the-art treatment for those longing for a more youthful appearance.

Consider, for a moment, the different things that take a toll on your skin. Exposure to the sun is the largest offender. Smoking, pollution, environmental dryness, and wind also damage the skin. Wrinkles and age spots occur in the outer layer of the skin that is exposed to this hostile environment.

Several different chemicals are used as peeling agents. Phenol is a deep peel that usually causes the skin to become permanently lighter, and is the most effective chemical peel. During phenol chemical peels, the phenol is applied to the skin. Then the area is sealed with a surgical paper tape mask. At the end of 48 hours, the paper mask is removed and replaced by an application of antiseptic powder. The powder is applied for several days until a firm parchment-like mask forms. On the seventh day a lubricant is applied to the mask, and it begins to soften and fall away. The layer of new, fresh skin is revealed. The cells of this new epidermis are "plumper" than the skin that was removed. Thus its structure is more similar to the skin texture you enjoyed earlier in your life. The procedure can often be done in the office, and ideally you will spend your recovery period in a comfortable secluded after-care facility.

Other peeling chemicals such as trichloroacetic acid (TCA) are easier on the patient, and require less postoperative care. This milder peel has less risk of scarring and pigmentation changes. Since it is not as deep as phenol, TCA is not as effective in improving deep wrinkles. But it is an excellent choice to improve blotches, freckles, sun damage, fine wrinkles, and some types of acne scars.

TCA treatment can be done in the office. The skin usually stings and burns for two to three minutes after the chemical is applied. There is no other discomfort. The skin turns dark and tight, then cracks and peels. There are no scabs, bandages, or bleeding. Cleansing agents and ointments are applied during the healing process. The peel can be repeated as necessary for the desired results.

Not everyone is a good candidate for a chemical peel. It is also important that you understand what the treatment can and cannot accomplish. What it CAN do is restore a youthful appearance by removing wrinkles and blemishes caused by increased thickening of the skin. It does not, however, remove *all* wrinkles. There is no change in facial structure or features. The facial grooves of the face, or the lines of expression, are not altered. It is also important to note that the treatment will not remove scars or facial hair. However, crinkles, wrinkles (such as "crow's feet") and age spots *will* be decreased. These beneficial changes from the treatment are long lasting. Of course your skin will resume aging from the point of treatment on. It's rather like turning back the hands of a clock. While the clock *is* turned back, it *does* continue to run. Being cautious about sun exposure will greatly extend the benefits of your treatment. In addition, you may have any problem area retouched if you desire.

There are several things you need to know and do prior to your treatment date. If you are planning to have hair removed from your face, it should be done at least 2 months before the procedure. Active acne should be treated ahead of time as well. If you are overweight and plan on loosing weight, discuss this with the doctor.

Since the procedure is usually cosmetic and elective, insurance will not pay. (They may allow payment, however, if skin cancer is present.) You may certainly claim your treatment as a tax deduction under medical. You will probably be asked to sign a financial agreement, a consent for the procedure, and a photograph release. (The photo release is optional.)

There are several things you need to be aware of after your

treatment is complete. Your new skin is delicate. Itching is normal, but do not pick at or rub your face. Sleep on your back. Swelling the first day or two is normal. Your face may feel flushed when you bend over. During the healing process avoid steam, wetting your face, and sweating. Use your cleansing agents, lotions, and antibiotic pills as directed. If you ever have any questions or problems, call your doctor.

Be very careful about sun exposure. You should wear a broad-brimmed hat and sun screen for even the shortest exposure (such as walking to the car or mailbox). After about two months, you may resume your normal activities. However, you should continue to use sunscreen and keep sun exposure to a minimum to extend the benefits of your treatment.

The eyelids and skin are your first line of defense against eye disease and injury of deeper structures. The tears are also a defense system. Learn more about them, and more, in the next chapter.

CHAPTER 9

Tear System and External Eye

ELIZABETH Martin slammed shut the book she was reading and mopped at her eyes with a handkerchief. "I can't even *read* anymore!" she thought angrily. Her husband looked at her sympathetically. "Eyes too watery again?" he asked.

Mrs. Martin nodded. "The tears just stream down my face every time I read, sew, or do anything up close," she said.

"Let's call the eye doctor," suggested Mr. Martin. "Maybe you need your glasses changed."

Two weeks later, Dr. Todd told Mrs. Martin that her eyes were watery because they were dry. "That just doesn't make sense," Mrs. Martin protested. "They water all the time!"

It doesn't seem to make sense, does it? The tear system of the eye is an intricate set-up of production and drainage that can have unique problems of its own. Likewise, the external eye is subject to growths and conditions you need to know about. We'll explore them together in this chapter.

Tear System (see Figure 9-A)

Canaliculitis

- Do you have tenderness in the corner of your eye next to your nose?

In the upper and lower lid at the corner of the eye are tiny openings, called puncti, where the tears drain out of the eye. The puncti lead to tiny tubules called canaliculi (just one is called a canaliculus). If an infection occurs in the canaliculi, this is known as canaliculitis.

Canaliculitis causes tenderness and sometimes redness in the area of the lid next to the nose. There may be excessive watering if the tears can't drain properly.

Antibiotic drops are used to treat this condition. Be sure to use

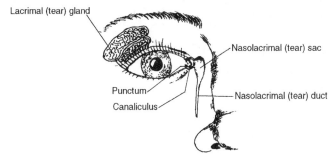

Figure 9-A The lacrimal system.

the medication as long as your doctor advises: don't just quit when the eye feels better. Warm compresses help with comfort and circulation.

Dacryocystitis (Tear Sac Infection)

- Do you have pain, swelling, and redness right below the corner of your eye (next to your nose)?

Tears drain off the eye and collect in the tear sac. From there they go through the nasolacrimal duct and dissipate at the back of the throat. Normally the tears wash bacteria out of the sac, but if drainage is stopped, then bacteria can multiply. Thus, an infection of the sac (dacryocystitis) may occur if the duct becomes blocked. The sac swells and becomes painful. That is the signal to see your doctor.

Treatment

Warm, moist compresses are usually recommended, along with an antibiotic ointment (or sometimes drops). Follow your doctor's instructions carefully. You will also be given an antibiotic to take by mouth. It is important for you to take every tablet. Don't stop the pills when you start feeling better.

Dacryocystitis usually clears up with the above treatment. Sometimes, however, the infected tear sac must be lanced. First the area is numbed with an injection (local anesthetic). Then the sac is pierced and drained. This usually gives immediate relief. Since the procedure creates a small wound, be very careful to use warm compresses and ointment as directed.

Once the infection has calmed down, the doctor will determine the cause of the blockage. You may have an irrigation test (described in Chapter 18) to see if the duct is still blocked.

Dry Eyes

Dry Eyes Survey

Risk factors:

- Do you live in a hot, dry climate?
- Do you have rheumatoid arthritis?
- Do you use antihistamines and other medications to dry up your sinuses?
- Do you often sit or work with air blowing on your face?
- Do you smoke, or are you exposed to smoke?
- For women, do you have a hormone (estrogen) deficiency?
- For women, are you going through, or have you already gone through menopause?

Symptoms:

- Do your eyes water a lot?
- Do you often have the sensation of having sand or grit in your eyes?
- Do your eyes itch and burn?

Did you know that watery eyes can actually be a sign of dryness? That sounds backwards, doesn't it? When the eye gets dry, it sends an S.O.S. message to the brain. Then the brain sends a message to the tear gland, telling it to produce tears. However, the tear gland often over-reacts, and you end up with tears streaming down your face. Unfortunately, these tears are of a poor quality, and do not actually help much.

The usual cause of dryness is the general decrease of body moisture that occurs as we age. But you might be surprised by some of the other causes of dry eye. Arthritis, for example, may be accompanied by very painful dryness in a condition known as Sjögren's Syndrome. An estrogen/hormonal deficiency in women has also been linked to dry eye. Thus, it occurs more often during and after menopause. Also, many sinus and cold medications dry the eyes as well as the nasal passages. In any case, either the eyes do not produce enough tears, or the tears that *are* produced are not of the proper quality.

The tear film of the eye actually has three layers. The outer layer is oily. Its purpose is to slow tear evaporation. The middle layer is watery, and washes away foreign particles. This layer has a germ-controlling property as well. The inner mucus layer is in direct contact with the cornea (the clear covering over the pupil and iris). It seems to play a role in the nutrition of the cornea.

If any one of these layers is under-produced, or if total tear production is low, problems will result. The eyes will feel dry and burn. You may also have a scratchy, gritty feeling as if there's sand in the eye. This is caused as the eyelid rubs raw, dry spots on the cornea. Your eyes may also burn, itch, and get red. These symptoms will be worse in warm, dry weather, since the heat tends to evaporate tears quickly. Air conditioning and ceiling fans also tend to aggravate the problem.

Poor blinking habits may contribute to the dryness. If you are concentrating on something, you may "forget" to blink. This most often happens when reading, watching TV, or during hobby work. Once the dryness reaches a certain level, your eyes begin to burn, blur, and water. You may even have to stop what you are doing because of the discomfort.

If the eyelids don't close completely, areas of the cornea can dry out. This condition is called exposure keratitis. Causes include:

1. nerve palsy where the nerve supply to the eyelid muscle is too weak to close the lid all the way
2. sleeping with the eyes partially open at night (Of course, this is unintentional. Have someone check to see if your lids are closing all the way as you sleep.)
3. lid deformities from birth, injury, or surgery
4. eye protrusion (exophthalmus)

Without enough tears to lubricate and wash the eye, the eyelids may develop a low-grade infection called blepharitis (or "granulated eye lids").

Dry eyes can lead to more severe problems. Debris and germs that would normally be rinsed away tend to hang around. So it's easier to get eye infections. Also, if the front of the eye gets too dry, the tissues can begin to break down and cause problems with vision.

To top it all off, sometimes there may also be an allergy involved. Yet over-the-counter eye drops used for allergy-type symptoms may have chemicals in them that dry the eye even more.

Dry eye is usually diagnosed strictly from the symptoms. Sometimes a tear test may be done.

Treatment

In general, this condition cannot be cured but only controlled. The main goal is to replace the moisture. Treatment usually consists of one or more of the following:

- Use tear supplement drops frequently. There are many kinds on the market, and they are all over the counter. Be sure you get "tears" and not something for allergies or redness. Ask your eye doctor for samples of different types of "tears," then use each one for three days in a row. After you have tried several, stick with the brand that works best. Use the drops at least four times a day. The more often you use the drops, the better off you will be. You will continue to use the tear drops indefinitely.
- Artificial tear ointment is recommended in more severe cases. This over-the-counter item is best used at night, first because it blurs vision and second because it stays on the eye longer. This is needed because the eyes tend to dry even more at night.
- Studies have shown that Vitamin A is of help in treating dry eyes. We recommend 10,000 units of Vitamin A per day. Your pharmacist can help you get the right amount of these over-the-counter vitamins.
- Use a moist-air humidifier in your bedroom at night. Since you don't blink while you sleep, the humidity in the air will help keep your eyes from drying.
- Avoid exposing your eyes to moving, blowing air. If you are out in the wind, wear glasses to keep your eyes from being dried.
- Avoid cigarette smoke as much as possible.
- For blepharitis, you need to cleanse and treat the lids as described in Chapter 8.
- In case of allergy, prescription eye drops may be given.
- If you tend to stare when you're concentrating, use the tear drops before you start your activity. This may moisten them

enough to prevent stinging. Also make a conscious effort to blink more often.

- Slow-dissolving time-released inserts are available for severe cases. A tiny pellet is placed inside the lower lid once or twice a day. This system has the advantage of constant lubrication. The draw-backs include: they are expensive, they are tiny and may be difficult to handle, some patients find them irritating, and they may blur the vision.

- In extreme cases, your physician may recommend moisture chambers, side shields, or goggles. These are designed to reduce tear evaporation.

- If the eye lids don't close completely, it may be necessary to tape the lids shut at night.

- If the eye and vision are threatened by severe drying, surgery to partially close the eye may be needed. The procedure is called a tarsorrhaphy. After numbing, the inner and/or outer edges of the lids are sewn and allowed to heal together. Ointment is used during recovery. A tarsorrhaphy can be reversed later. In extreme cases, an eye may be sewn totally shut temporarily. (The edges are not allowed to heal together as in a tarsorrhaphy.)

- The tear-drainage ducts in the lid may be sealed off. Tears are produced in the lacrimal gland (under the brow) and other tiny glands in the conjunctiva (membrane over the white of the eye and lining the inner lids). Since tears drain off the eye through the puncti, plugging or sealing these tiny openings helps keep the tears on the eye. Tiny plastic plugs can be inserted into the puncti as a temporary measure. Permanent sealing is done by cautery (heat) or laser.

When cauterizing the puncti, numbing injections are used first. Then the hot probe tip is touched to the openings. The scarring from this procedure seals the puncti. There may be some mild discomfort when the anesthetic wears off. Your doctor will prescribe some antibiotic drops and/or ointment to use during healing.

Laser works like cautery in that it burns and thus seals the puncti by scarring. Numbing drops are often all that is needed. The drops may be placed on tiny cotton wads which are placed in the eye directly on the puncti for several minutes. For the laser procedure, you will put your head in a headrest with your chin in a cup and your forehead pressed against a bar or band at the top. An assistant may hold your head in place, or a strap may be used to help you keep still. The laser is attached to a microscope, so the ophthalmologist has a good view of the area. The laser is aimed at exactly the right spot. It takes several bursts from the laser to seal the puncti. The entire procedure takes only a minute or so. There may be some mild discomfort after the numbing drops wear off. Your doctor will prescribe some antibiotic drops and/or ointment to use to help the area heal.

Obstruction (Blockage)

Obstruction Survey

Risk factors:

- Do you seem to keep getting eye infections?

Symptoms:

- Does the eye seem to water almost constantly?
- Do you have swelling and/or tenderness in the corner of your eye next to your nose?

Blockage of the tear system always refers to the tear *drainage* system. The tears are produced in the tear gland under your brow. Tears are pumped out of the gland as you blink. The tear gland does not get plugged.

A blockage *can* occur in the tear draining (nasolacrimal) system. If you plug up your sink and let the water run, eventually it will overflow. That's what happens in the eye. If the drainage system is obstructed, it's like plugging the sink. Eventually the tears overflow, spilling down the cheek. Blockage of the tear system may be caused by something mechanical or a narrowing of the openings. Any injury that damages the system by tearing the canals or scarring the openings can also create a barricade.

Recurrent infections can result from an obstruction. It is easy for an infection to begin because there is no way to flush the germs out. This is comparable to a stagnant pond choked with overgrowth and slime. The canals, the sac, and/or the entire eye could develop an infection. The most troublesome of these is repeated infection of the sac (dacryocystitis).

Loss of muscle tone can cause a situation that mimics obstruction. If the lower lids have become too lax, the puncti may be turned away from the eyes. Tears cannot reach the puncti to be drained away. The most severe situation of this type is ectropion, where the entire lower lid turns outward.

Evaluation and Treatment

The physician can use several methods to evaluate blockage. First, he/she will examine the openings in the lids using a microscope called a slit lamp. Other tests may be done to see if fluid is actually getting through (see Chapter 18, *Nasolacrimal Evaluation*).

If a blockage is indeed present, the physician will consider treatment. The first thing the doctor may try is nasolacrimal irrigation. After the puncti are numbed with drops, a slender tube is inserted into the puncti. A mild salt solution is pushed through the tube. The idea is to flush out the blockage.

Another option is to insert a silicone tube to hold the system open. This can be done under local or general anesthesia. A slender wire is inserted down through the tear draining ducts. Then the tube is passed through the upper and lower canaliculi, through the lacrimal sac, and into the nostril. The tubing is then tied, and the end allowed to slip up into the nostril. After the procedure, you will be using some antibiotic eye drops and nasal spray. The tube is usually removed in the office within six months. If successful, no further surgery may be needed.

The surgery to correct an obstruction of the tear sac has a long name: dacryocystorhinostomy. Just call it a DCR for short! A DCR can be done under local or general anesthesia. (See Chapter 15 for general information on surgery.) This procedure creates a new drainage route from the tear sac into the nose. A hole is made in the underlying bone, creating a place for the tears to go. Some surgeons also insert a piece of tubing through the puncti as described above. This tubing is used to hold the new drainage place open during healing, and is later removed.

Post-operative care following a DCR is simple. The main rule is: don't blow your nose! You will probably be given decongestants to reduce nasal secretions. An antibiotic may also be prescribed to fight off infection.

Tear Gland Prolapse

• Is there a yellowish or pink soft mass on the white of the eye under your upper lid?

The tear gland is normally found under the brow area). But as the tissues relax, the tear gland may drop down (prolapse) between the conjunctiva (membrane that covers the sclera) and the sclera (white of the eye). There is no pain or change in tear formation. Usually the only problem is the alarm of discovering a "tumor" that wasn't there before. Of course any mass that is new, or an old growth that begins to change needs to be examined by your eye care physician.

External Eye(see Figure 9-B)

Anisocoria (Unequal Pupil Size)

• Check some old photographs of yourself. Are the pupils equal?
• Have you had a head injury?
• Are you using eye drops with a red top in only one eye?
• Are you using eye drops with a green top in only one eye?
• Have you had an eye injury?

Unequal pupil size is normal in 2–5% of the population. At one time or another, approximately 20–40% of the population may have a difference in size between the two pupils. If you notice a size difference in yourself, check some old photographs to see if it actually existed before...you may just now be noticing something that has been there a long time. Other than this normal variation in some people, any difference between the pupils that is *new* should be checked out.

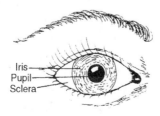

Iris
Pupil
Sclera

Figure 9-B The external eye.

Certain eye medications change the pupil size as part of their action. If placed in only one eye, this will cause a difference in pupil size.

Drops that enlarge the pupil usually have a red cap. They are used in the eye doctor's office to dilate the pupils. They are sometimes prescribed for home use after surgery, injury, or in some cases of inflammation. Some types are stronger than others, and may last up to seven days. The weaker kind last only for a few hours. If used in just one eye, that pupil will be larger than the other.

Other drops act to make the pupil smaller. These drops usually have a green top, and are used in treating glaucoma. If placed in only one eye, that pupil will be smaller than in the untreated eye.

Even if you are not putting drops in your eye, you can accidentally dilate yourself. Skin patches used to prevent motion sickness contain medication that dilates the pupil. When you apply the patch to your skin, some of the drug may remain on the fingers. If you then rub one eye, that pupil may become dilated.

Once, a patient of ours accidentally dilated his right eye with dilating drops. But he wasn't using them himself. His dog had had cataract surgery, and our patient was putting dilating drops in the dog's eye. Obviously, the drops had gotten on his fingers, and when he rubbed his eye he dilated that pupil.

Some oral medications can affect pupil size, but usually both pupils would be dilated. Some chemicals and chemical fumes can have the same result. The residue from some plants can dilate. When doing yard work, wear gloves and keep your hands away from your face.

An attack of angle closure glaucoma can cause one pupil to be larger than the other. There is usually redness, pain, and blurred vision in the affected eye.

Injury can damage either the muscles of the iris or the nerves that control it. So can surgery. During some types of eye surgery, the surgeon may be working inside the eye through the pupil. If the pupil is not large enough, the doctor may have to use instruments to stretch it. Normally this does not cause a problem, but occasionally the muscle might be torn or stretched, causing a large or irregularly shaped pupil.

Inflammation inside the eye (which can accompany infection, appear after surgery or injury, or occur on its own) often causes the pupil of that eye to be smaller. There is often redness and light sensitivity as well.

Problems with the nerve supply on one side can cause pupil size to be unequal. A paralysis (palsy) of the 3rd nerve of the brain will cause a dilated pupil on that side.

A smaller pupil can be caused by a condition called Horner's syndrome. Horner's affects only one side of the face. Besides the smaller pupil, the eyelid on the affected side is drooped, and that side of the face does not perspire.

Unequal pupils may accompany a migraine headache. Other possibilities include Hodgkin's disease, tumors, neurological disease, and trauma to the neck.

Diagnosis and Treatment

If the difference between the pupils is new, and no obvious cause can be found, your eye doctor may request that you see a neurologist (doctor who specializes in conditions involving nerves). If you are being treated with dilating or constricting drops for some reason, the difference in pupil size is something you will have to put up with until treatment is over.

Conjunctivitis (Pink Eye)

Conjunctivitis is an inflammation of the conjunctiva, the membrane that lines the inside of the lids and covers the sclera (white of the eye). Conjunctivitis can be caused by allergic reaction or infection, but the common symptom is redness. There may be a discharge of sticky matter or clear watery tears.

Allergic Conjunctivitis

The conjunctiva reacts to allergy with mild to moderate redness, swelling, and stringy white matter. This is not a contagious condition. It is sometimes difficult to find the exact cause, but we will discuss several of them.

Any medication used in the eye has the potential for causing an allergic reaction. Many people are allergic to sulfa, which is used in some eye medications. Preservatives used in drops and ointments may cause an allergy as well. You can see how tough it is to figure out what is causing the problem. Be sure to tell your eye doctor any drug allergies that you are known to have before he/she prescribes anything for you. If you are taking a medication and seem to be having a reaction to it, contact your eye physician.

Any allergy you have to the environment (dust, pollen, grass, animal hair, etc.) can affect the eyes. The redness, watering, and itching that goes along with allergies and hay fever has caused a boom in the over-the-counter eye drop market. While steroid drops would probably give quick relief, they are not generally prescribed for allergies (it is not good to use steroid drops for an extended period of time, or at random). Over-the-counter drops that "get the red out" may make the eyes look better, but don't really give any relief. Plus some of the chemicals used in these type of preparations can actually cause dryness . . . creating an additional problem. Your eye doctor can prescribe some anti-allergy drops for you. Some of these are used more frequently at first until the symptoms are under control, then used once or twice a day as a maintenance dose.

In rare instances where the eyelashes are infested with lice, an allergic conjunctivitis may occur. The eye is really reacting to the waste products of the insects, which are toxic and irritating to the eye. In addition to treating the allergy symptoms, your physician will prescribe treatment to eradicate the lice.

Bacterial Conjunctivitis

Conjunctivitis caused by bacteria usually causes marked redness. There is a sticky discharge, and the lids are often matted together in the morning. Matter may continue to form during the day. The conjunctiva may also swell, causing an appearance of fullness. The eye may feel irritated as if something is in it. The area in front of the ear (there is a lymph node here) may be swollen and tender.

The bacteria that cause conjunctivitis are the same ones that cause flu, pneumonia, strep throat, colds, bronchitis, etc. So conjunctivitis may develop after any of these infections. "Pink eye" can come suddenly and hit hard, or be milder and linger or recur. In addition, the bacteria can move from the conjunctiva to infect the cornea and/or eyelids.

Once your eye doctor has decided that you have a bacterial infection, he/she will prescribe eye medication for you. Antibiotic ointment or drops are used, sometimes in a steroid combination. Use as directed, and be sure to keep follow-up appointments. If you are being treated for conjunctivitis in one eye, and it seems to be spreading to the other eye, call your doctor's office for permission to begin treating the fellow eye.

Following several simple rules of hygiene will help you keep your germs to yourself!

Do:
1. wash your hands before and after using eye medications
2. wash your hands after touching your eyes or face
3. avoid close facial contact (such as hugging) until the infection is cleared up
4. try to keep your hands away from your face and eye

Do Not:
1. share towels and/or wash cloths with anyone
2. share pillows with anyone
3. touch the dropper tip to your eye or eyelids
4. touch the dropper tip with your fingers
5. wear contact lenses until the doctor says it's okay

In some cases, the doctor may also prescribe an antibiotic to take by mouth. Be sure to take every pill, even if you feel the infection has cleared up before the medicine is gone.

Usually, treatment is started by using an antibiotic known to be effective against many types of bacteria. If the infection does not respond to treatment, the doctor may want to do a culture. Some bacteria are best treated with certain antibiotics. Once the bacteria is identified, your doctor will treat you with the medicine specific for that type of germ.

Chemical Conjunctivitis (see *Burns* — Chemical in chapter 16)

Viral Conjunctivitis

Conjunctivitis caused by viruses usually has moderate redness. The conjunctiva swells and looks "full." If there is any discharge, it is usually watery. The area in front of the ear, where there is a lymph node, is often swollen and tender. The cornea may become infected as well.

The viruses that cause conjunctivitis can also cause colds, sore throats, flu, etc. So conjunctivitis can follow any of these infections. Some viruses can also be spread by bugs. (Every summer here in the South, a type of viral infection goes around that has been unofficially named "Gnat Conjunctivitis." This brand of conjunctivitis seems to occur after a gnat has gotten into the eye.)

Another type of conjunctivitis that has earned its own name is epidemic keratoconjunctivitis. Also known as "ship yard eye," this infection lasts about 3–4 weeks and is highly contagious. Both the cornea and conjunctiva become involved.

Herpes simplex, the same virus that causes cold sores, can also cause conjunctivitis. This is especially troublesome if the cornea also becomes affected. Herpes zoster, which causes shingles, can cause conjunctivitis as well.

Treatment depends on the cause. Viruses are difficult to culture, so the physician usually depends on your symptoms and an examination to decide what type of virus is involved. Most viral conjunctivitis is treated with a combination antibiotic and steroid. The antibiotic prevents bacteria from infecting the eye along with the virus. The steroid helps decrease inflammation and increase comfort. Cool compresses may also help.

Viral conjunctivitis caused by either of the Herpes viruses is *not* treated with steroids, however. An anti-viral drop is used. It is important to let your doctor examine you to determine the cause and treatment. Don't use eye drops you may have on hand without first checking with your physician.

Viruses are contagious, just like bacteria. So follow the hygiene notes listed above to avoid spreading the infection.

Episcleritis (Inflammation Of Tissue Between Conjunctiva and Sclera)

Episcleritis Survey
  Risk factors:

- Do you have rheumatoid arthritis?
- Do you have shingles (Herpes zoster)?
- Do you have gout?
- Are you a woman?

  Symptoms:

- Do you have a red, raised nodule on the white of your eye?
- Do you have a pink-red or purplish area on the white of your

eye? Does your eye have a deep throbbing pain? Is it worse at night?

• Is your eye uncomfortable?
• Is the eye watering?
• Are you light sensitive?

A red eye should be examined by your physician. Episcleritis is not usually serious. But only your eye doctor can determine why an eye is red and painful. For example, a glaucoma attack can also cause an eye to throb at night, be red, and water. SEE YOUR DOCTOR!

The episclera is a thin layer of fiber-like tissue that covers the sclera (white of the eye). Episcleritis occurs when the episclera becomes inflamed.

The simple form of episcleritis is more common in women, and tends to occur in the forties. One or both eyes may be involved. The eye becomes red and may be uncomfortable, with tearing and light sensitivity. The condition may clear up and then come back.

In nodular episcleritis there is redness and discomfort as above. But the area involved seems to be a swollen bump or nodule on the eye. This type of episcleritis may be associated with rheumatoid arthritis, shingles (Herpes zoster), or gout.

Episcleritis is not an infection, and may not require any treatment. An eye drop that reduces redness may be prescribed. In other cases, the physician may choose to prescribe a steroid drop. (Side-effects from steroid drops are usually minimal when used for a short time. Always follow your doctor's instructions.) In more severe cases oral steroids may be used as well.

Exophthalmus (Protruding Eye or Eyes)

* other names: exophthalmos, proptosis

Exophthalmus is an abnormal protrusion of one or both eyes (see Figure 9-C). However, abnormal lid positions can mimic exophthalmus. For example, if the right upper lid droops more than the left upper lid, the left eye may seem to be protruding because it is opened more. Such a lid droop is common following eye surgery.

In true exophthalmus, an eye doesn't just look as if it's protruding; it actually is. Graves' disease, sometimes called thyroid eye disease, is the most common cause of protrusion of one or both eyes. Cellulitis, injury, and tumors are other causes. An abnormal-

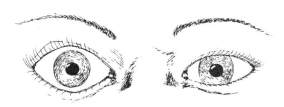

Figure 9-C Exophthalmus, right eye.

ity in the shape of the skull at birth can cause one or both eyes to be prominent.

A protruding eye in and of itself does not cause damage unless the lids do not meet to cover the cornea (clear window over the front of the eye). If the lids cannot cover the cornea, the cornea may dry out, causing a condition known as exposure keratitis. An exposed, dry cornea is treated similarly to dry eyes. The eye may need lubricating ointment at night. In some cases it is necessary to tape the lids shut to keep them closed during sleep. During the day, tear drops are needed to keep the cornea moist. In severe instances, surgery to partially close the eyelids may be necessary.

A protruding eye may be pushed out of alignment with the other eye, causing double vision (diplopia). This occurs more frequently if the exophthalmus develops rapidly. The doubled image may be beside, above, or diagonal to the other.

Diagnosis And Treatment

If you feel that one or both eyes protrude (when they did not before), take along some old photographs of yourself when you visit your eye doctor. The photos may show a progressive bulging which you have not been aware of.

Eye protrusion is measured with an exophthalmometer. This painless procedure (called exophthalmometry) tells how much an eye protrudes. Of course, every eye protrudes some. A normal measurement is anywhere from 16 to 21 millimeters. If there is a difference of more than 2 millimeters between the two eyes, the doctor will suspect exophthalmus.

Thyroid tests are usually ordered, since Graves' disease is the most common cause of exophthalmus. A B-scan ultrasound, CT scan, and/or X-Ray may be done as well. These are needed to help determine the cause of the protrusion.

If the protrusion is caused by a tumor, the physician may do a biopsy by withdrawing some tumor material through a fine needle. Treatment of a tumor will depend on what type of tumor it is, and where it is located. Surgery or radiation may be necessary in some cases.

Growths

- Is the growth a fluid-filled or blister-looking sac on the white of the eye? (see *Conjunctival cyst* below)
- Is the growth a small yellow, pink, or white bump on the white of the eye at 3:00 or 9:00? (see *Pinguecula* below)
- Is the growth a flesh colored triangle of tissue that is growing from the white of the eye onto the cornea (clear window on the front of the eye) at 3:00 or 9:00? (see *Pterygiula* below)

These are the three most common benign growths that occur on the eyeball. Any growth should be checked by your eye care physician.

Conjunctival Cyst

A conjunctival cyst is a painless, benign fluid-filled pocket in the conjunctiva. It can be present at birth, occur without apparent reason, or result from injury. If it becomes too large or is irritating, your eye physician can drain it. This can usually be done using only numbing drops.

Pinguecula

Pinguecula are very common benign growths on the eye (see Figure 9-D). They may become more yellow-colored with age. No treatment is necessary unless the pinguecula becomes red and inflamed. Then a weak steroid drop is sometimes prescribed to quiet the area. Pinguecula are not usually removed unless they become so large as to cause irritation. Surgical removal is usually done with a local anesthetic (numbing injection to the area). Stitches may be needed to close the wound. Antibiotic ointment is generally used afterwards because the ointment helps soothe the eye. Drops may be prescribed as well. Although a pinguecula is not cancerous, any growth removed from the eye is sent to the lab for biopsy just to be sure all is well.

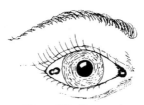

Figure 9-D Pinguecula.

Pterygium

A pterygium is a triangular, fleshy-colored tissue that runs from the white of the eye onto the cornea (usually on the nose side but sometimes on the ear side, see Figure 9-E). It is thought to be response to irritation, such as ultraviolet rays of the sun, dryness, and dusty environments.

A pterygium is benign and painless, but can cause problems if it grows across the cornea and toward the pupil. If the pterygium enlarges enough, it can block the vision. So an eye physician usually likes to check on a pterygium every six months or so. If growth is occurring, surgical removal is necessary. It is best to remove the pterygium before it gets too close to the pupil, because removing it will leave a scar. This causes little problem if the scar is at the edge of the cornea, out of the main line of sight. But if a pterygium is allowed to grow too far, the scarring after removal may be in the center of the vision. In this case a corneal transplant may be necessary.

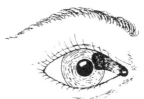

Figure 9-E Pterygium

Removing a pterygium is usually done under local anesthesia (use of a numbing injection). There will be stitches in the conjunctiva (membrane over the white of the eye). Usually the eye will be patched over night. You will be given antibiotic ointment and/or drops to use. The eye will be red for several weeks. The tissue is sent to the lab for a biopsy just to be sure that it is benign.

The most common complication after pterygium removal is that it can grow back. Some doctors treat the area with radiation to help prevent recurrence, but there is some debate about whether this really works. A pterygium can recur even after a corneal transplant has been done. This is because the pterygium arises from the conjunctiva, not the cornea. Avoiding dust and wearing sunglasses that filter out ultraviolet rays may help in preventing recurrence.

Scleritis (Inflammation of the White of the Eye)

Scleritis Survey

Risk factors:

- Do you have gout?
- Do you have rheumatoid arthritis?
- Do you have lupus?
- Do you have tuberculosis?
- Do you have sarcoidosis?

Symptoms:

- Does the eye have a deep boring ache?
- Is the eye ball tender to the touch?
- Is there redness or a purplish area on the sclera?
- Is the eye light sensitive?
- Does the eye tear?
- Has the vision decreased (perhaps only slightly)?
- Does the eye seem to bulge out?
- Is it difficult to move the eye?
- Is there swelling around the eye?

The sclera is the white of the eye. Scleritis is the condition where the sclera has become inflamed. It is not an infection, although an eye weakened by scleritis may later develop an infection. About 50% of the time, both eyes are involved. Scleritis is more common in women, and usually occurs in the 40–60 age range. Fortunately it is rare.

The affected eye may be red, purplish, or not red at all. There is usually pain, which may be severe and described as a deep boring ache. The eyeball itself may be tender and swollen. Sometimes the vision is slightly blurred. Often light sensitivity and tearing occur. When deeper, more serious inflammation is present, there may be swelling around the whole eye area. The eye may protrude and be difficult to move.

Scleritis may be associated with rheumatoid arthritis, shingles (Herpes zoster), gout, lupus, tuberculosis, and sarcoidosis. Your physician may order lab work, including blood work, urinalysis, and a chest X-Ray. To detect deep inflammation, a CT scan or ultrasound may be needed.

Scleritis can begin gradually or suddenly. It may occur once never to return or become a recurrent problem. Sometimes the cornea (clear window over the front of the eye) can be affected. Another problem is that other parts of the eye can become inflamed. Scleritis can be a serious condition that threatens sight. Advanced or long-standing cases may cause the sclera to thin and weaken.

Treatment

In treating scleritis, the focus is on the inflammatory response of the entire body. In some cases, oral steroids are used as anti-inflammatory agents. Or non-steroidal anti-inflammatory medication may be tried. If the inflammation is deep and severe, hospital admission may be needed so that steroids can be given by IV. Steroid drops are frequently used to quiet the eye. It may be necessary to use the steroid drops over a long period of time to prevent the inflammation from recurring.

Part of the function of the tears and eyelids is to protect the cornea. The cornea is a highly complex tissue with distinct conditions and diseases. We'll examine them in the next chapter.

CHAPTER 10

Cornea

IMAGINE that your house has only one window. Suppose you get up one morning and discover someone has covered your window with non-removable paint.

Or suppose that this window is made from very old glass . . . the kind that warps. Every time you look outside, all you can see are distorted shapes.

That's what corneal disease can be like. The cornea is like the window of the eye (see Figure 10-A). If the cornea is scarred, clouded, thinned, or warped, vision is decreased or distorted.

Abrasion (Scratch or cut)

* see cuts – cornea in Chapter 16

Dystrophy

Corneal Dystrophy Survey

Risk factors:

- Are you female? If yes, are you over 50?
- Is there a history of corneal dystrophy in your family?

Symptoms:

- Has your vision gradually decreased?
- Do you see halos around lights?

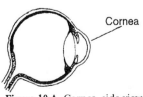

Figure 10-A Cornea, side view.

The term "corneal dystrophy" covers a variety of conditions involving a breakdown in the structure of the cornea. The problem tends to run in families, and especially affects women. At least seventeen kinds have been described. The most common type is Fuchs' corneal dystrophy (pronounced "fyukes").

Corneal dystrophy disrupts the internal chemical balance of the cornea. As the corneal tissue breaks down, the cornea becomes less clear. This, in turn, causes decreased vision. There is no way to predict the rate or severity of the degeneration. The vision may be barely decreased and never worsen. In the most severe cases, the cornea becomes totally clouded.

Treatment depends on the type of dystrophy and the type of breakdown that is occurring. Early treatment often includes sodium chloride (salt) drops and ointments made especially for the eye. The sodium chloride helps restore the chemical balance of the cornea.

If the tissue breakdown affects the outer layer of the cornea (the layer exposed to the air), painful blisters may result. A soft contact lens may be used as a sort of "bandage" to cover the blister.

If the vision becomes extremely poor, a corneal transplant may be considered. This is not always successful because over time the graft itself may develop corneal dystrophy.

Edema (Water-Logged Or Swollen Cornea)

Corneal Edema Survey

Risk factors:

- Do you have corneal dystrophy?
- Have you had angle closure glaucoma?
- Have you had eye surgery? Injury?

Symptoms:

- Do you see halos around lights?
- Has your vision decreased?

Edema is swelling caused by extra fluid in a tissue. Special cells in the cornea normally pump out any extra fluid. But if these cells don't function, or there is an overload of fluid, edema occurs. This causes the cornea to become hazy. Vision may be blurred. Also, the fluid acts like a prism and breaks white light down into colors, causing halos. (If you've ever been swimming a long time and open your eyes under water, you may have noticed halos due to corneal edema.)

There are several causes of corneal edema. First, some corneal dystrophies may damage the pumping cells. This also happens in angle closure glaucoma. Trauma from surgery or injury may also cause edema, usually temporary. Inflammation inside the eye, and some corneal infections can cause it as well.

Vision may be decreased only slightly, or significantly. Corneal edema is painless unless the outer layer of the cornea is involved.

Treatment

Treatment depends on the cause. If the edema is from angle closure glaucoma, the eye is treated to lower the pressure. Inflammation or corneal infections must also be treated in and of themselves. If the cause is relieved, the edema usually clears up. 5% salt drops or ointment may be used to draw the extra fluid out of the cornea. If conservative treatment doesn't help and vision is significantly reduced, a corneal transplant may be considered.

If the eye is uncomfortable, a bandage contact lens may be suggested. Surgery to cover the cornea with a flap of conjunctiva (membrane covering the white of the eye and lining the lids) may be used to "bandage" the sore cornea. The flap can be removed later. Cautery (heat) may be used to seal the raw spots. (This is done after the eye has been numbed.) As with any surgical procedure, carefully follow your doctor's directions for medications and appointments.

Infective Keratitis (Infection)

Corneal Infection Survey

Risk factors:

- Do you have "pink eye" (conjunctivitis)?
- Do you have dry eyes?
- Do you have granulated eyelids (blepharitis)?
- Have you recently had a cold, sore throat, sinus, or respiratory infection?

Symptoms:

- Does your eye hurt, as if there is something in it?
- Is your vision blurry?
- Is the area right in front of your ears swollen and sore?

If you suspect that you may have a corneal infection, see your eye doctor at once. *Do not* use someone else's eye drops or any drops that you may have on hand. Some types of medication can make certain infections worse. Only your eye doctor can determine what type of infection you have and what type of medication to use.

Corneal infection (infective keratitis) can be caused by virus, bacteria, or fungus. Your physician may order a culture to determine what type of germ is causing the infection. Once the cause is found, treatment is chosen for that particular germ.

If the eyes are already dry, tears are not available to wash away germs and debris. This makes the cornea more susceptible to infection. In blepharitis, bacteria are already on the eyelid. It is an easy jump to infect the cornea. The same situation occurs in conjunctivitis.

Keratitis can cause small infected ulcers and raw spots on the cornea. Both of these are painful. Every time the eye blinks, the lids rub over the sore spot, causing the sensation that something is in the eye.Regardless of the cause, your eye doctor will want to examine your eye until the infection is totally cleared up. Each time, a drop of fluoresceine dye will be used. This eye drop helps the doctor see the eroded places on the cornea when viewed with the microscope. Some infections tend to recur if treatment is stopped too soon. If not cared for properly, some infections can permanently scar the cornea, causing decreased vision. So it is vital that you follow your doctor's orders about medication and exams. Cool compresses, dim lighting, and over-the-counter pain relievers may increase comfort.

Many of these infections are contagious. Following several simple rules of hygiene will help you keep your germs to yourself!

Do:

1. wash your hands before and after using eye medications
2. wash your hands after touching your eyes or face
3. avoid close facial contact (such as hugging) until the infection is cleared up
4. try to keep your hands away from your face and eye

Do Not:
1. share towels and/or wash cloths with anyone
2. share pillows with anyone
3. touch the dropper tip to your eye or eye lids
4. touch the dropper tip with your fingers
5. wear contact lenses until the doctor says it's okay

Bacterial Infections

Many types of bacteria normally live on the skin. Even though they have the potential to cause an infection, most do not because the body's defenses fight them off. Bacteria are spread from one person to another by direct and indirect contact.

A bacterial eye infection is usually treated with antibiotics known to be effective against many common types of bacteria. If the eye does not get well, then a culture might be done. The doctor may also look at some tissue under the microscope to determine what sort of bacteria it is. (This is done by numbing the eye with eye drops, then gently scraping a little loose tissue from the ulcer.) If a specific bacteria is identified, the doctor will prescribe medication known to be effective against that particular germ.

The waste products from the bacteria may cause an allergic reaction in the eye. This may be treated with a steroid drop to relieve the symptoms.

In some cases, you might also be given an antibiotic to take by mouth. Be sure to take every pill, even if the infection clears up before they are gone.

Fungal Infections

Yeast infections sometimes occur in patients with lowered resistance. The cornea may be weakened by viral infection, long-term use of steroid drops, or severe dryness.

A fungus usually enter the cornea through an injury, for example a scratch from a tree branch or plant.

Both yeast and fungi can cause corneal ulcers, and are treated with special anti-fungal medications.

Virus Infections

There are several types of viruses that can attack the cornea.

Herpes Simplex Infection

The same virus that causes cold sores on the lips can cause corneal ulcers. (This is NOT the same type of Herpes that is a sexually transmitted disease. They are in the same family of viruses, but NOT the same thing.)

Herpes infection can be stubborn and hard to get rid of. Unfortunately, once the virus has gotten into the cornea, infection may recur. This virus can cause scarring of the cornea and inflammations deeper within the eye.

Treatment includes special anti-viral drops. It is vital that you use ONLY the eye medications that the doctor prescribes. Steroid drops are usually avoided.

Herpes Zoster Infection (Shingles)

Shingles is caused by another member of the Herpes virus family, Herpes zoster. Zoster occurs in people who have had chicken pox in the past, and more often among the senior population. The most common place for a zoster outbreak is in the skin, but the infection can extend to the cornea. In fact, the corneal infection may occur before the skin breaks out.

Corneal zoster is treated with anti-viral drops, and sometimes steroid drops. Steroid pills may be prescribed, along with a pain reliever, if necessary. An antibiotic drop may be added to prevent infection by bacteria.

Adenovirus Infection

The virus group that causes colds and respiratory infections can also infect the cornea. Some of these are highly contagious and can occur as epidemics. They can be spread to the eye by the infected person himself, or spread from outside sources (other people, bugs, etc.). The conjunctiva may be infected as well.

Treatment usually includes steroid drops. It may take a few days for the drops to "kick in" and help you feel better. If the drops are stopped suddenly or too soon, the infection may come back. Follow your doctor's instructions about doses and follow-up appointments.

Keratoconus

* other names: ectatic corneal dystrophy
The normal cornea is gently curved, like the back of a spoon.

In keratoconus, the cornea bulges like the end of a football or cone (hence the name) (see Figure 10-B). As you can imagine, this causes distorted vision.

Keratoconus progresses slowly. Most likely a person would have noticed changes in vision during their 20's. This gradually worsens until around age 60. It is unlikely that a person over 40 would be finding out they have keratoconus for the first time. But we are discussing it here for those of you who have lived with this condition, and need information about what has happened to your eyes and what can be done.

The cause of keratoconus in unknown. Heredity has been suggested. Keratoconus has been found in patients with cataracts, retinitis pigmentosa, optic atrophy, Downs syndrome, Marfan's syndrome, neurofibromatosis, and allergic disease. But no one can say that any of these condition caused the keratoconus. Some believe that constant rubbing of the eyes and eyelids triggers the condition in some cases. No one knows for sure.

The main problem in keratoconus is that it continues to get worse—distorting the vision more and more. The cornea is stretched thinner and thinner and may develop scars or edema.

Diagnosis and Treatment

The first symptom of keratoconus is blurred vision. The glasses need changing frequently . . . maybe every couple months. The correction needed for astigmatism gradually increases every time.

When the doctor suspects keratoconus, he/she will begin taking keratometry readings at each visit. The keratometer measures the cornea's curvature. An increasing curve at each visit suggests keratoconus. Once keratoconus is diagnosed, keratometry readings are taken frequently to monitor its progression.

Keratoscopy, corneal topography, and Placido's disk (each de-

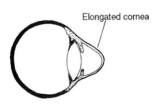

Figure 10-B Keratoconus.

scribed in Chapter 18) are also used to check the cornea's shape. In the normal eye, the reflection from these instruments will be round or slightly oval. In keratoconus, the reflection is grossly oval or broken. The keratoscope is attached to a camera, so a permanent record can be made.

There is no medication that can keep keratoconus from getting worse. Glasses may help to improve vision, but may need to be strengthened often.

Special contact lenses have been developed for patients with keratoconus. Only rigid contacts (such as hard or gas permeable) will work. Soft lenses generally cannot be used. (See Chapter 6 for general information on contact lenses.)

If the disease progresses to the point where contacts can no longer be worn, corneal transplant surgery can be considered. To be most successful, the transplant must be done before the edges of the cornea have been stretched too thin. Unfortunately, sometimes the graft itself will develop keratoconus after surgery. Please see page 193-200 for complete information on corneal transplantation.

Recurrent Corneal Erosion (see page 294)

Scar

Corneal Scar Survey
Risk factors:

- Have you had an eye injury where the cornea was penetrated?
- Have you had a virus infection in your eye?
- Have you ever had a foreign body in your eye that had to be removed by a doctor?

Corneal scarring is a result of injury, just like anywhere else in the body. Often there are no complications if the scar is faint or at the edge of the cornea. But a dense scar in the center of the cornea can cut off the vision in that eye. A scar that is near the center can cause distorted vision or halos.

Scarring can be the result of a laceration or cut. A scratched cornea will heal with no scar if it is not too deep. But if deeper layers are cut, scarring will follow.

Chemicals splashed into the eye can cause scarring as well. Chemicals and materials such as lye, lime, cement, mortar, and bleach are the most damaging. Any chemical splashed into the eye should be rinsed out immediately with water for at least 15 minutes.

Infections that cause corneal ulcers may leave scars. The most common is Herpes simplex. Other conditions, such as dry eye, in-turned lids (entropion), and in-turned lashes (trichiasis) can scar the cornea as well.

Treatment

Scars that are not blocking vision are not treated. Severe corneal scarring is treated with corneal transplant surgery. The scarred tissue is removed and clear, donor tissue is sewn in its place. The procedure is explained in detail in the next section.

Transplant Surgery

* other names: keratoplasty, penetrating keratoplasty, lamellar keratoplasty, corneal graft

Replacing the diseased cornea with a new cornea is like replacing a window. If the full thickness of the cornea is replaced, the procedure is called a penetrating keratoplasty. In a lamellar keratoplasty, only a partial thickness is replaced.

About 10,000 corneal transplants surgeries are performed each year in the United States.

What causes corneal opacities and distortion?

An opacity is any cloudy or hazy area on the normally clear cornea. There are a number of problems that could cause corneal damage. Corneal scarring was discussed above. Cloudiness can also result from edema following injury or inflammation such as iritis. Corneal dystrophy and keratoconus can progress to the point where a new cornea is indicated.

What is a corneal transplant?

In the penetrating type of procedure, the center part of the diseased cornea is removed (see Figure 10-C). The process is rather like using a cookie-cutter. Then the center of a clear, healthy donor cornea is cut out with the same cutter. This cut-out, called a "button", is usually about half the size of a dime. The button is sewn into the eye, to replace the diseased portion that was removed.

If only the top layer of the cornea is clouded, the lamellar pro-

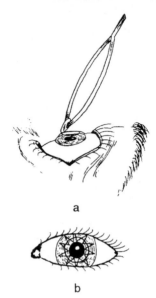

a

b

Figure 10-C (a) Scarred corneal tissue is removed and (b) donor graft is sewn into place.

cedure is used. The cloudy layer is removed with the cutter. A layer of donor cornea is stitched in place.

The diseased cornea that is removed is sent to the lab for evaluation. This is routine procedure for *any* tissue removed from the body, to check for malignancy. The report is later sent to your surgeon. (You may get a separate bill from the pathologist who examined the tissue.)

Where does the donor tissue come from?

Donor tissue comes from people who were generous enough to donate their eyes after death. The tissue is refrigerated and/or specially preserved according to strict regulations. Information about the donor is taken carefully. Data such as cause of death, medications used, eye problems, and diseases are recorded. Lab work is done to be sure the person didn't have any contagious diseases. If there is ever any doubt about the health of the donor, the tissue is not used.

The tissue itself is examined, and detailed records are made. The cornea is evaluated by microscope. A cell-count is also done (described in Chapter 18). Not all tissue meets the rigid standards required for use in corneal transplantation.

Physicians prefer to use young tissue for corneal transplants. The reason is that the endothelium, or inner-most layer of the cornea, is more healthy in a young person. (The cells of the endothelium do not regenerate, and are responsible for keeping the cornea clear.)

When your surgery is scheduled, the ophthalmologist calls the eye bank. These banks are under regulation by the state with strict guidelines about handling and dispensing the tissue. The doctor gives the eye bank information about your case, and your name is placed on a waiting list. Tissue is used within a few days of obtaining it. A cornea is usually available by surgery day. In rare instances surgery may have to be postponed if a good graft is not available.

It may seem strange to think about having tissue from someone else placed into your body. This idea bothers some people. But please understand that donating is voluntary...no one is forced to contribute. By accepting the transplanted cornea, you are fulfilling the last wishes of someone who wanted very much to give you the gift of sight.

Am I a good candidate for a corneal graft?

A corneal graft won't help everyone with a corneal disease or problem. Pre-operative testing, discussed below, helps determine if the eye can handle a transplant. If the cornea is too thin or has a lot of abnormal blood vessels growing into it, a graft may not be recommended.

I also have a cataract. Can I still have it removed?

When a cloudy cornea co-exists with a cataract, the surgeon may suggest combination surgery. Even if the cataract is not too advanced, it may be wise to remove it during the corneal transplantation procedure. This avoids having two separate surgeries. This saves time and money, and lowers the risks involved.

If a corneal transplant is done and the cataract is not removed, the vision will only improve as far as the cataract will allow. Vision will again decrease as the cataract worsens with time, regardless of having a clear corneal transplant.

In combination surgery, the cataract is removed in the normal way (see Chapter 11). An intraocular lens (IOL) is implanted into the eye. In routine cataract surgery, the eye is measured before surgery to find the correct power for the implant. These measurements may be impossible to perform on a diseased cornea. For that reason, the surgeon may use measurements from the other, non-diseased, eye to estimate the IOL power. While the IOL power may not be exact, this is the best that can be done.

After the cataract is out and the IOL is in, the corneal transplant procedure is done.

I had a corneal transplant that failed. Can I have a new transplant?

A corneal transplant can often be repeated, even several times if necessary. The cloudy button from the first surgery is removed then replaced with a new donor button.

The outcome of a repeat transplant may not be as good if the first graft was rejected. In this case, special testing may be used to try to match the donor tissue more closely with the recipient. (These tests are not required under normal circumstances.)

How well will I see after surgery?

Your vision depends in part on the health of the rest of the eye. If the only problem is a cloudy cornea, then your vision may improve to the level you enjoyed before the cornea became clouded.

However, if you have problems with other parts of your eye, only portion of the blurred vision that was caused by the cloudy cornea will be improved. For example, if you have macular degeneration that has decreased your central vision, you will still have this problem after surgery.

There is no way to accurately determine post-operative sight. (And of course, no surgery comes with any guarantees.) Your ophthalmologist, who is familiar with your case, is best able to predict the extent of your improvement.

Your vision also depends on how well your eye adjusts to the graft. It usually takes several months to a year to get your best vision. In addition, there is usually some astigmatism after corneal transplantation. The amount of post-operative astigmatism affects the vision as well.

What is required in preparation for surgery?

Having a corneal transplant requires a lot of leg-work before you ever go into the operating room, but most of it is simple and quick.

Much of the pre-operative testing is done while you are in the office. Depending on your case, your doctor may elect to do all or none of the following:

- cell count—Your diseased cornea is examined with a high-powered microscope, called a specular microscope, that can see a single layer of cells. This may be done for documentation (as evidence that the surgery was needed) or to provide more information about the area that will receive the donor tissue.
- pachymetry reading—The pachymeter measures the thickness of the cornea. The physician may want to know the thickness of the cornea where it will be joined to the graft. If this edge is too thin, surgery may be impossible. In addition, readings from the center of the cornea help to document that surgery was necessary.
- B-scan ultrasound—If the cornea is so cloudy that the doctor cannot see into the eye, there is no way to be sure that the retina and other internal parts are healthy. The B-scan provides a picture of the eye's interior. If there are severe problems inside the eye, the corneal transplant will not improve vision much (if any).
- photographs- The physician may want slit lamp pictures of your cornea to help support the need for surgery or for research purposes. If the photo includes facial features that could identify you, you will probably be asked to sign a photograph release. This means that you give permission for your picture to be published. You may decline this consent if you wish. Photos of your eye, where you cannot be identified, may be used without a consent.

Each of the above tests are described in detail in Chapter 18. Please refer to Chapter 15 where we discuss eye surgery in general.

What is it like to have a corneal transplant?

Corneal transplant surgery is done as an out-patient. On the average, the surgery takes anywhere from thirty minutes to two hours. If the procedure includes cataract removal, it may take five to fifteen minutes longer.

After surgery, your eye will be cleansed and patched. In most cases you are not to remove the patch yourself. So go home and prop up your feet! Bed rest with bathroom privileges are the order of the day. Do not eat a heavy meal. Take a nap. Consider yourself on holiday. Most people have very little discomfort. If you develop severe headache or eye pain, contact your physician at once.

I can't stand to have my face covered. Can I still have the surgery?

Yes. There is a way to tape the drape to the microscope so that it isn't on the patient's face (see *claustrophobia*, Chapter 15).

What can I expect after surgery?

First, you should know that recovering from a corneal transplant takes time, sometimes up to a year. You will need to be patient.

Most likely your eye will feel scratchy. This is due to the stitches. Your surgeon will have prescribed some ointment for you to use to ease this discomfort. Some redness and light sensitivity is also normal.

Your eye may water a good bit. That is normal. But if the tears are thick, notify your surgeon.

These symptoms should gradually decrease as the eye heals. If any of them flare up again after they had started improving, contact your doctor at once. (Please also see the next section on *rejection*.)

Your vision will be very blurry, and may improve very slowly. Vision fluctuates during the entire healing period, so you may notice that your sight is better one day, and worse the next. This is normal. However, if your vision falls way down, contact your physician right away.

You will be using eye drops and ointments which will include antibiotics and steroids. Follow your doctor's instructions carefully. If you run out of a medication, get it refilled. DO NOT discontinue any medicine until you are told to do so. If you have any questions, call the office.

To protect the eye, you will need to tape a shield over the eye at night. (The surgeon will tell you when you can stop.) Wear your glasses during the day.

Certain activities are not allowed for a period after surgery. These include heavy lifting, bending and stooping, swimming, and bowling. Your doctor may have other restrictions as well. Do not get water in your eye, and do not rub the eye.

Driving after surgery depends on the vision in the other eye. Ask your doctor if and when you can get behind the wheel again.

He/she can also advise you about working and hobbies. Just give the physician an idea of the tasks you perform during a routine day.

You will get to know your doctor very well, because transplant surgery requires a lot of follow up. Each exam will probably include vision, pressure check, slit lamp examination, keratometry, and refraction. In general, you will be examined the day after surgery, then several times a week during the first month. Your visits will taper from every week to every two weeks, etc. Keep your appointments faithfully!

The stitches in your eye may be removed gradually during the healing period. A numbing drop is used, so there is no discomfort. You will sit up to the slit lamp microscope, and an attendant will hold your eyelids open. Open both eyes and relax. It only takes a few seconds.

Stitches that remain in the cornea may break later (sometimes years later). If this happens, your eye will feel scratchy, as if there is something in it. Notify your surgeon, who can trim the stitch.

What is rejection?

Rejection occurs when the body repels the donor tissue because it does not recognize the button as "self." It can occur within the first days after surgery or many years later. Symptoms of rejection are redness, light sensitivity, decreased vision, and sometimes pain. Your surgeon will evaluate your eye with the microscope, checking the cells of the graft and looking for signs of inflammation.

Often times rejection can be stopped and/or reversed. The key is to recognize the problem early and begin treatment right away. Steroid eye drops may be used frequently at first (maybe even every hour), then tapered off during the weeks and months that follow. In more severe cases, a steroid injection may be used. Another treatment option is oral steroids. While steroid use has gotten some bad press because of its possible side effects, using them is generally considered worth the risk in treating graft rejection.

Will I need glasses after surgery?

Usually the answer is yes. It is common to have astigmatism after a corneal transplant, and you will need glasses to correct this. You may be given a prescription to change your glasses several months after surgery. Complete healing may take about a year, though, so you may need to change lenses a time or two during the recovery period.

A contact lens may be needed if there is a large difference between the two eyes, or if there is a lot of astigmatism. Sometimes astigmatism can be corrected with refractive surgery (see *Refractive Surgery*, Chapter 6).

Will the transplant ever need to be replaced?

If healing has gone well, the transplant is good for the rest of your life. However, certain corneal diseases sometimes recur in the graft. Two examples are keratoconus and corneal dystrophy. Also, if corneal rejection runs its full course and the graft clouds over, a new graft may be attempted. In the majority of cases, however, one graft is all it takes to provide sight for life.

What are the risks of corneal transplant surgery?

While it is unlikely that any of these would occur, it is possible that a cataract, glaucoma, or retinal disease could develop after surgery. In some cases these developments would have occurred anyway, and are not related to the surgery. Other possibilities include graft rejection (above), loss of vision, and high nearsightedness, farsightedness, or astigmatism.

Ulcers see Infective Keratitis, in this chapter

The cornea is not the only structure of the eye that must be window-pane clear. The lens of the eye is like a second, internal, "window". Read the next chapter to learn what happens when this second window needs "cleaning" . . . because of cataracts.

CHAPTER 11

Cataract

A BOUT 95% of everyone age 65 or older has some degree of cataract. Just because you fall into a certain group or have some of the following symptoms doesn't mean that you have a cataract that needs surgery. In fact, some of the symptoms can occur with other eye problems as well. But if you answer yes to any of the symptom questions, check with your eye doctor.

Cataract Survey

Risk factors:

- Are you over 65?
- Do you have a family history of cataracts?
- Do you take steroids, Mevacor™, or gout medication?
- Do you smoke, or have you been a smoker?
- Are you grossly over or under weight?
- Do you have diabetes?
- Do you have hypothyroid?
- Have you had a severe electrical shock?
- Have you had a blunt or penetrating injury to the eye?
- Have you had inflammation of the eye (this is different from a simple eye infection)?
- Have you ever had an angle closure glaucoma attack?

Symptoms:

- Do you find you can now read without glasses (when you needed them before)?
- Has your vision gradually decreased?
- Do you have a problem with glare (sunlight, or headlights at night)?
- Do you have poor night vision?

- Have straight edges begun to appear wavy or curved?
- Has your color vision changed?
- Has your depth perception diminished?
- Do you see halos around lights at night?

What is a cataract?

The lens is behind the pupil, and focuses what we see. The focused image then falls on the retina.

A cataract occurs when the lens of the eye becomes cloudy (see Figure 11-A). It is not a growth, but a haziness in the lens itself. If the lens is not clear, the vision is blurred (see Figure 11-B).

What are the symptoms of cataracts?

Looking through a cataract is like looking through waxed paper or frosted glass. Some patients describe this as a skim, fog, or film over their vision. There seems to be a general blur over everything. Glare may also be a problem. Difficulty driving at night is a common complaint.

Another symptom is called "second sight." This occurs when you can read close-up without your glasses . . . something you probably haven't done in years. Although this seems to be a change for the better, it is a sign of cataracts. "Second sight" is only temporary, lasting several months, then diminishing as the cataract progresses. It is sometimes called the "honeymoon" stage of cataracts, because

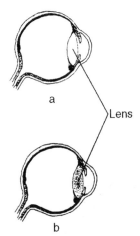

Figure 11-A (a) Clear lens, (b) cataract (cloudy lens).

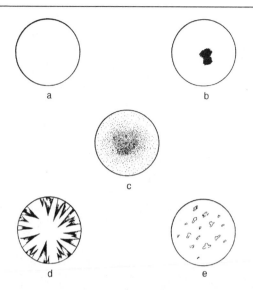

Figure 11-B (a) Clear lens, (b)–(e) types of cataracts.

things seem great (or even better than before) and no work needs to be done!

Yet another indication of cataract is seeing halos around lights. Traditionally, halos have been associated with glaucoma. But more often it is due to cataracts. This occurs because the cloudy material in the lens scatters light.

Sometimes a person with cataracts will notice a change in color vision. There may be a brown or yellow tinge on objects. Family members may complain because you constantly try to adjust the color on the TV when nothing is really wrong. Or you might have disputes with friends over whether or not your clothes match!

A cataract can cause double vision in the affected eye. Distortion can also occur. Straight edges may appear wavy or curved. Depth perception may be altered.

What causes cataracts? Can they be prevented?

Some evidence indicates that ultraviolet (UV) light can cause cataracts. Ultraviolet light is invisible radiation from the sun that causes skin cancer. Researchers say that exposing the eye to UV light over a long period of time can cause the lens to cloud. (Because of this possibility, many eye care specialists add ultraviolet protection to every patient's glasses prescription.)

Certain drugs have been known to trigger cataracts. Most notable of these is steroids. Sometimes the medical need to use a drug outweighs its possible risks. Your medical doctor is best able to advise and monitor your condition if you must use steroids. He/she may advise you to continue the steroids, and to visit your eye care physician every six months. Not everyone who uses steroids will develop cataracts.

New evidence seems to indicate that malnutrition can cause a higher rate of cataracts. Taking a daily multivitamin, or one of the new vitamins especially for the eyes, is a great idea. Other than this, be wary of any claims that a device or drug can prevent or slow cataract formation.

Blunt or penetrating injury to the eye can also cause a cataract to form. Use common sense and eye protection (such as goggles) when hammering, grinding, sawing, etc. A cataract can form following an attack of angle closure glaucoma.

The tendency to form cataracts does seem to be hereditary. Sometimes a baby is born with cataracts. But most often the cause is aging. Cataracts occur primarily in the population over age 60. In fact, some researchers say that everyone will develop a cataract if they live long enough. It's a matter of a person's "chemistry." While one person may live to age 90 and have only early cataracts, another may have significant cataracts at age 55 or younger. With improved health care, Americans are living longer than before. Thus cataracts are becoming more and more common.

In some studies, diabetes seems to cause cataracts to mature earlier. Therefore diabetics often need cataract surgery at a younger age than the rest of the population.

How are cataracts detected?

Your regular doctor or eye care physician has several ways of detecting cataracts. Occasionally a cataract may be seen with nothing more than a flashlight. More often, the doctor uses an instrument called an ophthalmoscope. The ophthalmoscope allows the doctor to see into the eye. This is best done with the pupils dilated. Cataracts are easily visible with this method.

Your eye care physician has an additional instrument not found in most general medical offices. This instrument is a highly specialized microscope called a slit lamp. Cataracts are best examined in this way. With the slit lamp, the doctor can see the various layers of the lens. He/she can tell how severe the cataract is, and its location. The rate at which the cataract is progressing can be evaluated over a period of time.

What is the treatment for cataracts?

In the past, a strange array of potions and drugs claimed to prevent, delay, or reverse cataracts. This country's strict drug regulation laws have prevented most of these quack remedies from plaguing us. At the present time, the only method of treatment is surgery. Cataracts cannot be removed with laser.

During cataract surgery, the cloudy lens is removed through a small incision in the eye. A clear plastic intraocular lens implant (made of polymethylmethacrolate) is then placed inside the eye. This implant (known as an IOL) is considered permanent (see Figure 11-C).

The history of the IOL is interesting. Pilots during World War II occasionally got plastic from a shattered windshield imbedded inside the eye. To the doctors' surprise, the eye simply healed! There was no infection, no rejection, and little affect on the vision. From the discovery that the eye can tolerate implanted plastic de-

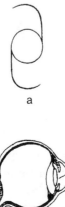

Figure 11-C (a) Intraocular lens implant (IOL), (b) IOL in place inside eye.

veloped the idea of implanting plastic lenses to improve vision after cataract surgery.

An IOL functions to focus incoming light, much as the natural lens does. Before the development of the IOL, the only option a patient had was thick cataract glasses. These glasses look like the bottom of a bottle. They cause distortion and can be difficult to fit properly.

Later on, contact lenses became available. Using contact lenses got rid of the thick glasses, but brought problems of their own. Contacts must be handled: inserted, removed, and cleaned. This is often difficult or impossible for an elderly patient who has arthritis or shaking hands. Also the risk of infection was increased.

The advent of the intraocular lens implant changed cataract surgery almost over night. It is now the most popular method of restoring sight after cataract removal. Each lens has a specified "power" designed to meet the visual need of the patient. The success of cataract surgery depends on proper pre-operative diagnosis, lens selection, and surgical skill.

What is this new type of cataract surgery I've been hearing about?

The most up-to-date cataract extraction procedure available is known as phacoemulsification (phaco for short). Phaco uses precise ultrasonic vibrations to break up the cataract into small particles. These particles are then removed by suction through a tiny hollow tube. The special surgical equipment needed for this procedure is not available at all hospitals and clinics.

The traditional method of extraction requires a surgical incision of about half an inch. The incision needed for the phaco procedure is only one fourth of an inch. An IOL that folds up is inserted into this smaller opening. For the patient, this smaller incision potentially means better vision without glasses after surgery. The larger the incision, the greater the risk that the cornea (clear covering over the eye) will become irregular. This could cause astigmatism, possibly reducing post-operative vision. Since it is less traumatic to the eye, the new procedure also reduces the risk of retinal detachment and intraocular hemorrhage. Post-operative discomfort and recovery time are reduced as well, allowing a quicker return to a normal schedule. Often no stitches are needed and the incision is allowed to heal on its own. Without stitches, recovery time is shortened and discomfort is decreased.

Cataracts can still be safely removed by methods used before phaco. In this case, the cataract is removed whole through a larger wound. Stitches may be needed to close the incision. If stitches are used, this type of surgery can cause increased astigmatism. With experience and careful trimming of stitches, the problem of astigmatism can be reduced.

In some cases, the surgeon may feel that the cornea is not healthy enough to undergo phaco. Traditional surgery may then be the best choice for the patient.

Can cataract surgery correct my astigmatism?

It is possible. First, the surgeon must give careful attention to the measuring process (described on page 211). Proper selection of IOL power is the starting point.

In traditional cataract surgery using stitches, the incision is usually made at the top of the eye. When the operation is over, the surgeon stitches the opening tightly to prevent leakage. The tight stitches pull on the cornea, the clear covering over the front of the eye. This tugging distorts the cornea and creates astigmatism. If a patient has natural astigmatism before surgery, then the stitches from the surgery could make it worse. The newer no-stitch cataract surgery does not distort the cornea as much.

For patients with moderate astigmatism, there is a method of placing the cataract incision so as to reduce astigmatism. The tors work together to counter-balance the astigmatism.

Where there is a good bit of astigmatism before cataract surgery, an additional step is required. One or two "relaxing incisions" are made at the edge of the cornea during the cataract procedure (arcuate keratotomy). These incisions do not cut all the way through, but are only partial-depth. They are placed to allow the cornea to "relax." This flattening effect greatly reduces or eliminates the astigmatism.

I have cataracts and glaucoma. Can I have my cataract removed?

This is another area where ophthalmology has made great strides in recent years. Traditionally, the problems had been treated separately. Now, when surgery is needed, it is common to treat both conditions at the same time.

Glaucoma occurs when the aqueous (fluid inside the eye) does not drain out properly. Pressure builds up inside the eye as the fluid collects. This pressure damages the optic nerve. Untreated, glaucoma can lead to blindness. It is usually controlled with eye drops, but sometimes surgery is desirable or necessary. (For details on glaucoma, see Chapter 14.)

In modern combination surgery the cataract is removed, an IOL inserted, then a draining system created. The cataract is removed in one piece, or by phacoemulsification (as discussed above). The glaucoma portion of the surgery is called a trabeculectomy. The trabeculectomy allows the fluid inside the eye to filter out more easily, thus lowering the pressure inside the eye. Often a person will no longer need to use glaucoma medications after surgery. Those persons who still need to use glaucoma medications usually need fewer than before.

My eyes are crossed (strabismus), and I need cataract surgery. Can both problems be corrected?

If your eyes have drifted a little because of poor vision in the eye with the cataract, removing the cataract may stimulate the eyes to pull straight. But if your eyes have been crossed for many years, surgery will be needed to straighten them. Most surgeons prefer to handle these problems separately: one surgery for the cataract, and then some weeks or months later another surgery to straighten the eyes.

It is possible to combine cataract and eye muscle surgery. There are six muscles attached to each eye. The blood supply to the front of the eye travels through the muscles. Operating on two or more muscles along with a cataract removal would increase the risk of infection. In addition, the blood supply to the front of the eye might be decreased, causing the tissues to break down. For this reason the combined procedure can only be used if just one muscle will be involved. If further straightening is needed, traditional eye muscle surgery can be done after the eye has healed. (A copy of the journal article on the combined technique is available by writing the authors.)

I have a cataract, but also need a corneal transplant. Can they be done at the same time?

In most cases, yes. The cataract portion of the surgery (often called a "triple procedure") is done pretty much as described below. Please refer to *Transplant Surgery* in Chapter 10 for details on corneal transplant surgery.

When should a cataract be removed?

In years past it was necessary to wait until a cataract was "ripe" before performing surgery. With the newer surgical methods, a cataract can be removed at any time. Nowadays the decision to operate is based on the patient's ability to function. When a patient is unable to do the things he/she wants and needs to do because of poor vision, it is time to remove the cataract. Likewise, if glare and poor night vision is a problem for the patient, surgery can be performed at once. The determining factor is geared more toward patient need than it was in years past.

Until recently, the only means of documenting a patient's vision was the traditional eye chart. The eye chart uses black letters on a stark white background, providing a great deal of contrast. Most of the things we normally see are not of such strong contrast, but blends of shades and hues. Thus, vision as recorded from the chart is better than actual vision. A patient will say, "I don't care how good your chart says I can see. I can't recognize the faces of my friends until they get real close to me!" Basing the decision to operate based on the patient's vision as per the eye chart can be invalid.

Fortunately, a better method has come along. This latest technology is known as the contrast sensitivity test. It measures the eye's ability to distinguish variations of shades. Failing the test is grounds for performing cataract surgery, regardless of the vision according to the eye chart. (See Chapter 18, *Contrast Sensitivity Test*, for more details.)

Cataract surgery is occasionally performed as an emergency procedure. If a cataract causes the lens to swell, the pressure inside the eye increases. This increased pressure, or glaucoma, damages the optic nerve. When this condition is identified, surgery is done immediately. Glaucoma caused by a cataract is usually cured by removing the cataract.

How well will I see after cataract surgery?

Your vision after cataract removal depends in large part on the condition of the retina (inner lining of the eye). The retina is like the film in a camera. Even if you have an expensive lens for your camera, you will not get good pictures if the film is bad. Likewise, in the eye, removing a cataract will not give perfect vision if the retina is diseased. Cataract surgery will restore only the vision that has been blurred because of the cloudy lens.

It is important to remember that good vision depends on the health of all the structures of the eye. If there are other problems in addition to the cataract, this may affect your vision after surgery.

There used to be no way to predict what vision would be after surgery. Now, however, it is possible to estimate post-operative vision by use of a potential acuity meter (PAM) or interferometer. These instruments project letters, numbers, or patterns to the back of the eye by by-passing the cataract. The results of these tests let the surgeon know what vision to expect after surgery, in spite of the retina's condition. Both of these tests are described in Chapter 18.

Will I have to wear glasses after surgery?

As intraocular lens implants came into popular use, the misconception that glasses would not be needed after surgery also grew. Although it is true that some post-operative cataract patients do not require glasses, most need them for clearest vision at distance and/or near. The important thing to remember is that these glasses will be rather thin, unlike the bottle-bottom cataract glasses of the past.

The need for glasses after surgery can be virtually eliminated by a technique known as monovision. This method is usually used when both eyes will have implants. The power of each IOL is chosen to make one eye see up close and the other eye see at a distance. Patients who choose this method report that they quickly learn which eye to use for a particular activity. They also adjust their sense of depth perception. Once the orientation period is over, they don't even think about which eye is doing what. Glasses can still be worn if desired, but are not necessary.

Patients with monofit IOL's can drive without glasses if the vision in the "distant" eye meets the state's driving requirements. There may be a problem when taking the vision test to renew the license, however. The trouble occurs when you are asked to read at a distance with the "close-up" eye. Since this eye is focused at near, it might fail the distance reading test. In this case all that is required is a note from the eye surgeon. The license will then be issued (assuming that the "distant" eye passes).

What is required in preparation for cataract surgery?

Several eye measurements are needed in order for the doctor to choose the proper implant for your eye. First, the curvature of your cornea is measured using a *keratometer*. Then the length of your eye is measured using a sophisticated instrument called an *A-scan*. The A-scan utilizes sound waves, much like sonar, to obtain this critical measurement. The third element in choosing an implant is a *refraction* (testing you for glasses). The diameter of your cornea (the length across it) may be measured as well, usually by holding a small ruler close to the eye. Each of these tests is painless.

In some instances, the cataract may be so cloudy that the doctor cannot see through it to examine the retina. A B-scan ultrasound bounces sound waves off the structures of the eye's interior. It creates a picture of the eye (including the retina) on a TV-like monitor.

Another factor to be considered is the health of the cornea. Previously, a doctor could only wait and see how the cornea healed. Now, using a specular microscope, it is possible to view the cells of the cornea. Knowing the health and number of cells assists the surgeon in deciding whether a diseased cornea can withstand surgery. Most cataract surgery is done without this test, known as a cell count.

Please refer to Chapter 15 and read about pre-operative physicals, lab work, medications, consent forms, etc.

If you normally use eye drops for glaucoma, your doctor will advise you about their use before surgery. Any drop with a green top makes the pupil small. The pupil needs to be large during the procedure. Your surgeon will probably have you stop the drop a few days prior to surgery. If you use the drops in both eyes, continue to use them in the eye NOT having surgery. If you have any questions, contact your eye doctor.

What is it like to have cataract surgery?

Cataract surgery is now an out-patient procedure. This means that you do not have to spend the night in the hospital. In fact, most insurance companies will only cover out-patient cataract surgery (see Chapter 19). Your physician will advise you if you have any questions about being an out-patient.

Chapter 15 discusses all aspects of surgery, including preparation, IVs, anesthesia, operating room, recovery, and post-operative care. However, there are several details of cataract surgery that are different from other types of eye surgery.

To lower the pressure inside your eye before the procedure, a small heavy bag is placed over the closed eye. The pressure from the bag, applied from the outside, lowers the pressure on the inside of the eye. The bag is placed on the eye for ten to thirty minutes. This shouldn't be uncomfortable because the eye is already numbed.

When the surgeon is ready to start, the room lights are dimmed. The phaco instrument makes a soft whirring noise. The machine that draws out the pieces of cataract may make an electronic musical sound like a video game.

The actual surgery takes anywhere from ten to forty minutes. When the procedure is finished, the eye is patched. After surgery, you will go to the recovery room. When you are ready to leave, you will be taken to the car by wheel chair. (Even though you feel great, hospitals are required to "wheel" you out.)

Go home and take it easy. Most people have very little pain, if any. Some folks have a mild headache after the procedure. You might notice some numbness, coldness, or tingling of the face and scalp. This is from the anesthetic. If you have any discomfort, you may take a non-aspirin pain reliever. If this doesn't help, call your physician. If you have severe pain, notify your physician at once.

When doing research for this book, we asked hospital and operating room staff what they wish folks knew about cataract surgery. Their overwhelming response was "Don't worry!" Don't listen to "spook" stories about someone else's surgery. Ask questions. If you don't understand something, keep asking until you do.

I'm claustrophobic. Can I have surgery without my face being covered?

Yes. See *Claustrophobia*, Chapter 15.

What can I expect after surgery?

The vision is usually blurred right after surgery. Best vision is realized at eight to twelve weeks after surgery. During that eight to twelve week period, your vision will be changing. It is not unusual to see a little more clearly one day, and not quite as well the next.

These slight fluctuations will gradually level off as your eye heals. If your vision suddenly decreases a lot, phone your eye doctor.

It is not uncommon to have a little tenderness in the bony area around your eye. This is usually due to the injection given to numb the eye, and fades in a few days.

Your eye may be red. This should gradually diminish as the weeks pass. Notify your surgeon if the redness increases dramatically.

The eye will usually drain some during the first day or two. If drainage increases again later on, call your doctor.

It's not unusual to be a little light sensitive after surgery. Your cataract was cloudy, and prevented light from entering your eye. Now that the cataract is gone, everything seems brighter. You may notice a bluish tint. Colors will be much brighter. All this is normal. Wear sunglasses outside to cut down on the discomfort from the glare. You may also wear sunglasses indoors for the first few days if room light seems too bright. This light sensitivity generally fades with time.

It is not unusual to notice little specks, like gnats, floating around in your vision. But if these floaters get larger, or you see a sudden shower of them, notify your surgeon. You should also call your doctor if you begin to see light flashes.

After the patch is removed, wear your regular glasses during the day. This helps protect your eye. The lens in your glasses over the eye that had surgery isn't correct any more, but it will NOT damage your eye to wear it. The idea is to prevent anything from getting into the eye. Please be careful when you put your glasses on, so that you don't poke your eye with the temple.

The eye might feel a little scratchy if stitches were used. Your physician may have prescribed eye ointment for you to use after surgery. Use a little of the ointment when your eye feels irritated. Report any severe discomfort to your eye care physician.

Restrictions after cataract surgery are minimal, and every physician has his/her own list of do's and don'ts. While we can give some general guidelines here, please follow the advice of your doctor.

You may be told not to stoop or bend over. In this case, you may kneel to pick something up, but don't lean over from your waist so that your head dangles down. It is okay to incline your head to read.

There is often a limit on the amount of weight you may lift for a week or so after surgery. Avoid any type of exertion. If you find that you are constipated, take a mild laxative to avoid straining.

Other common (and temporary) restrictions include:

1. Sleep on the side opposite the eye that had surgery
2. Do not rub the eye
3. Driving: Ask your doctor when you can drive again. This depends on the legal driving vision in your state, and how well you see.
4. Working: Again, ask your surgeon. It will largely depend on what you do for a living. Someone who works at a desk may get back to the office much earlier than a person who works in a dusty environment, or who must do heavy lifting.

You will be scheduled for a number of follow-up appointments following surgery. Often the surgeon will see you. In some cases, you may be seen by an associate or the optometrist who referred you for surgery. The timing of these follow-up exams varies, but generally a person who is doing well will be seen 1 day after surgery, then on post-operative weeks 1, 4, and 8. A new lens for glasses is usually prescribed four to eight weeks after surgery. Please follow your ophthalmologist's requests, and keep each of your appointments.

Every time you are examined after surgery, you will be told how to use your medications. Ideally this should be written down. Follow your medication schedule carefully. If you have any questions or need refills, call your doctor. **Do not stop using a medication just because you have run out of it, unless your doctor has told you to do so.**

Will I need laser surgery after cataract surgery?

The lens of the eye is encased in an envelope. When a cataract is taken out, the front of this membrane is removed with the cataract. The back of the membrane is left inside the eye to support the plastic lens implant (see Figure. 11-C).

Although the membrane is polished during surgery, it occasionally turns cloudy in later months. This causes symptoms similar to cataract: decreased vision, halos, glare, and "ghost" images. Until

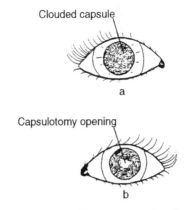

Figure 11-D (a) Cloudy capsule, (b) capsule opening after laser capsulotomy.

the early 80's, this problem had to be corrected by surgery. Nowadays a special laser, called a YAG, is used. The YAG makes an opening in the center of the membrane (called a capsulotomy), thus restoring clear vision. The outer portion of the membrane remains to support the implant (see Figure 11-D).

What is it like to have YAG laser surgery?

Before having the laser, you will be asked to sign a consent stating that you understand the treatment and that your questions have been answered. This is merely a standard requirement. No physical is required. Your doctor may have the laser in his office, or you may have to report to the hospital for treatment. You will not be admitted, since the laser is an out-patient procedure.

Laser surgery is truly unique. The eye is not cut as in regular surgery. The light beam is aimed precisely at the structure needing treatment and passes safely through the eye until it reaches that point. Since the eye is not surgically opened, there is virtually no risk of infection or bleeding.

Your pupil will probably be dilated with eye drops. You may also be given a numbing drop before the treatment starts. The laser is attached to a slit lamp microscope. Your chin and forehead will be in a headrest. The treatment is usually painless and takes only a few minutes. You may be asked to remain at the office to have your eye pressure checked after the laser.

Your physician will prescribe one or more eye drops for you to use after the laser. A follow-up exam will be scheduled to measure your vision and eye pressure. Now and then the eye pressure will rise after laser treatment. If this happens, your physician will ask you to use some additional eye drops until the pressure comes down. This is usually a temporary condition.

Many people notice an immediate improvement in their vision after the laser. Others observe visual recovery after the dilation wears off. Some find that their glasses need changing again after the laser.

There are no restrictions following laser surgery. If you have difficulty driving with your pupils dilated, you may want someone to drive you home.

A few rare cases of retinal detachment, fluid buildup, or glaucoma have been reported. It is unlikely that any problems will occur. If you should notice any large floaters, a curtain over your vision, or flashing lights, notify your doctor at once.

Sometimes a capsule opacity is referred to as a "secondary cataract." This name is not really correct. Since the cloudy vision of a capsule opacity is similar to the foggy vision of cataracts, though, it seems as if the cataract has returned. Once removed, however, a cataract cannot come back. Because laser is used on the cloudy capsule, the rumor developed that a *cataract* can be removed with laser. Researchers are working on it, but as yet a cataract cannot be removed with laser.

Miscellaneous Questions

Can the cataract grow back?
    No.

Is the eyeball removed during cataract surgery, then put back?
    No.

What kind of charges can I expect?
    This is a tough question to answer because fees vary so much. Your physician or someone in the billing department should give you the details. (see Chapter 19)

My cataract isn't ready to be removed. Or, I can't have my cataract removed right now. How can I cope until surgery?
    Use plenty of light when you read. Use large print if necessary. Avoid driving at night if glare is a problem. Ask your eye doctor if having your glasses changed would improve your vision at all. (Even-

tually cataracts progress to the point where changing glasses *won't* help.)

I had my cataract removed several years ago and didn't have an intraocular lens implant (IOL). Can I have an IOL now?

The situation of having no natural lens or IOL is called aphakia. An IOL may be implanted unless there is some eye disease that makes this unwise. The measurements needed for an IOL are basically the same whether you are having cataract surgery or just an implant.

Once my cataract is removed, do I need to be concerned about damage from ultraviolet (UV) rays?

In addition to causing cataracts, UV rays have also been suspected of damaging the retina. Most modern IOL's have been treated to filter out UV light. Ask your surgeon about your implant. If there is no UV protection in the IOL, have the UV dye put in the lenses of your glasses. If you don't wear glasses all the time, wear sunglasses that protect against UV rays when you're in the sunlight.

What are the risks of cataract surgery? How likely is it that anything like this will happen?

Like any surgery, there are risks involved with having a cataract removed. (Statistically, you are more likely to be involved in a car accident than have any problems from cataract surgery.) When you discuss surgery with your doctor or the office staff, they will explain all possible risks to you. Here are the most common:

1. **Rise in the eye's pressure—**If pressure in the eye rises and stays elevated for a period of time, the optic nerve can be damaged. However, your pressure is checked at every post-operative visit. If the pressure does rise, eye drops are given to lower it. Such a pressure elevation is almost always temporary. You may need the drops for a few weeks. FOLLOW YOUR DOCTOR'S INSTRUCTIONS ABOUT MEDICATION USE!
2. **Hemorrhage inside the eye—**Since the eye is cut during surgery, there is the possibility of bleeding. In rare cases, the bleeding can cause decreased vision. This usually clears up with time, as the blood is reabsorbed.
3. **Infection—**Symptoms of infection, which occurs very rarely, include pain, redness, discharge, and/or blurred vision. Most infections are handled with eye drops and oral antibiotics.

4. **Retinal detachment—**The risk of retinal detachment is present in nearly all eye surgery procedures. Although it is very unlikely to happen, these are the symptoms to watch for: an increase in the number or size of floaters, flashes of light, decreased vision, and/or a veil or curtain over the vision. If any of these occur, contact your eye physician at once.

I have astigmatism caused by previous cataract surgery. Can anything be done to reduce or eliminate this?

This may be possible. Earlier, we discussed a technique for handling astigmatism DURING cataract surgery by using relaxing incisions. These same incisions (called arcuate keratotomy) can be done later, apart from cataract surgery. This surgery is done in the office or hospital as an out-patient. Depending on the severity of the astigmatism, the procedure lasts only 2–20 minutes. A numbing drop is the only anesthetic necessary. (See *Refractive Surgery*, Chapter 6 for more details.)

The lens of the eye has one major function: to bring light to a focus on the retina. We'll examine the retina and other structures inside the eye in the next chapter.

CHAPTER 12

Internal Eye and Retina

DO you remember Sharon Watson? We met her in the Introduction. One day she had floating specks and light flashes and later found out she'd had a retinal detachment. Her neighbor, Jim Matthews, had the same symptoms a few months later. Warned by Sharon's experience, he went to see his eye doctor right away.

"You've had a posterior vitreous detachment," his doctor said. "Nothing serious."

The doctor went on to explain the condition, and how it differs from a retinal detachment. *Golly*, thought Mr. Matthews, *There's a lot more to the inside of the eye than I thought!*

The retina is a thin membrane lining the inside of the eye (see Figure 12-A). It contains the light receptor cells that are responsible

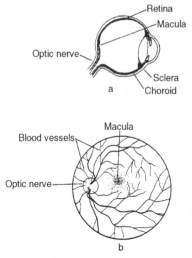

Figure 12-A (a) Side view showing location of retina, (b) fundus (view through ophthalmoscope).

for vision. Like the film in a camera, the retina gathers light. These light impulses are transmitted to the brain, which interprets what is seen.

Diabetic Retinopathy

The term "diabetic retinopathy" refers to retinal damage caused by diabetes. These conditions can include retinal hemorrhage (bleeding), growth of abnormal blood vessels, and leakage of fluids from the blood vessels into the retina. Please read *Diabetes* in Chapter 7 for more information.

Hemorrhage (Bleeding)

Retinal Hemorrhage Survey

Risk factors:

- Do you have diabetes?
- Do you have high blood pressure?
- Have you had surgery or injury to the eye?
- Do you take blood thinners?
- Are you a free-bleeder?
- Are you taking chemotherapy?

Symptoms:

- Have you had a shower of floaters?
- Has your vision decreased suddenly?

Retinal hemorrhage is bleeding from the blood vessels in the back of the eye. If the hemorrhage is small and in an outlying area, the vision may not be affected. Small hemorrhages usually resorb on their own without decreasing the vision. Larger hemorrhages may obscure the vision. If there is a lot of blood inside the eye, the eye pressure may rise, causing secondary glaucoma. Another complication can be retinal detachment.

Treatment

The doctor may order a fluoresceine angiography (dye study) of the eye. This photographic test shows which vessels are bleeding.

If there is a lot of blood inside the eye, the doctor will not be able to see the retina. Yet it may be important to know certain things about the retina right away (such as, is it torn or detached?). The physician may order an ultrasound, which gives a computer picture of the retina using sound waves.

There is no medication for a hemorrhage, but you may be asked to sleep with your head elevated. Once the blood has cleared up enough for the ophthalmologist to see the where the blood is coming from, the eye may be treated with laser to seal the bleeding blood vessel.

Hypertensive (high blood pressure) retinopathy

See *High blood pressure (hypertension)* in Chapter 7.

Iritis (Inflammation of the Iris)

* other names: anterior uveitis

Iritis Survey

Risk factors:

- Have you had a recent eye injury?
- Have you had recent eye surgery?
- Have you had iritis before?
- Do you have sarcoid?
- Do you have tuberculosis?
- Have you had an angle closure glaucoma attack?
- Are you using any type of eye drop with a green top?

Symptoms:

- Is your eye red?
- Is your eye painful?
- Are you light sensitive?

Iritis is an internal inflammation of the iris (colored part of the eye). The condition causes pain, light sensitivity, and redness. Usually the entire eye is not red, just the edges next to the iris. Vision is not affected much at first, but if the condition is not treated, vision can decrease. (These same symptoms occur in other eye conditions as well. Only your eye doctor can determine the cause of a painful red eye.)

When the iris becomes inflamed, cells and debris are released into the aqueous (the watery fluid inside the eye). Some of this material clumps together and sticks to the back of the cornea. If cells clog the aqueous drainage area, pressure inside the eye can rise, causing secondary glaucoma.

Iritis is usually a response to injury. Any type of trauma, even just a gentle bump to the eye, can cause an inflammatory reaction. Iritis can occur as part of a general inflammation that is going on in the body as a whole. This is the case in tuberculosis and sarcoidosis.

Certain eye drops used to treat glaucoma (especially angle closure glaucoma) may cause iritis, but this is rare. The drops in question have a green cap. In most instances, the benefits of using these drops to control glaucoma far outweigh the small risk of iritis.

Treatment

Since steroids are ideal for fighting inflammation, the first treatment is usually steroid eye drops. They are used more often at first then gradually tapered off. If you stop the drops too soon, you may suffer a relapse.

In more severe cases, oral steroids may be used as well. These are also discontinued step-by-step. Finally, in rare cases a steroid injection may be necessary. (These are given after the eye has been numbed.)

Steroids have gotten a bad reputation because of their side effects. But in short-term use to treat iritis, the risks are minimal and outweighed by the benefits of healing.

A second medication often used in treating iritis is dilating drops (these medications have a red top). When the pupil is not dilated, the iris constantly moves to adjust to incoming light. This causes pain because the iris is inflamed. Dilating the pupil holds it still. In addition, dilating temporarily paralyzes the muscle that focuses the lens of the eye. This muscle is attached to the base of the iris, so deactivating it increases comfort as well.

The side effects of being dilated are a large pupil and blurred vision (usually for close-up). There may be some light sensitivity, so wear sunglasses if you are uncomfortable. These symptoms will go away once your doctor discontinues the medication.

Ischemic Optic Neuropathy (Tissue Death from Blocked Arteries in the Optic Nerve)

* other names: papillitis

Ischemic Optic Neuropathy Survey
Risk factors:

- Do you have giant-cell (temporal) arteritis?
- Do you have high blood pressure?
- Do you have diabetes?
- Do you have high cholesterol?

Symptoms:

- Do you have periodic episodes where your vision (one eye or both) goes out then returns?
- Have you had a sudden visual loss?
- Do you have headache or tenderness in the temples?

The optic nerve contains nerve fibers which conduct visual images from the eye to the brain. The nerve also contains blood vessels. In ischemic optic neuropathy (ION), there is blockage of the arteries that nourish the optic nerve and choroid (layer under the retina). Without a blood supply, these tissues begin to break down. Vision loss is usually sudden. There may be periods of vision loss that come and go before the major loss occurs. There is usually no pain. Blind spots may occur in the peripheral vision. The pupil of the affected eye may be larger, or may not respond normally to light. In rare cases there may be double vision. Headache in the temples may occur, depending on the cause of the blockage. If both eyes are not affected to begin with, the other eye usually becomes involved later (anywhere from a few hours to 2–3 years later).

Diagnosis and Treatment
Vision improvement depends on the cause of the blockage. To diagnose the cause of ION, your physician will order some blood work. Depending on the results of the blood tests, your eye doctor may refer you to another doctor for a biopsy of the temporal artery or other arteries. This is done by numbing the area and taking a sample of tissue for the lab.

Treatment is usually started right away by taking steroid pills.

The amount of steroid taken is usually larger at first to get the problem under control, then gradually decreased over several months. You have probably heard some bad things about steroids. These side-effects are always possible, but usually occur after using steroids for a long period of time. In the case of ION, the benefits of taking the steroids is considered worth the risk of any side-effects. Report any problems to your eye doctor and follow directions carefully.

If you also have diabetes, anemia, high blood pressure, or glaucoma, you will need to be careful to control these problems. If you need any type of surgery while you have ION, be sure to get an okay from your eye doctor. It may be best to delay non-emergency surgery until the eye has settled down.

Laser Surgery

The term "laser" used to make us think of space ships firing at each other. But modern medicine has brought laser closer to home . . . first into the hospitals, then right into the doctor's office. Eye care has been no exception. The use of laser surgery has brought incredible advances in treating eye disease.

When laser is used, the eye is not cut as in regular surgery. That means there is no risk of infection or bleeding. Most laser treatments are painless and quick. The light beam is aimed precisely at the area needing treatment, passing safely through the eye until it reaches that point. Then the laser accomplishes its task of sealing or dissolving.

Some aspects of laser surgery are similar, regardless of the condition being treated or the type of laser being used. When laser treatment is recommended, the physician or an assistant will explain the procedure. Once all your questions have been answered, you will be asked to sign a consent form.

Your eye will be numbed with eye drops. If the doctor is treating your retina, your pupil will be dilated.

You will be asked to place your head in a headrest with your forehead against a bar and your chin in a cup. Someone may gently hold your head in place, or sometimes a strap is used to help you hold still.

Depending on the type of treatment, the doctor may place a special lens on your eye. This should not be painful. In fact, if you

Table 12-1 Retinal Treatment with Argon Laser.

Problem	Procedure	Approximate Time
hemorrhage (diabetes, high blood pressure, injury, etc.)	focal photo-coagulation (treats specific area)	5 minutes
abnormal growth of blood vessels (diabetes)	panretinal photo-coagulation (treats broad area)	Usually done in several sessions of 20 minutes
retinal hole	focal photo-coagulation	5 minutes
macular degeneration	focal photo-coagulation	5 minutes, may need repeating

can keep from squeezing your eyes, you probably won't be uncomfortable at all. Keep both eyes open as much as possible. (It is okay to blink now and then.) The doctor may ask you to look at a light or other object to help keep your eye still.

The Argon laser is used for most retinal surgery. The time it takes to do laser surgery depends on its purpose. (see Table 12-1 for details).

There are no restrictions after laser surgery. Your vision may be blurred from being dilated or feel a bit scratchy from the lens used during the laser. You may use artificial tears for relief. In most cases this irritation will be gone the next morning. If it is not, notify your doctor.

You may be given some eye drops to use following the procedure. Be sure to use them as directed and keep your appointment for follow-up exams.

Recently, a new instrument has been developed called the ophthalmic laser microendoscope. The endoscope combines a light source, video transmission, and laser in one handpiece. The endoscope probe is inserted through a very small opening in the eye. A magnified view is transmitted from the probe tip onto a TV-like screen. Thus, portions of the eye that have not been visible before (in a living eye) can now be seen. In addition, the interior of the eye is visible to the probe even if there is a cataract or other obstruction. Any area needing laser is treated using the same probe. Retinal procedures that can be done using the endolaser include treating retinal holes and detachments as well as certain disorders of the blood vessels. This device is experimental and available only in a few locations. We expect it will eventually be approved and come into common use.

Macular Degeneration

 * *other names: age-related macular degeneration, senile macular degeneration*

Macular Degeneration Survey

Risk factors:

• Do you have a family history of macular degeneration?

Symptoms:

• Has your reading vision slowly decreased?
• Is your near vision distorted (straight lines appear curved or solid lines appear broken)?
• Are parts of your reading vision blank or blotted out?

The above symptoms can indicate problems other than macular degeneration. But if you answered "yes" to any of them, you should see your eye care professional.

The macula is the center of the retina, and is the area of sharpest vision.

Macular degeneration is the leading cause of permanent vision loss in the elderly. It is thought to be caused by hardening of the arteries in the layer of the eye beneath the retina. This can lead to slow break-down of the macula. Sometimes new blood vessels are formed, creating a network beneath the retina. The new blood vessels can bleed or leak fluid into the macula, causing loss of function. This lost vision cannot be restored.

Total blindness does not occur. Macular degeneration causes loss of central vision, but enough side vision remains to allow performance of tasks that don't require good central vision. Thus a person with macular degeneration may have trouble reading and recognizing faces, but still be able to get around and care for himself.

A dilemma occurs when a person with macular degeneration also has cataracts. Each of these conditions causes vision loss. But because the health of the retina is in question, it can be hard to predict just how much the eyesight will improve after removing the cataract. The interferometer and potential acuity meter (both described in Chapter 18) can help determine how much vision has been lost because of macular degeneration, and how much from the cataract. If the macular degeneration is severe, removing the cataract may not improve the fine reading vision very much. But it may increase side vision and allow the patient to get around better. This could mean the difference between being able to care for oneself or being totally dependent on others.

Treatment

Many physicians recommend that their patients with macular degeneration take specific vitamins to nourish the retina. Experts have found that taking these vitamins can slow the degenerative process and/or restore some of the lost vision. The recommended vitamins and their recommended daily doses are:

Vitamin A: 100 IU's
Vitamin C: 1,000 mg
Vitamin E: 400 IU's
Zinc: 50 mg

Many over-the-counter daily multivitamins do not contain enough of these four vitamins. You may purchase each vitamin separately. Several companies now make a multivitamin especially for the eye (see *Nutrition* in Chapter 17). Ask your pharmacist to help you.

We often recommend that a patient with cataracts and macular degeneration take the vitamins for six weeks, then return to the office for another vision check. This way the retina is in optimum health before cataract surgery is done.

Laser treatment may be beneficial if a network of new blood vessels has formed beneath the retina. Only vessels *outside* the macula can be treated by laser. The laser treatment causes a small scar inside the eye. If this scar is in the macula, the scar would cause decreased vision. The treatment does not improve vision, but seems to help prevent continued loss in some cases.

Monitoring

Your physician watches for any further degeneration by checking your vision (especially your near vision) every time you come in for an exam. It is important that you report any changes you have noticed since your last visit.

A special photography technique, called fluoresceine angiography, is also used to monitor macular degeneration. A special dye is injected into a vein in the arm. Photographs are then taken of the eye's interior as the dye enters the eye's blood vessels. These photographs will demonstrate the network of vessels, if they are present, as well as any progression of the degeneration.

You can help your physician keep track of your macula by using an Amsler grid at home (see Appendix G). Several times a week, look at the grid through your glasses just as you would normal reading material. Cover one eye with your hand and focus on the dot in the center of the chart with the uncovered eye. If you notice that the blocks in any area of the grid are distorted or blurred (and they were clear before), call your ophthalmologist immediately.

Coping

Regular glasses seem to work best. You may need to use a hand-held magnifying glass as well. However, if vision becomes extremely poor, other magnifying aids may be helpful (see *Low Vision Aids*, Chapter 17). These include telescopic lenses and special magnifying glasses.

Macular Edema (Fluid on the Macula)

* other names: cystoid macular edema

Macular Edema Survey

Risk factors:

- Are you diabetic?
- Have you had a lens implant?
- Have you had uveitis?
- Have you had a retinal vein occlusion?
- Do you take any of the following drugs: hydroxychloroquine, chloroquine, quinine, nicotinic acid?
- Have you had a cataract removed *without* an intraocular lens implant AND do you use eye drops containing epinephrine (for glaucoma)?

Symptoms:

- Is your central vision blurred in the affected eye?
- Do things appear smaller than they really are with that eye?
- Do straight lines appear bowed or curved when viewed with that eye?

The macula is the area of finest central vision. Macular edema occurs when fluid seeps into the tissues of the macula, resulting in distorted and blurred vision. Edema may be caused by diseases, conditions, or drugs that affect the blood vessels of the retina. In rare cases, macular edema has been linked to intraocular lens implants (IOL's).

The decrease in vision may be very mild, causing a slight blur or distortion. In other instances, legal blindness may result. Total blindness does not occur. While the central vision is blurred, side vision remains. This allows a person to see well enough to get around.

Testing and Treatment

The most common test to evaluate macular edema is the fluoresceine angiogram. Other tests include the photostress test (see Chapter 18) and dilated examination of the inside of the eye.

Steroid eye drops and/or steroid pills are the usual medications used to treat macular edema. In recent years some non-steroid eye drops that reduce inflammation have been developed that may be used instead. What ever your physician prescribes, be sure to use it as directed. Do not discontinue use until told to do so.

If the edema is due to diabetes, it may be treated with laser. If the problem is found to be due to an IOL and medications fail to help, your surgeon may consider removing the implant. However, this is a very rare occurrence.

Recovery

Recovery depends on the cause of the edema. In diabetes, the vision does not normally recover. The goal of laser treatment is slowing vision decrease. Macular edema from other causes may show slow vision improvement over a 2–12 month period. In some cases, the vision may not recover totally.

Optic Atrophy (Deterioration of Optic Nerve)

Optic Atrophy Survey

Risk factors:

- Does anyone in your family have optic atrophy?
- Have you had, or do you have, glaucoma?
- Have you had, or do you have, inflammation of the optic nerve (papillitis)?
- Have you had, or do you have, recurrent swelling of the optic nerve (papilledema)?
- Are you an alcoholic?
- Do you smoke?
- Are you malnourished?

Symptoms:

- Have you developed a loss of color vision?
- Do you have blind spots in your vision? (This is different from floaters.)

Optic atrophy is deterioration of the nerve fibers in the optic nerve. Nerve fiber death can cause a general decrease in vision and/or blind spots. Once a nerve fiber is dead, it cannot be restored.

There are three basic types of optic atrophy

1. Hereditary optic atrophy runs in families, usually starting in childhood. Males are more often affected. Vision loss is almost always permanent, although total blindness does not usually occur. There is no treatment, and recovery is rare.
2. Diseases—Certain conditions can trigger optic atrophy. These include: alcoholism, smoking, malnutrition, tumors, drug reaction, and trauma.
3. Optic nerve problems—Optic atrophy may occur as a complication of inflammation (papillitis), or swelling of the optic nerve head (papilledema). Atrophy due to these conditions usually occurs only when the swelling or inflammation goes on for a long time.

Treatment

Optic atrophy itself is not treated, but the condition causing it may be. Treatment depends on the cause. Obviously alcohol and tobacco use need to be stopped. A well-balanced diet with vitamin supplements is necessary. Optic atrophy caused by malnutrition may recover if detected and treated early enough. Sometimes steroids are used in cases of papillitis. Papilledema is considered an emergency and requires hospitalization. If optic atrophy goes on for a long time, chances for improvement decrease.

Optic Neuritis (Inflammation or Degeneration of the Optic Nerve)

* other names: retrobulbar neuritis, papillitis, neuroretinitis[†]

Optic Neuritis Survey
Risk factors:

- Do you have multiple sclerosis?
- Does anyone in your family have multiple sclerosis?
- Do you take chloramphenicol, streptomycin, sulfa drugs, Diabinese[R], or oral contraceptives (birth control pills)?
- Are you diabetic?
- Are you an alcoholic?
- Do you smoke?
- Do you suffer from malnutrition?

Symptoms:

- Has your vision blurred, or does it come and go?
- Do you have eye pain?
- Is there a blind spot in your vision?

Optic neuritis is inflammation of the optic nerve, usually occurring in only one eye. The optic nerve extends from the back of the eye to the brain. It carries all the nerve fibers from the retina, as well as blood vessels. Often the cause of optic neuritis is unknown. If no cause is found in an adult, there is a 40% chance that multiple sclerosis will develop . . . usually within 2 years of the neuritis. Other causes include viruses, injury, radiation, lead poisoning, sarcoid, lupus, high blood pressure, vascular disease, leukemia, and thyroid eye disease.

---

† There is some disagreement about the names of these conditions. It depends somewhat on what part of the optic nerve is affected.

Pain is usually the first symptom. It may be mild or severe, and can take many forms. There may be a dull ache behind the eye, the eye may be sore to the touch, or there may be a sharp stabbing pain when the eye is moved.

Vision often decreases over a 2–5 day period, beginning one or two days after the pain starts. Or there may be episodes of blurred vision that lasts a few minutes to a few hours. Color vision and depth perception are decreased as well. A blind spot may appear in the center of the sight, or anywhere in the vision. Side vision may diminish. Light may seem dimmer in the affected eye.

Treatment and Testing

In severe cases, or if the condition is known to be caused by multiple sclerosis, steroids (oral or even IV) are used. Otherwise, unless a specific cause is found, there is no treatment. The condition merely has to run its course.

Because central blind spots are so common in optic neuritis, your physician may order a visual field test. This maps out the side vision and any areas of missing sight. Repeating the test later, during recovery, will show any changes that have occurred. Color vision testing and stereo testing (both discussed in Chapter 18) can monitor color vision and depth perception in the same way.

Because optic neuritis is often associated with multiple sclerosis or other central nervous system disease, your eye doctor may refer you to a neurologist (physician specializing in diseases and conditions involving nerves). Periodic MRI scans may be ordered to monitor for the onset of multiple sclerosis.

There is also a slight chance that the inflammation is caused by a growth pressing on the nerve. To investigate this, your physician may order an X-Ray, a CT scan, or a visually evoked response (see Chapter 18).

In addition, you may need a lumbar puncture (also called a spinal tap), where a small amount of fluid is drawn from the spinal column. The lumbar puncture is done with the patient lying on one side. You may be asked to curl up (this widens the space between the bones of the back). A numbing injection is given in the area below the waist above the buttocks. Once the area is numb, a very fine needle is used to draw some fluid off the spine.

Recovery

Pain rarely continues for more than 10–14 days. Vision usually begins to recover in one to four weeks. The process can be slow, however, taking from seven months to over a year. Color vision and depth perception improve at the same time. One study reports some vision improvement in 75% of cases.

Blind spots gradually shrink and side vision slowly expands. In 51% of cases, normal side vision returns in about seven months.

Recurrence is not unusual.

Papilledema (Swelling of the Optic Nerve Head)

Papilledema Survey

Risk factors:

- Have you had a recent head injury?
- Do you have rheumatic or congenital (from birth) heart disease?
- Have you had a recent infection of some sort (such as infected sinuses, lung abscess, ear disease)?

Symptoms: (Note: If you are highly nearsighted or have optic atrophy, papilledema cannot occur.)

- Do you have episodes of blurred or blacked-out vision that lasts less than one minute?
- Have you developed double vision?
- Has your side vision seemed to close in?
- Do you have headaches that have increased? Are they worse in the morning, or when you cough or sneeze?

Papilledema is swelling of the optic nerve head (the place where the optic nerve enters the eye). It is caused by elevated pressure inside the head ("intracranial") and spinal cord. This elevated pressure squeezes the optic nerve, blocking messages traveling along the nerve fibers. Extra fluid is also forced into the nerve, causing more pressure. The swelling usually begins one to five days after the intracranial pressure rises. In the case of a head injury with internal bleeding, however, swelling starts within two to eight hours.

Elevated intracranial pressure can occur on its own, without anything being wrong. Other causes of pressure elevation include tumor, abscess, bruising, aneurysm, and malignant hypertension (a rare form of high blood pressure that has resulted in kidney damage). It occurs most often in overweight women in their forties. Papilledema is a major emergency requiring immediate hospitalization.

Papilledema often occurs in both eyes, but may be present in only one. In 25% of the cases, papilledema causes brief episodes of blurred or lost vision. When the episode is over, normal vision comes back. There may be double vision. As the nerve is pinched side vision may decrease. The normal blind spot may get larger. Headaches may occur, but this varies. The headaches may be sudden or occur off and on over a period of time. The pain may be mild or severe. Often the headache is worse in the morning. Coughing, sneezing, or straining may make the pain more intense. There may be nausea and vomiting.

If optic atrophy is already present, papilledema cannot occur. However, if papilledema continues for a long period of time, optic atrophy may develop.

Testing

When papilledema is discovered, a CT scan or an MRI may be ordered. The goal with either procedure is to get a view of the brain.

In cases where a tumor is suspected, an electroencephalograph (EEG) may be needed (see Chapter 18). The EEG records electrical brain waves, which will be abnormal if a growth is present.

If it has been determined that the elevated pressure is due to an abscess, the physician will look for infection. A chest-X-Ray will probably be ordered. To help identify the bacteria or germs causing the infection, blood and spinal fluid will be collected for cultures.

Treatment

The main goal in treating papilledema is to lower the intracranial pressure. A spinal tap may be done to drain spinal fluid, thus lowering the pressure. Medications to lower the fluid content of the body (diuretics, or "water pills") may be used. Depending onerlying cause of the pressure, steroids may be prescribed. In the case of infection, antibiotics are ordered.

Recovery takes six to eight weeks from the time that the intracranial pressure goes down to normal.

Papillitis (Inflammation of the Optic Nerve Head)

The optic nerve head is the part of the optic nerve that the physician can see when he looks into the eye. Papillitis involves swelling of the optic nerve head due to inflammation, fluid seeping into the nerve tissue, or problems with the blood vessels in the nerve. There is always vision loss. Two types of papillitis are ischemic optic neuropathy and optic neuritis. (Please refer to these sections for detailed information.)

Posterior Vitreous Detachment

Posterior Vitreous Detachment Survey

Risk factors:

- Are you over age 60?
- Are you near-sighted?
- Have you had a blow to the eye?

Symptoms:

- Do you see "specks" in your vision? (These may be small dots, hairs, or a net.)
- Do you see flashing lights (especially in the dark when you move your eyes)?
- Do you see a light resembling a half-moon?

The vitreous is a gel-like substance in the inside of the eyeball. It is normally in contact with the entire retina (inner lining of the eye). Age, injury, and disease can cause the vitreous to become more fluid-like. Then fibers of protein, membranes, and clumps of cells may become visible and appear in the line of vision. These "floaters" may look like cobwebs, spots, dust, or strands of thread.

As the vitreous becomes partially or completely fluid, it may be

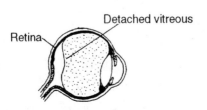

Figure 12-B Posterior vitreous detachment.

stripped away from the retina in one or more areas. This is called a posterior vitreous detachment (PVD) (see Figure 12-B). PVD occurs in half the population over 60 years of age. In addition to floaters, symptoms of PVD include seeing a large spot or ring, and light flashes (especially when moving the eye quickly). Vision is not significantly affected. There is no way to predict its occurrence, but it is generally not serious. For the most part, the diagnosis is made only after you develop symptoms.

You should contact your eye doctor if symptoms of PVD occur. In itself PVD is not an emergency. However, as the vitreous pulls away from the retina, the retina may be detached or torn. Your doctor will perform a dilated examination to see if this has occurred.

There is no treatment. The symptoms gradually disappear, although the vitreous detachment itself remains. The other eye may have a similar episode within months. After being diagnosed with a PVD, you should be checked by your doctor promptly if there is an *increase* in the number of spots or light flashes, or if a "curtain" appears over your vision. Both of these occurrences are symptoms of retinal detachment. Let's talk for a moment about the normal floaters that are common to nearly everyone. These are the "spots" that you see, especially when looking at a clear blue sky or a blank wall. They scoot around when the eyes are moved. Floaters are caused by clumps of protein in the vitreous and do *not* indicate any problems or detachments. They often settle below the line of vision, and rarely cause any problems. Having your vision corrected (getting glasses, or having your glasses updated) may make it harder to see the floaters, but it won't make them go away.

Retinal Artery Occlusion (Blockage of Arteries in Retina)

Retinal Artery Occlusion Survey
Risk factors:

* Do you have giant-cell (temporal) arteritis?
* Do you have arteriosclerosis (hardening of the arteries)?
* Do you take oral contraceptives (birth control pills)?

Symptoms:

* Have you had a rather sudden and painless loss of vision? (May be total loss, or so dim that you can only detect light.)

- Have you had a sudden flash of light followed by a loss of vision?

Like blood vessels anywhere in the body, arteries in the retina can become blocked. This is usually caused by debris (emboli) in the blood which clog the tiny retinal arteries. Retinal artery occlusion is an emergency situation, so if you develop the symptoms, call your eye doctor at once.

Treatment

It is important to get treatment right away. Even though breathing itself is not affected, you may be given oxygen. The eye itself may be gently massaged. An IV may be used to administer medication to lower the pressure in the eye. These three things are done to increase blood flow and hopefully wash the emboli through, thus opening the artery.

Some physicians recommend drawing off some of the watery fluid (aqueous) from inside the eye. In this procedure the eye is numbed (usually with drops) to reduce discomfort. A tiny needle and syringe are used to remove some of the aqueous.

If not treated promptly (within a few hours), irreversible retinal damage and vision loss occurs.

Retinal Detachment (see Figure 12-C)

Retinal Detachment Survey

Risk factors:

- Have you had surgery or injury to the eye?
- Are you very nearsighted?
- Have you had cataract surgery *without* an intraocular lens implant?
- Have you had a posterior vitreous detachment?

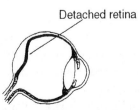

Detached retina

Figure 12-C Retinal detachment.

Symptoms:

- Do you have episodes of flashing lights?
- Have you had a sudden shower of floaters, new floaters, or an increase in the size or number of floaters?
- Does there seem to be a curtain over your vision that doesn't blink away?

The retina is the lining inside the eye that gathers light and sends images to the brain. In retinal detachment, part or all of the retina has been stripped away from the back of the eye. The retina may tear or get holes in it as well. When the retina pulls, flashes of light occur. These may be more noticeable in dim light or when moving the eye.

The torn or detached portion of the retina no longer receives light rays. Thus there may be blind spots in the vision. It may seem as if an entire half of the side vision (horizontal OR vertical) is missing. This may have the appearance of a curtain that seems to float back and forth or up and down. Or the entire vision may black out. There may also be floaters (specks in the vision) because of cells and other debris floating around inside the eye.

A retinal detachment or tear may occur without any injury or other condition. People who are very nearsighted are more likely to have a detachment or tear. This is because their eyeball is longer than normal, and the retina tends to be stretched out.

Retinal detachment may develop as a complication of retinal hemorrhage, or following surgery or injury. It is considered an emergency situation, so report any symptoms to your eye doctor at once. (Be sure to tell the receptionist about your symptoms. If you just call and ask for an eye exam, she won't know about your problem and may put you off for a few weeks. If you describe your symptoms to her, she will recognize them and have you come in right away.)

Diagnosis

To detect a retinal detachment, your physician will dilate your pupils then examine you with the ophthalmoscope. By looking inside the eye with this instrument, he or she can actually see any detached or torn areas.

Another test that can be used is the B-scan ultrasound. This uses sound waves to produce a picture of the eye's interior, revealing detachments and holes.

Treatment

The goal in retinal detachment treatment is to reattach the retina to its basement structure (the choroid). In one type of surgery, the physician draws off fluid between retina and choroid, hopefully pulling them together. Once they touch, cryo (a cold probe) is used to cause the retina to re-attach. Another reattachment surgery involves use of a band made of silicone (called a buckle). The buckle pushes the sclera (white of the eye) and choroid inward. Once the choroid and retina make contact, air, gas, or oil may be injected into the eye to flatten the retina. These procedures are done under local anesthesia. This means that you are awake but very relaxed, and do not see or feel anything.

Laser surgery is used to seal holes by "welding" the retina to the choroid. Laser surgery is done using only numbing eye drops.

Retinal Scar

A scar in the retina may have many sources. Injury, diabetes, and certain viruses can scar the retina. Laser treatment also causes scarring, but in this case the scars are part of the cure. Some retinal surgeries (such as for retinal detachment) also scar the retina.

There are no retinal light receptor cells in scar tissue, so each scar is like a blind spot. This may not cause much problem during the day if the scarring is on the outer edges of the retina. Scarring in the periphery may cause problems with night vision, because this outer area contains the light receptor cells that function in the dark. However, if the scar is on or near the macula, then the central vision is affected.

Scars from injury and laser are usually stable (don't change). Other scars, such as those caused by viruses, are "active," or can get larger. Sometimes these active scars can be removed by surgery or treated with laser.

Retinal Vein Occlusion (Blockage of Veins in Retina)

Retinal Vein Occlusion Survey
  Risk factors:

- Do you have high blood pressure?
- Do you have diabetes?
- Do you take oral contraceptives (birth control pills)?
- Are you over 50?
- Do you have cardiovascular disease?

  Symptoms:

- Have you suddenly developed a blurry spot in one eye, or blurred vision in one eye?

Like veins in any other part of the body, it is possible for the retinal veins to become blocked. High blood pressure is the most common cause. With the blood flow stopped, there can be a build-up of fluid causing swelling (edema), leakage of fluid into the tissues, bleeding inside the eye (hemorrhage), and/or growth of new abnormal blood vessels.

Treatment
  Medications are not usually helpful. Of course, controlling the blood pressure is important. Your eye care physician may order a special dye test, a fluresceine angiogram, to better examine the blood vessels. In certain cases Argon laser may be done. In this procedure, the laser is used to treat a wide area of the retina to help dry up leaking fluid and/or stop the abnormal blood vessels from growing. Vision will improve on its own in a few cases. Unfortunately, most will have a permanent loss of central vision.

Uveitis (Inflammation of the Uvea)

Uveitis Survey
  Risk factors:

- Do you have, or have you had, shingles (Herpes zoster)?
- Do you have, or have you had, Herpes simplex, especially in the eye?
- Have you had cataract surgery *without* an intraocular lens implant?

- Do you have toxoplasmosis?
- Do you have histoplasmosis?
- Have you had a penetrating eye injury?
- Do you have rheumatoid arthritis?
- Do you have ankylosing spondylitis?
- Do you have sarcoidosis?
- Do you have tuberculosis?
- Do you have chronic bowel disease?
- Have you had eye surgery?

Symptoms:

- Do you have pain in the eye?
- Is the eye red?
- Is your vision blurred?
- Are you light sensitive?

"Uvea" refers to three connected structures in the eye: the iris (colored part), the ciliary body (at the root of the iris), and the choroid (layer of blood vessels and pigment that lies between the retina and sclera). Any or all of the three parts of the uvea may be involved. If only the iris is inflamed, the condition is usually called iritis. There are so many causes and types of uveitis, we are only giving general information here.

Uveitis may occur suddenly or gradually, and usually involves one eye. The inflammation may be a response to eye injury or the result of a condition involving the entire body. Symptoms may include light sensitivity, pain, redness, and blurred vision. Since there are many eye conditions that have these characteristics, it is vital to see your eye care physician for diagnosis.

Complications of uveitis can include cataracts, macular edema, corneal edema, secondary glaucoma, and retinal detachment.

Testing and Treatment

If it seems appropriate, you may be tested for tuberculosis, toxoplasmosis, or histoplasmosis.

Steroids are very effective against uveitis. Eye drops or ointments are used, often on a decreasing dose. While steroid use can have side effects, the benefit of using them in uveitis outweighs the risks. Oral steroids may be used as well. Do not discontinue drops or pills except as directed by your physician. In some cases, an injection of steroids is used. This is given after the eye is numbed with drops, to reduce the discomfort.

Anti-inflammatory drugs that are not steroids are sometimes used. These include common aspirin.

You may be asked to use an eye drop to dilate the affected eye. Dilating helps prevent the iris from forming adhesions to other eye structures. Side effects of being dilated include blurred vision and sensitivity to light. These problems go away once the drop is discontinued.

If secondary glaucoma develops, you will be given drops to lower the pressure inside the eye. Continue to use them until told otherwise by your physician.

In cases where cataract or retinal detachment has occurred, the physician will generally prefer to clear up the inflammation before attempting surgery to repair these problems.

Recovery depends on the type and cause of uveitis. Some will clear up with treatment in a few days to weeks. Other types may linger on. It is common for the problem to occur again.

For the last five chapters, we've looked at each section of the eye . . . inside and out. But that's not the end of the story. In order for vision to function properly, the eyes have to be looking in the right direction! Find out how they do it in the next chapter.

CHAPTER 13

Muscles and Nerves

FRANK Holly woke up that morning just like any other day. His dog, Kelcey, nuzzled his hand, urging him to get up and produce breakfast.

"Okay, okay. I'm coming, Boy!" he said good-naturedly, without opening his eyes. "What time is it, anyway?" He rolled over to look at the clock. He looked, rubbed his eyes, and looked again. The clock-face was doubled! He looked at Kelcey. "Great," he said in an attempt to be light-hearted. "Just what I needed. Two dogs!" He swung his feet over the edge of the bed and patted the dog on the head. "Kelcey, we've got to call the eye doctor to see if he can get rid of your twin!"

Double vision is just one symptom of problems involving the nerves and muscles. We'll look at others, too (see Figure 13-A).

Blepharospasm

* other names: jumping eyelid, tic

A twitching eyelid can be aggravating. There is no pain, just a tickling sort of feeling as the eyelid jumps. Blepharospasm can be as mild as a corner of the lid jumping, or as severe as the entire

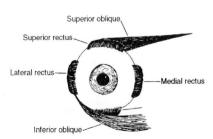

Figure 13-A External muscles of the eye.

eye squeezing shut. The tic can come and go over a period of hours or it can be permanent.

The twitch may occur in one eye or both, and is more common in older people. It may be a response to irritation, pain, or trauma to the eye itself or to the nerve that activates the eyelid. Other causes include stress, too much caffeine, and fatigue.

Treatment

If the tic is caused by stress, caffeine, or lack of sleep then it is obvious to remedy those situations. Your eye care physician should examine for anything that might be irritating the eye and causing the lid to jump (such as a foreign body, in-turned eyelashes, or infection).

When a blepharospasm does not go away, an injection of dilute botulism toxin may be tried. This stops the twitching by paralyzing the muscle, and lasts from 3 to 6 months. Injecting alcohol into the eyelid to paralyze the muscle is a rarely used treatment, because it destroys tissue.

Surgery may be done to weaken the eyelid muscle, thus decreasing the strength of the spasms. This is done under local anesthesia (numbing injections). Another type of surgery, also done under local anesthesia, actually removes the nerve that runs to the lid. For general information about surgery. (see Chapter 15)

Nerve Palsies

A "nerve palsy" is partial or total muscle paralysis caused by a disruption in the nerve messages to a muscle. Different diseases, conditions, and injuries can cause a palsy. They can also be present at birth. (We will be discussing the non-birth type.)

The nerves have numbers (given according to the order in which they leave the brain) and names. We have listed them here according to number. Although we explore each nerve palsy individually, a palsy can occur which involves more than one nerve.

Third Nerve Palsy

*   *other names: oculomotor nerve palsy*

Third Nerve Palsy Survey
Risk factors:

- Do you have diabetes?
- Do you have multiple sclerosis?
- Do you have high blood pressure?
- Do you have migraine?
- Have you had a head injury?
- Have you had a recent viral infection, especially of the inner ear or sinus?
- Do you have myasthenia gravis?

Symptoms:

- Have you developed double vision?
- Is one pupil larger than the other?
- Has the upper eye lid drooped?
- Is your reading vision blurred in the affected eye?

The third nerve affects many structures of the eye. Of the six muscles attached to the eye, four of them are controlled by the third nerve. The third nerve also sends messages to the muscle in the iris (colored part of the eye) which closes or constricts the pupil. The muscle that opens the upper lid is supplied by the third nerve as well. Finally, the muscle inside the eye that focuses the lens is under the power of the third nerve.

The causes of a third nerve palsy include diabetes, high blood pressure, tumors, inflammation, aneurysm, multiple sclerosis (and related disorders), infection, migraine, and injury.

The effects of a third nerve palsy depend on what part of the nerve has the problem. One eye or both may be affected, and symptoms often develop rapidly. One eye may be turned outward. The vision is doubled, usually with side-by-side images. Turning the head to left or right may make the images come together. The pupil of the affected eye may be enlarged. The upper lid on that side may be drooped down, even far enough to cover the pupil and block vision. Those over age 60 will generally not notice a change in vision, even though the focusing muscle is involved. (This is because the ability to focus is already lost by this age.)

Your physician may order a CT scan or MRI to determine if the palsy is due to something within the brain. Treatment of the problem causing the palsy is the first step, if a cause can be found.

Recovery may occur over a six month period. During this time, you may patch one eye or the other to eliminate the double vision. Some doctors may recommend putting prism in the glasses to bring the images together. If no improvement has occurred after six months, surgery may be suggested. Surgery may be needed to lift a drooped lid or straighten the eyes.

Fourth Nerve Palsy

* other names: trochlear nerve palsy

Fourth Nerve Palsy Survey

Risk factors:

- Have you had a head injury?
- Do you have multiple sclerosis?
- Do you have myasthenia gravis?

Symptoms:

- Have you suddenly developed double vision where the images are diagonal to or up and down from each other?

The fourth nerve is connected to a single eye muscle, the superior oblique. The superior oblique muscle helps move the eye in a down and outward direction. A problem with the nerve supply to this muscle causes double vision. The images are usually diagonal, but may vertical. Tilting the head toward one shoulder or the other often reduces or eliminates the double images. The most common cause of fourth nerve palsy is a head injury. Other possibilities include tumor or aneurysm.

Depending on the cause, no treatment is often suggested for a period of six months. This time is necessary to see how much improvement will occur on its own. Patching one eye during this time will eliminate the double vision. Putting prism in the glasses may bring the images together as well. After the waiting period is over, surgery may be considered.

Sixth Nerve Palsy

* other names: abducens nerve palsy

Sixth Nerve Palsy Survey

Risk factors:

- Are you diabetic?

- Have you recently had a viral infection, especially of the inner ear or sinuses?
- Do you have high blood pressure?
- Do you have migraine?
- Do you have hardening of the arteries (arteriosclerosis)?
- Have you had a head injury?

Symptoms:

- Have you suddenly developed double vision where the images are side-by-side?

The sixth nerve runs to a single muscle (the lateral rectus) that moves the eye outward. Double vision results when there is a problem with the sixth nerve. The images are usually side-by-side. Turning the head to the right or left may bring the images together. Diseases affecting the blood vessels, Lyme disease (caused by small ticks), tumor, and an increase in the pressure inside the brain are possible causes besides those listed in the survey.

The first six months are spent watching and waiting. Some sixth nerve palsies begin to improve on their own within 3 months. If there is no improvement after six months, eye muscle surgery may be considered. During the six months, one eye may be patched to eliminate double vision. In some cases putting prism in the glasses can eliminate the double images.

Seventh Nerve Palsy
* other names: bell's palsy, facial palsy, facial nerve palsy

Seventh Nerve Palsy Survey
Symptoms:

- Have you developed a weakness or droop on one side of your face?
  Bell's palsy is a paralysis due to problems with the facial (or seventh) nerve. It almost always affects only one side of the face. Often the cause is unknown, although it sometimes occurs after dental procedures. The condition may begin with pain behind the ear, followed by paralysis of the face within several hours. This facial weakness may be slight or total. The face has no expression on the affected side.

If there is any question about the cause of the condition, the doctor may order a CT or skull X-Rays. Bell's palsy is usually easy to diagnose, however, and no testing is required.

The seventh nerve controls the muscle that closes the eye. If the eye cannot close properly, the cornea may dry (see *exposure keratitis, page* 168). Lubricating drops and ointments, as well as taping the eye shut at night, are usually recommended. Vision is not affected unless the dryness causes the cornea to become cloudy.

In cases of partial paralysis, total recovery may occur over a period of several months. If that side of the face is totally paralyzed, recovery depends on the part of the nerve involved.

Nystagmus

* other names: dancing eyes, jiggle eyes, jerking eyes

Nystagmus Survey
Risk factors:

- Do you have multiple sclerosis?
- Do you have severe inner ear problems?
- Do you take barbiturates (sedatives)?
- Do you use alcohol?
- Do you take medication to prevent convulsions, as in epilepsy?
- Do you have myasthenia gravis?

Symptoms:

- Have others told you that your eyes seem to jerk?
- Has your vision decreased?
- Do objects seem to move?

Nystagmus is a rhythmic jerking of the eyes. The eye movements are usually left to right, but can be in other directions as well. The eyes may dance all the time, or jerk less if you look in a certain direction. In most cases of nystagmus, a person is born with it.

Many factors work together to keep the eyes aligned and steady. The eye muscles, nerves, inner ear, and brain each play a role. Weakness or disease in any one of the parts (especially inner ear and brain) can cause nystagmus to occur suddenly in adulthood.

Nystagmus blurs the vision because the eyes are not able to hold still. The constant movement blurs the image. Everything may seem to be moving. This is an optical illusion created by the jerking.

Diseases of muscle weakness, such as myasthenia gravis and multiple sclerosis, may be accompanied by nystagmus. Other possible causes include stroke, problems with the brain stem, and tumor of inner ear or brain. A jerking pattern may occur if only one eye has vision and it is losing its sight.

Tests And Treatment

A CT or MRI may be ordered to see if the problem is originating in the brain. A special test to evaluate eye muscle movements, an electromyography (see *EMG*, Chapter 18), may be done as well.

If nystagmus is suspected to be caused by an inner ear problem, an irrigation test may be done. Cold or warm water is gently run into the ear canal while the doctor or assistant watches the eye movements. Any change in the jerking may indicate that the problem is due to degeneration or irritation of the inner ear.

If the cause of the nystagmus can be found, it is treated. In some types of nystagmus, medications can help. Putting prism in the glasses may be of benefit in some situations.

Strabismus

* other names: crossed eyes, wall-eyed, squint

There are six muscles attached to each eye. They must all be in balance to hold the eyes straight. If just one muscle or its nerve is stronger or weaker than it should be, it can pull that eye out of line. This is usually present at birth, but can result from injury or nerve palsy (see Figure 13-B).

A person whose eyes have crossed since childhood has learned to use only one eye at a time. If one eye is used more than the other, amblyopia ("lazy eye") may develop. Usually there is no double vision in an adult whose eyes have crossed all his or her life.

Surgery may be done to straighten a crossed eye. Sometimes this is performed in hopes of getting both eyes to work together. Other times it is done only for the sake of appearance.

There are two basic procedures in eye muscle surgery. One method tightens a muscle, the other loosens it. Depending on the problem, these techniques may be done alone or in combination to

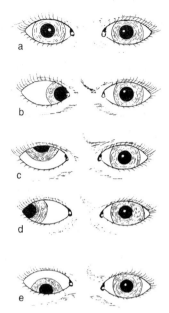

Figure 13-B Types of strabismus (a) normal, (b) esotropia (one eye turned in), (c) hyperopia (one eye turned up), (d) exotropia (one eye turned out), and (e) hypotropia (one eye turned down).

straighten the eyes. In some cases only one eye needs surgery. In other circumstances, both eyes may need it.

Measurements are done before surgery to give a record of how much the eye(s) are out of line (these are painless tests). Photographs are also taken.

Muscle surgery is done as an out-patient . . . you do not have to spend the night in the hospital. Chapter 15 discusses the details that apply to most eye surgery.

Adults having muscle surgery are not put to sleep for the operation. The surgeon may ask you to look at a light or some other object during surgery to help him judge how far to move the muscles. You couldn't do that if you weren't awake!

The time it takes to do the surgery depends on how many muscles must be fixed, and whether one eye or both are involved. Often a problem is over-corrected on purpose, because with time the muscles tend to relax a little. By over-correcting, the eyes end up in the right place once healing and loosening takes place.

You will be using some eye drops and/or ointment during the

healing period. Follow directions carefully. Do not discontinue a medication until told to do so. Call the surgeon's office if you have any questions.

Most likely the eye that had surgery will be red. In some cases the entire white of the eye may look blood-red. Although this may be alarming to look at, it is just the normal bruising (called a subconjunctival hemorrhage) that goes along with the procedure. Sometimes the red area spreads and gets larger for a day or two. It may take a week or more to completely clear up.

Any discomfort is probably due to stitches. If your surgeon has prescribed ointment, use it to relieve the scratchy feeling. You may also notice a pulling sensation, especially when you roll your eyes around. This tugging will go away as the muscles adjust to their new position. If you experience pain that is not relieved with over-the-counter pain medication, call your eye care physician.

Some patients have double vision after surgery, but this depends on many factors. Your physician may be able to predict whether or not your vision will be doubled after surgery, and how long it will last. In cases of temporary double vision, patching one eye will restore single vision. This also works well in instances where you are waiting for the eye to heal enough so you can get prism in your glasses.

Your surgeon will usually want to examine you the next day. In some types of muscle surgery, the stitches need to be adjusted twenty four hours later. This is done in the office. Be sure and keep your follow-up appointments. The muscle balance of your eyes will be tested and measured at each visit. This enables the physician to monitor your progress.

Eye muscle surgery is not an exact science. It is impossible to know exactly how much or how little to move a muscle, no matter how experienced the surgeon is. In some cases another muscle surgery is required to straighten the eyes further.

This finishes our tour of the eye's structures. You've learned that certain problems have certain symptoms, and that most symptoms can have many possible causes. But can something happen to your eyes without your knowing? In the next chapter you'll find out.

CHAPTER 14

Glaucoma

DICK Langley was troubled as he hung up the phone. His older brother had just called with disturbing news. His eye doctor told him he had glaucoma. "You'd better get checked, too, Dick," his brother urged. "My doctor says glaucoma can be hereditary."

Mr. Langley remembered an elderly aunt who had gone blind. No one ever knew what was wrong with her eyes. Was his brother going to be blind, too? It was a solemn thought. *And what about me,* he wondered. *Will I get glaucoma, too?*

Can something happen to you without you knowing it? Glaucoma can. Glaucoma causes blindness so gradually that it goes unnoticed until severe damage has occurred. In fact, glaucoma is the second leading cause of blindness in the U.S.

There are many different types of glaucoma. We will discuss the three main types in this chapter. These three categories of glaucoma are different in that they arise from different causes. But they are similar in that they all involve increased pressure inside the eye.

Open Angle Glaucoma

* other names: chronic open angle glaucoma, primary open angle glaucoma, simple glaucoma, wide angle glaucoma, chronic simple glaucoma, glaucoma

Glaucoma Survey

Risk factors:

- Are you over 35?
- Do you have a family history of glaucoma?
- Are you black?

Glaucoma occurs when abnormal pressure builds up in the eye

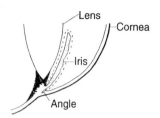

Figure 14-A The flow of aqueous.

(see Figure 14-A). The front of the eye is filled with a watery fluid called aqueous. The aqueous is constantly being formed. It circulates inside the front of the eye, bathing all the inner structures. Then it drains out to make room for more. This creates a pressure inside the eye, known as the intraocular pressure (IOP). If proper aqueous drainage does not take place, a build-up of the fluid occurs inside the eye. It's similar to a hose with a knot in it. If the water is turned on, pressure builds up behind the knot. A leak will develop if there is a weak area in the hose. Increased pressure in the eye does not lead to leakage, but the pressure transfers back throughout the entire eyeball. This eventually begins to harm the delicate optic nerve (see Figure 14-B).The damage to the optic nerve causes blindness starting at the outside edge of the side vision and gradually closing in. Left untreated, it can cause tunnel vision and even blindness.

The most common type of glaucoma is called "open angle" glaucoma. In fact, when the term "glaucoma" is used, it almost always means this type of glaucoma. In open angle glaucoma the drainage area is open but not functioning properly.

Did you notice that the survey above did not include symptom-related questions? This is because there *are* no immediate symptoms, since vision loss occurs gradually.

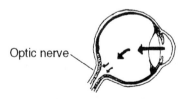

Figure 14-B Pressure transfer in glaucoma.

Some studies have shown that this type of glaucoma can be inherited, so anyone with a family history of glaucoma should be checked. Glaucoma also seems to occur more often in the black population. It is more common after age forty. (Just one more reason why an annual eye exam is so important.)

How is Glaucoma Detected?

Fortunately, glaucoma is easy to detect. Making a diagnosis of glaucoma involves three items.

1. Tonometry: An instrument called a tonometer painlessly measures the IOP. This takes only a few seconds per eye. Checking the pressure with a tonometer should be a part of every complete eye exam. "Normal" pressure is considered to be 22 or less. Anything over 22 is suspicious for glaucoma.

   However, just because the IOP is 23 doesn't mean that a person has glaucoma. Eye pressure, like everything else in the body, can vary from one individual to the next. Thus a person might have an eye pressure higher than 22 and not have glaucoma. However if pressure is over 29, it would be unlikely for this to be "normal," even for that particular person.

2. Examination of the optic nerve: Every complete eye exam includes an examination of the eye's interior. The pupils are usually dilated, and the doctor uses an ophthalmoscope or a Hruby lens to look inside the eye. If the eye pressure was found to be high, the physician looks at the optic nerve very carefully for damage (see Figure 14-C).

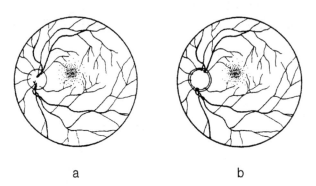

a   b

Figure 14-C (a) Normal optic nerve, (b) optic nerve in glaucoma (note larger, dug out appearance).

3. Peripheral vision examination: During a routine eye exam, the doctor or assistant may make a rough check of your side vision. This "confrontation" test is usually all that is necessary for most exams. But if the pressure has been found to be high and/or there is evidence of optic nerve damage, your physician will want a more detailed test. This is done by visual field testing, which is described in detail in Chapter 18. The visual field test creates a map of the peripheral vision. Glaucoma causes certain patterns of change in the map.

Diagnosing glaucoma involves a three-step process. Most doctors agree that any two of the three items should be present in order for the condition to be labeled "glaucoma."

There are several "in-between" conditions. First, if the pressure is high but there is *no* nerve damage and *no* field loss, it is called *ocular hypertension* or *glaucoma suspect*. In this case, the doctor will want to examine you one to three times a year. If the IOP is high enough, some doctors will go ahead and give medication to lower the pressure. The idea is to prevent damage to the nerve from ever beginning. Once you start on medication, your eye doctor will want to check you every couple months. Ocular hypertension can be caused by nearsightedness, diabetes, heart and blood vessel disease, and heredity. If you have ocular hypertension, you are at a higher risk for developing glaucoma.

Second, if the pressure is normal but there *is* damage to the nerve (with or without visual field loss), the condition is termed *low tension glaucoma*. (Other names are *normal pressure glaucoma* and *low pressure glaucoma*.) The physician may give medication to lower the pressure even more to prevent further damage.

How is Open Angle Glaucoma Treated?

Medications

Open angle glaucoma cannot be cured, but it can usually be controlled. Often using prescribed eye drops several times a day is all that is required to lower the IOP. Sometimes pills are used. Using the prescribed medications may be all that is required to bring the pressure down. These drugs cannot restore any vision that has already been lost, but if properly used they go a long way toward preventing any further loss of sight. In fact, all things considered, the only thing between you and blindness may be using the medications correctly.

Proper use of glaucoma medications is the key to pressure control. Follow your physician's directions to the letter. You may want to use the medication chart (Appendix F) to record your dosage times. Do not run out of your medication. If you run out, call your physician for a refill, or have your pharmacy call. If you have a problem paying for your medication, notify your physician. He or she may have samples or know of another way to help.

Sometimes a patient will not use their medicine on the day they have an eye exam. They think the doctor will want to know what their pressure is without the medicine. This is exactly the opposite of what your doctor wants. He or she is seeking to reduce your IOP with the drops or pills, and won't know how well the medicine is working if you don't use it the day you come in. So unless you are told otherwise, take your medicine according to schedule even on appointment days.

If your doctor makes a change in the type, strength, or dosage of your medication, you may need to be checked again sooner than usual. This is because the physician needs to monitor for any change.

For a list of glaucoma medications and their possible side effects, please (see Appendix A).

Laser

While medication is the first choice to lower pressure, sometimes things aren't so simple. The medication may not lower pressure enough, or the side effects may be too troublesome. Laser is considered by some to be the second line of defense. Laser uses intense, focused light. Since the eye is not cut, there is virtually no risk of infection or hemorrhage.

In open angle glaucoma, laser can be used to reopen the drainage areas (trabecular meshwork) to siphon off the excess fluid. The procedure is called a *laser trabeculoplasty,* and is done with an *Argon laser.*

Before the procedure is done, the doctor or an assistant will explain the surgery. You will be asked to sign a consent form stating that you understand the risks and benefits, and that you have no further questions.

A numbing drop will be placed in your eye. You will sit up to the laser machine with your chin and forehead in a headrest. An assistant may help hold your head in place. Sometimes a strap is used to brace your forehead against the headrest. The ophthalmologist will gently place a lens against your eye. (The lens is used to aim the laser beam.) This may feel odd, but it should not be uncomfortable. It is important that you keep *both* eyes open and look exactly where the doctor tells you. It is okay to blink now and then, but do not squeeze your lids. An Argon laser trabeculoplasty usually takes only minutes to complete. When the laser is done, your eye may be gooey from the solution on the lens. Wipe your eye gently, since it is still numb.

There are essentially no restrictions following laser surgery. You will be required to use some eye medications for a few days. Use them as directed and be sure to keep your follow-up appointments. Your vision may be a bit blurred, and your eye may feel a little scratchy, for a few hours after the laser. If you experience any severe discomfort, see spots or flashes in front of your eyes, or your vision completely blacks out, call your surgeon at once.

Some researchers feel that the IOP-reducing effects of the Argon are temporary, lasting only several months. Others report longer results. Often some glaucoma medications must still be used. Laser surgery is not as aggressive or risky as traditional surgery, and may be chosen for those reasons.

Surgery

Trabeculectomy

Traditional glaucoma surgery, called a *trabeculectomy*, involves making an incision into the eye and creating a new drainage system. The aqueous is then allowed to drain into a sort of "bubble" created by using the eye's own tissue. The bubble, called a bleb, is usually hidden under the upper lid. A trabeculectomy can be done as a procedure by itself, or combined with cataract surgery.

When you and your doctor make the decision to have surgery, the procedure will be explained to you in detail. Chapter 15 covers the details of most eye procedures, so you should read over it carefully. Follow your doctor's instructions. You may be instructed to stop some of your glaucoma medications before surgery. Be sure you understand what you've been told to do! If you use glaucoma drops in both eyes, continue to use them as usual in the eye

NOT having surgery. If you have any questions about using your drops, call your surgeon's office and ask.

Surgical trabeculectomy is done on an out-patient basis. The surgery itself takes about 10 to 15 minutes, maybe longer. When the procedure is over, you will be taken to the recovery room. After a while you will be allowed to go home. You will need someone to drive for you. When you get home, take it easy. Eat a light meal and take a nap.

The eye will be patched. Don't remove the patch unless your doctor has told you to. Use your glaucoma medications in the other eye as usual. In most cases, your doctor will see you the day after surgery. Follow his/her advice about medications and follow-up appointments . . . this type of surgery generally requires a lot of care afterwards.

Since there are stitches in the eye, you may experience some scratchiness. If your doctor has prescribed ointment, you may use this to relieve the discomfort. Sometimes there is a slight brow-ache. If you have any pain that is not relieved by over-the-counter pain medication, notify your eye care physician.

Your eye may be red and light sensitive. Some people notice a non-painful sensation of fullness. Your vision may be a little blurred. All of this usually clears up with time.

Filtering Implants

In an individual whose body tends to produce a lot of scar tissue, the bleb may scar over and stop functioning. Until recently, there was nothing else an ophthalmologist could offer such a patient. With the development of a new implant (sometimes called a valve), there is new hope.

The implant consists of two parts. The first is a tube which is placed into the eye to act as a drain for the fluid. The second part is a plastic ring. This ring is implanted under the eye tissues and should prevent the bleb from collapsing, even in the presence of scarring. Please read Chapter 15 for a description of what it's like to have eye surgery.

Laser Microendoscope

The ophthalmic laser microendoscope was described on page 225. In glaucoma, laser is applied to the ciliary body (structure that forms the aqueous) to decrease the amount of fluid inside the eye. The surgery is called a cycloablation. This can be done as a single procedure or combined with cataract surgery (see below).

Combined Cataract/Glaucoma Surgery

A cataract is a clouding of the eye's natural lens, causing blurred vision. Cataracts are treated by surgically removing them. (For a detailed discussion, see Chapter 11.)

When a person with glaucoma also has a cataract that needs to be removed, some decisions must be made. In the past, each condition was treated with separate surgeries. It has now become possible to do a single surgery which combines techniques to treat both problems.

In combined surgery, the cataract is removed and an intraocular lens implant inserted. Then a trabeculectomy or laser cycloablation (both described above) is performed.

The most up-to-date cataract extraction procedure available (known as phacoemulsification, or "phaco") has been adapted for patients with glaucoma. Phacoemulsification uses precise ultrasonic vibrations to break up the cataract into small pieces which are then removed by suction through a small hollow needle. The small phaco incision can be used as an entry-way for the trabeculectomy. The combined "phaco-trabec" procedure treats cataracts and glaucoma at the same time, using a smaller incision than previously.

First, the cataract is removed through a small incision in the sclera (white of the eye). After the intraocular implant is in place, the incision is enlarged and a bleb created. Or the incision can be used as the entry-way for a laser probe during laser cycloablation.

The small incision required for the cataract portion of the surgery allows for a larger drainage area. This means that more aqueous can drain out. In the past, the larger opening required for cataract removal weakened the eye's structure, and a smaller drainage opening had to be used. Phaco allows for a larger filtration opening, decreasing the eye's pressure even more.

Even the placement of the phaco incision offers advantages. Because the incision is made through the sclera (white of the eye), the cornea is not stretched as it may be in traditional cataract surgery. This leads to better vision after surgery, and a lower chance of developing astigmatism.

The results of combined surgery done in our clinic have been impressive. Without surgery, it may take several different medications to control glaucoma. After this combined procedure, more than half the patients no longer use any glaucoma medications at all. In one case, a patient had been using four different eye drops to control his glaucoma before surgery. Now he uses none. For details on the procedure, please write the authors.

While not everyone who has the surgery can stop using glaucoma medications altogether, most of those who still require medications need fewer than before. This is still a success story. For example, if you had to take three different eye drops before and only have to use one now, that's quite an improvement. It's more than just a matter of convenience or expense. Using fewer medications means there are fewer side-effects and fewer drugs to interact with other medicines you may take.

In combination cataract/glaucoma surgery, the laser microendoscope (see above) can also be used to treat the eye, instead of performing a trabeculectomy.

Angle Closure Glaucoma

* other names: narrow angle glaucoma, glaucoma attack, acute angle closure glaucoma

Angle Closure Glaucoma Survey
Risk factors:

- Do you have a family history of glaucoma attack?
- Are you farsighted?
- Are you diabetic?
- Do you have cataracts?

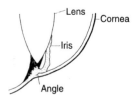

Figure 14-D Angle closure glaucoma.

Symptoms:

- Do you see colored halos around lights at night?
- Do you have eye pain?
     Does this occur in the evening or morning?
     Does this occur during or after you've been in dim light?
     Does it ever hurt so much that you feel nauseous, or vomit?
- Do you have headaches that center around one eye?
     Does this occur in the evening and/or early morning?
     Does this occur during or after you've been in dim light?
     Does it ever hurt so much that you feel nauseous, or vomit?
- Do you have episodes of a combination of eye pain, blurred vision, and redness?

A "glaucoma attack" usually sends the sufferer to the eye doctor's office or emergency room. This type of glaucoma is painful. It may start as a headache over, around, or behind one or both eyes. The pain may be so severe that the patient is nauseated and ill. The eye is usually very red, and vision blurs. This type of glaucoma is the one that causes halos to appear around lights at night. (Halos *without* pain are often caused by cataracts.)

A glaucoma attack is brought about by a defect in the structure of the eye(see Figure 14-D). The iris (colored part of the eye) actually folds back and blocks the aqueous fluid from draining out. Pressure builds up quickly, causing pain and blurred vision. If not treated promptly, the eye can go blind due to damage of the optic nerve. Even with treatment, the vision may not fully recover.

What conditions may cause the iris to block the drainage area? Anything that would make the pupil enlarge. The most common situation is being in the dark (during the night, or in a movie theater for example). Another possibility is medications that affect the nervous system and cause dilation (such as NeoSynephryn[R] nasal spray, other sinus/cold preparations, or scopalomine for motion sickness). This includes the drops used to dilate your pupils at the eye doctor's office, although this rarely happens. An examination with the microscope will usually reveal if an attack is likely to occur. Angle closure has also been known to occur after certain laser procedures or surgery for retinal detachment.

An attack can occur all at once and be severe as described above. Or small episodes can occur over a period of time. These "mini" attacks usually occur in the evening and are gone in the morning. During an episode, the eye is painful, red, and blurry. There are halos around lights. If you have been experiencing anything like this, notify your doctor at once. He or she may do a special test to help determine whether or not you are having angle closure attacks. For this test (called a "dark room provocative test"), you are asked to lie face-down in a dark room. Your pressure is checked before the test starts, then again after you've been in the dark for thirty minutes. If the IOP has risen over 3 mm during that time, you are considered to be at risk for having angle closure attacks.

Treatment

Modern treatment includes immediate medications to help lower the pressure. This includes eye drops, medication by mouth, and, in some cases, by IV. Once the IOP is lowered, laser surgery is needed to make a hole in the iris. A YAG laser or Argon laser can be used. The opening in the iris gives the aqueous a way to drain out even if the iris folds back. The procedure is called a laser iridotomy (see Figure 14-E).

Before surgery, the doctor or an assistant will explain the procedure, and you will be asked to sign a consent form. This also gives your permission for the procedure. The eye is numbed with drops. You will sit up with your chin and forehead in a headrest. Keep both eyes open and look exactly where the ophthalmologist tells you. There is usually no discomfort. A laser iridotomy takes only a minute or so to perform. You may have to use some eye drops afterwards for a few days. Be sure and keep your follow-up appointments.

An iridotomy usually "cures" the condition. Rarely will the iridotomy hole close, renewing the risk for an attack. Keeping your appointments with your eye doctor is your best defense: an examina-

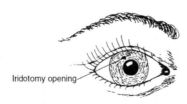

Iridotomy opening

Figure 14-E Laser iridotomy.

tion with the slit lamp microscope will easily show whether the iridotomy is still open or not.

While an attack cannot occur with an open iridotomy, the pressure may still be elevated. This may require standard glaucoma medications to control.

If small attacks occur over a period of time or a "big" attack is not treated promptly, the drainage area in the eye may be permanently blocked. In this case glaucoma surgery, as described above, may be needed as well.

An eye care physician can sometimes determine that a glaucoma attack may occur by the structure of the eye (more common in farsightedness). In this case, a laser iridotomy might be done to prevent an attack from ever happening. In other instances, specific glaucoma medication may be used to make the pupil small. If the pupil is very tiny, the iris is stretched out and drawn away from the drainage area. The disadvantage of these drops is that they have side effects, must be used daily, and do not cure the problem. In still other situations, the physician will warn the patient that an attack might occur. The doctor will explain how an attack happens, what might cause it, and what the symptoms are. The patient is warned to seek help at once if he/she has signs of an attack.

Have you ever noticed the warnings on some medications that patients with glaucoma should not use them? This is referring to angle closure glaucoma, *not* open angle glaucoma (discussed above). Those who have been warned about having an attack should consult their eye doctor before using such preparations. Those with an open YAG iridotomy can safely use them.

Secondary Glaucoma

Secondary Glaucoma Survey
    Risk factors:

- Have you ever had a blunt or penetrating injury to the eye?
- Have you had inflammation of the eye (this is different from a simple eye infection)?
- Do you have diabetes?
- Do you have rheumatoid arthritis?
- Have you had a stroke in the eye?

- Do you take steroids?
- Have you had surgery for retinal detachment?

"Secondary glaucoma" occurs when glaucoma stems from another problem in the eye, such as inflammation or injury. This type of glaucoma will often clear up once the problem causing it is gone. If an injury or surgery has damaged the fluid-draining structures of the eye, glaucoma may be permanent. Another type of secondary glaucoma is caused by a cataract. As the cataract worsens, it may swell and cause the IOP to increase. Surgical removal of the cataract, sometimes required as an emergency procedure, usually cures this type of glaucoma. Some medications, especially steroids, can cause glaucoma. Other drugs that sometimes change the eye pressure include amphetamines, reserpine, and some antidepressants. Discontinuing these drugs may restore the pressure to normal.

In cases where the cause of the glaucoma cannot be removed, the medication, laser, and surgery treatments are the same as described above under open angle glaucoma.

Many of the problems we've discussed in past chapters have described treatment that include surgery. What is it like to have eye surgery? What can you expect in the operating room? These questions and more will be answered in Chapter 15.

CHAPTER 15

Eye Surgery

A few years ago it was reported that 10% of all operations were eye surgeries. Cataract extraction with intraocular lens implant is the most common. Other procedures routinely performed on the eye include blepharoplasty (lid lift), glaucoma surgery (trabeculectomy), muscle surgery (to straighten crossed eyes), corneal transplant, retinal surgery, and plastic surgery (to restore looks or function). The details on these and other procedures are covered in the chapter that discusses the particular problem. (Check the Contents or Index.) In this chapter, we will look at some generalities that apply to most major surgeries. (For minor surgery, see pages 274-275.)

Out-Patient Surgery

Most eye surgery is done on an out-patient basis. This means that you do not have to spend the night in the hospital. In fact, most insurance will only cover out-patient cataract surgery. There has to be special reasons, and advance approval by insurance, in order to admit a patient before or after having most types of eye surgery. For instance, a person who has no one to care for him/her at home for the first twenty four hours following surgery may qualify. So might someone with severe diabetes or heart problems. All things considered, it is very rare these days for a patient to be admitted. Your physician will advise you if you have any questions about being an out-patient.

In-Office Surgery

The benefits of having your surgery in an office vs. hospital are numerous. The main blessing is a large reduction in the cost of the procedure itself. You also avoid the hassle of pre-admission and numerous insurance woes. Your fees often appear on one single bill, rather than being billed separately by the hospital, the surgeon, anesthesia, and others. Plus, an office may have a more homey atmosphere than a hospital setting. If the office staff mans the operating room, you may feel as if you're among friends.

Hospital Surgery

Not all offices have an operating room. Having your surgery done in the hospital has advantages of its own. A hospital operating room may be better equipped than an office, although this is not always true.

If your surgery is to be done at a hospital, find out if you need to be pre-admitted. This means that you go to the hospital's office a day or two before surgery to fill out papers and show your insurance cards. You can also arrange payment of any hospital fees that you will owe. This saves a lot of time and hassle on surgery day.

Be aware that you will receive a bill from the hospital, separate from your surgeon's bill. In addition, you may get a separate bill from anesthesiology, lab, pathology, and other professionals and/or services.

Scheduling and Preliminaries

Someone will fully explain the procedure and answer your questions. You may be given a brochure, or shown a video about the surgery. Then you will be asked to sign a consent form for the operation. This form (or there may be more than one) states that you understand the risks and benefits of surgery, and that your questions have been answered to your satisfaction. In addition, you give permission for use or disposal of any tissue that is removed. Other items may include allowing others to assist the surgeon, and video taping the procedure. You may also be asked to sign a release to allow before and after photographs to be published. This is an optional consent, and you may decline if you wish.

A physical of some sort is usually required before surgery. Some ophthalmologists perform the physical themselves. Others have doctors, nurses, or assistants on staff that do the exam. Yet others request that you see your regular doctor or internist for a checkup. You will be told what to do and given any necessary forms for the physical when your surgery is scheduled.

The guidelines for the physical are often set up by the hospital or in-office clinic. Generally, the doctor will listen to your heart and lungs, check your blood pressure, and evaluate your over-all health.

Depending on the procedure you are having, some lab tests may be needed as well. The number and type of tests required varies from doctor to doctor. The hospital or clinic where the surgery takes place has rules of their own about what lab work is needed. Some institutions do not request any tests. Others may want blood work and an EKG (heart trace). Other clinics may also require a chest X-Ray, urinalysis, or other tests.

The lab work may be done at the ophthalmologist's office, the doctor's office, private lab, or the hospital lab. In some cases there will be separate billing for this lab work. The person scheduling your surgery will tell you where to go and what tests are needed. He or she will also tell you if you need to pre-register at the hospital. Finally, you will be told what time to be at the hospital or clinic the day of surgery.

There is very little that you need to do to get ready for surgery. While we can give you a general idea here of what to expect, your doctor will tell you what you should do. Follow his or her directions exactly, and if you have any questions, call the office.

Generally, you are asked not to take aspirin or aspirin-containing products (see Appendix C) for two weeks before and one week after surgery. If you take a blood thinner, your doctor may want you to discontinue using it for several days before surgery. Since smoking causes increased bleeding, quitting for two weeks prior to surgery is helpful. If you tend to bruise or bleed easily, tell your doctor. If you are diabetic, your physician will advise you as to whether or not you should take your insulin or pill the morning before surgery. Normally, you would take any heart or blood pressure medication as you usually do. Ask your doctor or the staff. Take just enough water to swallow the pill(s).

For some procedures, the surgeon will ask you to begin using an antibiotic eye drop the day before surgery. You may also be instructed to take some other drops, ointment, or pills. You will be given a prescription for these medications. Some offices prepare a kit which contains the appropriate medicines.

You may find that you have instructions to use one or two medications before surgery, but have prescriptions for three or four. The "extra" ones are for after surgery. Your doctor will tell you how to use them on your first visit after surgery.

The night before surgery you should bathe and wash your hair. Do not eat or drink anything (not even juice or coffee) after midnight, except enough water to swallow medications you usually take in the morning (see above).

You will need to arrange for someone to drive you home after surgery. It is also best not to spend the first night alone if you had general anesthesia or IV sedation.

"Prep"

The day of surgery, report to the hospital or clinic on time. Leave all jewelry and valuables at home. (You may need to leave dentures or partial plates at home, too. Ask your surgeon's staff.) Do not wear any face make-up. Wear comfortable clothing that opens down the front and not a pull-over (not even a pull-over undershirt).

Check in at the hospital out-patient or clinic desk. At this point you may be asked to show your insurance cards or other papers. Then take a seat and relax until you are called by an attendant. Before taking you to the pre-operative room, you will probably be asked to leave your glasses, wallet, etc., with the person who came with you.

At pre-op you will be prepared for surgery. You will be asked to put on a hospital gown. Leave it open in the back. An attendant will help you if you need assistance. Some hospitals require that you remove all clothing. Others allow you to remain dressed from the waist down. If you are allowed to keep your shoes on, the attendant will put paper shoe covers over them. A paper "shower cap" is put over your hair.

While you are changing clothes is a good time to empty your bladder. You may use the bathroom at any time, but once you have had the anesthetic to numb the eye you will have to use a bedpan.

Once you are "dressed," the hospital staff takes over. You will be asked to lie on a stretcher or bed. The nurse or technician who prepares you for surgery will ask you about your medications and any drug allergies. You will be asked when you last ate, and if you took any medication that morning.

An IV will be started. If you wish (and hospital policy permits), you can ask for a numbing injection in the back of your hand before the IV is put in. You will be given medicine through the IV to help you relax.

You will be monitored carefully throughout the surgery. Several sticky pads will be placed on your chest. These are to monitor your heart. A blood pressure cuff and perhaps a pulse rate monitor will also be used. Your temperature will probably be taken several times.

Eye drops may be placed in the eye periodically. Before starting the drops, the nurse will ask you which eye is having surgery. In fact, NEARLY EVERYONE YOU COME IN CONTACT WITH AT THE HOSPITAL WILL ASK WHICH EYE IS HAVING SURGERY, even your doctor. They are not asking because they don't know. (They have your chart right there to tell them.) Please don't be alarmed or impatient with the constant questioning. This is a system of double-checking time and again to be sure that the correct eye is treated.

You should be comfortable with a pillow and sheet provided. If you are cold, ask for a blanket. If you experience discomfort in your back or neck, or have trouble breathing while lying on your back, tell the nurse. Sometimes the head of the bed can be raised a little. A calm and comfortable patient is easier to care for, and the staff will do all they can to help you relax.

You may be moved to a special holding area at this point. The paper "shower cap" is taped to your forehead. Your blood pressure and pulse will be checked again. The heart monitor will be hooked up. You may hear its gentle beeping. A small mask for oxygen may be placed over your nose and mouth.

The eye and the area around it will be cleansed. You may be asleep if this is done right after the eye is deadened. If you are not asleep or numb, the cleansing solution may feel cold, wet, and drippy.

Anesthesia

Elimination and control of discomfort is important to both you and the doctor. If you are uncomfortable in any way, tell the doctor or staff. In addition to anesthesia, medication for pain can be given in the IV (if there is one), injection, or mouth. You may also be given a mild tranquilizer if you need something to help you relax.

In general, there are three types of anesthesia: topical, local, and general.

Some procedures require only topical anesthetic (numbing drops). The drop usually stings the first time it is put in. The numbing occurs in a few seconds, so you generally don't feel any other drops after that. More drops can be applied during the procedure if necessary.

Local anesthesia consists of an injection of numbing medication to deaden only the area being worked on. This is similar to deadening a tooth before dental work. You may feel a slight prick followed by a mild stinging sensation when the anesthetic is injected. This type of local injection is commonly used in plastic, reconstructive, and lid surgery.

Local anesthesia for major eye surgery is done a little differently. Many surgeons give medication in the IV so that you are asleep for a minute or two while the eye is deadened. This is nice, because then you don't feel the discomfort from the injection. You wake up a few minutes later, and are often unaware that you slept. This injection numbs the area and also temporarily paralyzes the eye so it cannot move during surgery. When you awaken, you are aware of your surroundings, voices, and faces...but you are very relaxed. Vision in the numbed eye is decreased, as well. You may detect motion and light, but you will *not* be able to see the doctor "working" on your eye. Procedures that are performed using this type of anesthesia may include cataract, glaucoma, corneal transplant, and muscle surgery.

General anesthesia (being "put to sleep") is not used very often during eye surgery. In cases of severe injury, or an enucleation (removal of an eye), the emotional impact of surgery may be high. In these and similar instances, the surgeon prefers to have the patient totally relaxed and asleep during the procedure. Otherwise, the side effects and potential risks of general anesthesia may not be worth it.

A person who is nervous about routine eye surgery can generally be calmed with IV medication, rather than using general anesthesia. Even when local anesthesia is used, however, many ophthalmologists order "anesthesia stand-by." This means that a procedure scheduled to use local anesthesia can be changed to general anesthesia during surgery, if the situation warrants.

Remember that any type of anesthesia or medication can have side effects and risks. Be sure and tell your surgeon or staff if you have ever had a past reaction to any type of anesthesia.

The Surgical Procedure

When the surgeon is ready, you will be wheeled into the operating room (OR) and transferred to the table. The heart monitor will be attached again, and you will hear it beeping. The people around you will have on masks, caps, and surgical clothing.

A piece of wide surgical tape may be place across your forehead and around the table. This is to help keep your head steady. Some hospitals strap the hands down to prevent accidents.

OR's are often chilly. If you are cold, tell someone and they will bring you a blanket.

A plastic drape (it's like the napkin that dentists use) is placed over your face. The drape has a hole in it, which is positioned over your eye. If you don't want your face covered, the drape may be taped up away from the face. Although you won't feel it, a small instrument is placed to keep the eyelids open. Periodically, a nurse will put a drop in the eye to keep it moist. You may be aware that there is a bright light overhead, but the numbed eye cannot see any detail.

The surgeon brings the microscope above your face, and the procedure begins. The room lights may be dimmed. You will hear the staff talking to each other, and sometimes to you. Many doctors play soothing music in the operating room. And, of course, the heart monitor beeps gently all the time.

When surgery is over, your doctor leaves the room. But you won't leave the operating room just yet. The drape will be removed from your face and your eye will be cleansed. Depending on what type of surgery you had, the eye may be patched. You will be transferred from the table to your stretcher and wheeled into the recovery room.

Claustrophobia

Some dilemmas have a small range of influence, but are intensely important to the folks they affect. "Several years ago I had a patient who needed cataract surgery to restore her vision," Dr. Gayton recalls, "but she refused to have it done. We found out that she was claustrophobic . . . afraid to have her face covered with the drape during the surgery." He devised a way to keep her face uncovered by taping the cover to the operating microscope. Other physicians have developed alternate ways to keep claustrophobic patients comfortable.

Recovery Room

After surgery, you will go to the recovery room for an hour or so. Your blood pressure, pulse, and temperature are checked again. The IV and heart monitor pads are removed, and you are helped to dress. You may be given juice and crackers. You receive an instruction sheet that tells you exactly how to use your medications. You will also be told what time to report to the doctor's office for your first post-operative visit. When you are ready to leave, you will be taken to the car by wheel chair. (Even though you feel great, hospitals are required to "wheel" you out.)

Postoperative Care

Once you arrive home, prop up your feet! You may still feel relaxed from the medications you were given. Bed rest with bathroom privileges are the order of the day. This means you will not be doing any lifting or straining for the first twenty four hours. Restrict eating to light, non-greasy food for the first twenty four hours. Take a nap. Consider yourself on holiday.

Follow your written instructions on using medications. In some cases you are not to remove the patch yourself.

Most people have very little, if any, pain after surgery. Some folks have a mild headache after the procedure. You might notice some numbness, coldness, or tingling of the face and scalp. This is from the anesthetic. If you have any discomfort, you may take a non-aspirin pain reliever. Some physicians give a prescription for a mild pain pill when you leave the hospital. If this doesn't help, call your physician. If you have severe pain, notify your physician at once.

Minor Surgery

"There's no such thing as *minor* surgery if they're working on *me*!" quipped one patient. The term "minor surgery" usually refers to procedures with a relatively low risk, requiring only topical or local anesthesia, and taking only a short period of time. Examples include laser treatments, removing a growth, and freezing eyelashes. A physical exam and lab work is not generally required for this type of surgery. There is usually no need to have an empty stomach beforehand. IVs are not used. Minor surgery is almost always done right in the office, often in the exam room. You can drive yourself home afterward, unless you feel queazy or were given medication to help you relax.

Ideally, eye surgery is something that is planned to correct a problem that has probably been going on for some time. In the next chapter, we'll look at the unexpected.

CHAPTER 16

Injury and First Aid

ELSIE Meeks had no intention of becoming an injury statistic that morning. What could be safer than doing laundry in her own home? She struggled a little to remove the cap of a new bottle of bleach. When the lid finally gave, it came off with a jerk and some bleach splashed in her left eye. She washed it out right away, but an hour later the eye still hurt.

"I'm taking you to the eye doctor," Mr. Meeks said firmly.

She returned from that visit with her eye patched. "I have a chemical burn from the bleach," she explained to a friend. "Next time, I'll be more careful."

An Ounce of Prevention . . .

The best defense against eye injury is protection. Safety glasses should be worn during any activity that produces small particles at high speeds (such as grinding or sanding). Many cases of blunt trauma (causing broken bones, black eye, retinal detachment, etc.) occur during sports activities, as do corneal abrasions. Safety goggles are even better than glasses for sports, because there is no hinge. If you weld or use a sun lamp (both generate ultraviolet light), be sure to protect your eyes properly. Safety glasses should also be worn when handling any type of chemical.

First Aid Kit

Your home first aid kit can be expanded to include items for eye emergencies. You should be able to find any of these articles at the drug store.

- sterile gauze or eye pads
- sterile irrigating solution—Ask your pharmacist to help you

with this. Irrigating solution is non-medicated and comes in a stream bottle. It is *not* the same as "eye wash."

- artificial tear drops
- artificial tear ointment
- tape
- eye shield—An eye shield is used to protect an injured eye from further harm. You can buy one from the pharmacy or your eye doctor, but you can also make it yourself. To make a shield with a paper cup, cut the cup down to size so that there is only a 3/4 to 1 inch rim left at the bottom. Or, you could make a cone from a light-weight piece of cardboard. Tape the shield over the eye. The edges of the shield should rest on the bones of the face around the eye, NOT on the eye itself.

Coping with Treatment

Anesthetic (Numbing) Drops

Numbing drops are often used after an injury to make you comfortable enough to endure examination and/or treatment. You would probably love to have a bottle to take home, but that would spell disaster. Used once or twice in the office, the drops are harmless. Used frequently, they can actually damage the eye by interfering with the healing process and breaking down the tissues of the cornea.

Eye Patch

Many injuries are treated by patching the eye shut. In medical circles we call this a pressure patch, and if you've ever been patched you understand the name! The pad is taped on tightly to keep the eye closed. If the eye is open under the patch, the cornea may get scratched by the pad. Plus, the inside of the lid creates an even surface for the cornea to rest against while it heals, encouraging a smooth corneal surface.

Having one eye covered will make you appreciate the benefits of having two. Two eyes are required for stereo vision. Thus your depth perception will probably be impaired with one eye covered. Drive only if you must, and then with great care. Be careful when reaching for hot items. Walk and climb stairs slowly.

Pupil Dilation

As you know, dilating drops are used to examine the inside of the eye. But in some cases of eye injury, dilating the pupils is part of the treatment. Dilating holds the pupil and focusing muscle still. This makes the eye more comfortable. (A similar example would be putting a sprained wrist in a sling to hold it still.)

The doctor may dilate your pupil once, while you are in the office. In other instances you may be asked to use a dilating drop at home, too. Wash your hands after using the drops.

The effects of being dilated include light sensitivity and blurred vision. Wearing sunglasses will help ease any discomfort from glare. Once the drops are stopped, the dilation will gradually wear off. How quickly depends on the type of drop used. Some dilating drops wear off in a few hours. Others may take a week to completely clear up.

Dilating drops come in a bottle with a red cap. When you are finished with them you may keep them in the medicine chest, but tape the cap on. This will remind you that they are not to be used without a doctor's order.

Stitches

Stitches in the skin should be kept dry. If eyelid stitches rub and irritate your eye, contact your doctor. You may be able to use some ointment in the eye to "grease it up" and stop the scratching. Sutures in the eye itself may also cause irritation that can be eased in the same way. If you think a suture has come out, contact the surgeon's office. Don't try to remove stitches yourself.

Black Eye

The black eye is actually a combination of injuries caused by a blunt blow to the eyelids and eye. The most obvious symptom is bruising and swelling of the lids.

First Aid

It is best to seek treatment right away. After an hour or two the lids may be too swollen for a good eye examination. Put a shield over the eye and head for the emergency room or doctor's office.

Tests

In addition to vision testing, you will be checked with the slit lamp microscope. A dilated exam will also be done to check for internal eye injury. Your eye pressure will be checked by tonometry. If the physician cannot see the back of the eye, a B-scan ultrasound may be required. Photographs, X-rays, and/or a CT scan might also be ordered. These special tests are described in Chapter 18.

Treatment

Cold compresses are used at first to help reduce swelling. Pain reliever is used to lessen discomfort.

Possible Complications

Broken bones, subconjunctival hemorrhage, hyphema, iritis, torn iris, retinal detachment, retinal hemorrhage, retinal tear, secondary glaucoma, dislocation of the lens, traumatic cataract.

Broken Bones

It may seem strange to be talking about broken bones and the eye. After all, there are no bones in the eye itself. But the eye is set in a skull of bone. The brow bone can be broken, but it is pretty tough. Blunt trauma to the eye more often crushes the delicate bones at the bottom of the orbit (bones surrounding the eye). This is called a "blow-out fracture." When this happens, it creates a hole in the floor of the orbit. The muscles at the bottom of the eye can herniate or push through this hole, then become trapped. The most common symptom is double vision, because the trapped muscle prevents the eye from moving properly.

First Aid

Protect the eye from further injury. *Do not* press on the eye with hand, cloth, etc. Apply a shield. See your eye doctor at once, or go to the emergency room.

Tests

Your physician will probably order a set of skull X-rays. You may also need a CT scan. A slit lamp microscope exam and a dilated exam will be done to be sure that the inner structures of the eye have not been damaged.

Treatment

Most blow-out fractures do not need to be treated surgically. The ophthalmologist will usually wait two weeks or so before deciding if surgery is necessary. This gives the swelling a chance to go down, and the eye an opportunity to recover on its own.

The thin bones at the bottom of the orbit are also part of the sinuses. Thus, infection might spread from the sinus into the orbit. Do not blow the nose forcefully, as this could push germs from the sinuses into the area surrounding the eye.

Surgery, when needed, involves freeing the muscle from the bony trap and placing a bone or plastic implant over the fracture.

Possible Complications

Bruising, infection, subconjunctival hemorrhage, hyphema, iritis, uveitis, retinal hemorrhage, traumatic cataract, secondary glaucoma, retinal detachment, double vision.

Bruises—Lids

Bruising of the lids may follow surgery or an injury.

Treatment

If you have had surgery, or have had medical treatment for an injury, follow your doctor's advice about applying cold packs to the area.

Possible Complications

A bruise in and of itself usually poses no threat to the eye. However, the *cause* of the bruise may have its own set of complications. Please see the specific category (such as lid laceration, plastic surgery, etc.) for more information.

Bruises—Conjunctival (Subconjunctival Hemorrhage)

A subconjunctival hemorrhage (SCH) is a bright blood-red area on the sclera (white of the eye). An SCH is caused by bleeding from tiny blood vessels in the conjunctiva (membrane lining the sclera and inner eye lids). It is comparable to a bruise elsewhere on the body. Although it can look quite alarming, there are no other symptoms, and it is not serious. The redness may spread for a day or two, then gradually fade with time. It can take a week or so for all the redness to clear away.

Several things can cause an SCH. Heavy lifting and straining (as in constipation or vomiting), or hard coughing and sneezing can result in a subconjunctival hemorrhage. In some cases, high blood pressure or some other blood disorder can trigger it. For this reason you should consult your doctor if you have repeated episodes of SCH. Taking blood thinners or aspirin also tends to contribute.

Rubbing the eye can cause a blood vessel to burst, as can many types of injury. It is not unusual to have such a bruise after eye surgery. An SCH can also just "happen" with no apparent cause.

First Aid

None.

Tests

In the absence of obvious injury, no tests except a vision test and examination with the microscope are usually needed. Blood pressure may be taken. In the case of repeated SCH's with no obvious cause, blood work may be ordered.

Treatment

There is no treatment. Eye drops to "get the red out" do not really help an SCH go away any faster. You may use artificial tears if you have a scratchy feeling in the eye.

Possible Complications

An SCH has no known complications.

Burns—Chemical (Chemical Conjunctivitis)

First Aid For Chemical Burns

With any chemical splash, the first thing to do is irrigate *IMME-DIATELY.* Use an irrigating solution from your first aid kit, if you have it. If not, use whatever is at hand. A water fountain is great. Or fill the sink and dunk your face, holding your eye open in the water. Or pour cupfuls of water over the eye. Don't waste time trying to come up with a special solution that will "neutralize" the chemical. Use water! Continue irrigating the eye for fifteen minutes. Then seek medical attention. Redness, swelling, pain, light sensitivity, and watering are common following any chemical burn.

Acids

Acid splashes cause painful surface burns. Battery acid is an example. Other industrial acids include sulfuric, hydrochloric, nitric, and acetic acid. The lids and cornea are the most often affected.

First Aid

Irrigate immediately as above.

Tests

Your eye will be examined with the slit lamp microscope. A numbing drop may be given for comfort.

Treatment

The eye will be irrigated again when you get to the emergency room or doctor's office. If the cornea is burned, ointment and an eye patch will probably be applied. Follow your doctor's advice as to removing the patch. You will probably be using ointment and/or eye drops at home. You may be given oral antibiotics. Be sure to keep follow-up appointments.

Possible Complications

Lid: infection, scarring, entropion, trichiasis.

Cornea: keratitis, recurrent corneal erosion, edema, scarring, iritis.

Bases (Alkalies)

Burns from a basic chemical (alkali) are more serious than burns from an acidic chemical. This is because alkaline substances penetrate into the tissues. This spells extra trouble when the eye is involved. In addition to a painful surface burn, the penetrating alkali can damage internal tissues and structures.

Examples of alkaline materials include lye, bleach, mortar, lime, plaster of Paris, ammonia, white wash, plaster, and cement.

First Aid

Irrigate immediately, as described above. Seek medical attention at once.

Tests

The pH (acid/base balance) of the eye may be checked periodically to determine if the base has been diluted. For this painless test, a small strip of test paper is touched to the edge of the eye. The paper will change color according to the chemical balance of the eye.

If there has been corneal scarring, the physician may request a B-scan ultrasound (see Chapter 18) to determine if the inside of the eye has been damaged.

Treatment

When you arrive at the doctor's office or emergency room, the eye will probably be irrigated again. In fact, because of the penetrating nature of alkalies, the eye will probably be irrigated off and on for several hours. In severe cases, a special irrigating contact lens may be used. This lens is actually more like an eye cup with a tube on it. The tubing is connected to a bag of solution so that the eye is being bathed constantly.

If any foreign material is in the eye, it will be gently rinsed away and/or removed. You may be given an anesthetic (numbing) drop for comfort. (This anesthetic cannot be used many times, however, since it slows healing.)

Home care after an alkali burn usually includes steroid drops, drops to dilate the pupil, and drops to keep down the internal eye pressure. Do not discontinue any drop unless told to do so by your physician. If you run out of drops, call your doctor's office for a refill (even on the weekend). Some specialists prescribe Vitamin C eye drops for alkali burns. Follow your doctor's advice.

If the cornea is slow to heal, a bandage contact lens may be used as a "bandage." Another option is to temporarily sew the eyelids together (partially or totally) in a surgical procedure called a tarsorrhaphy.

Possible Complications

Keratitis, conjunctivitis, corneal abrasion, corneal edema, corneal scar, recurrent corneal erosion, iritis, uveitis, secondary glaucoma, angle closure glaucoma, entropion, dry eye.

Burns—Radiation ("Flash burn")

Radiation burns from ultraviolet light cause painful raw spots on the cornea. Sources of UV burns include welding arc, sun lamp, and reflected sun (from water, sand, or snow). All of these can be prevented with UV filtering glasses.

Often the burn does not begin to be painful until 6–12 hours after it occurs. Then the eye begins to water and feel gritty. The discomfort generally worsens according to the severity of the burn. Light sensitivity and swelling also occur.

First Aid

Patch the eye and seek medical attention.

Tests

The eye will be examined with the slit lamp microscope. The eye will probably be numbed with an eye drop so the exam will be more comfortable. Fluoresceine dye (in eye drop form) is used to help the doctor see the raw places and evaluate the seriousness of the burn.

Treatment

The doctor will put antibiotic ointment (and perhaps a dilating drop) in the eye and patch it shut. Your eye should be closed under the patch. Follow the doctor's instructions about taking the patch off.

Your eye will probably still be numb when you leave the doctor's office. This will wear off within half an hour. Your best bet is to go home, take your favorite pain reliever, and lie down in a dark room. Numbing drops cannot be prescribed for home use because they sabotage the healing process and can actually cause further damage.

The surface of the cornea, which is damaged by UV burns, is the fastest healing tissue in the body. Often over-night patching is all that is necessary. In severe cases, several days of patching might be indicated.

Once the patch is removed, you may be asked to use antibiotic and/or steroid drops. Healing usually occurs over 24 to 48 hours. If the doctor dilated the pupil when you were patched, it may take several days for the dilation to wear off. Symptoms of dilation include blurred vision and light sensitivity.

Possible Complications

Infection, iritis, recurrent corneal erosion.

Burns—Thermal (Heat)

Heat burns to the eye and lid may come from many sources. Splattering grease, tobacco ash, molten metal, and curling irons are common causes.

First Aid

Gently cover the eye with sterile gauze or an eye pad (no pressure). Tape on a shield and seek medical help.

Tests

You will be examined with the slit lamp microscope. The eye will be numbed with a drop if you are uncomfortable. A drop of dye may be used to evaluate corneal damage.

Treatment

A burn to the lids is treated with antibiotic eye ointment. A patch may be used if the burn is deep.

A corneal burn is treated with ointment and an eye patch. If the eye remains closed under the patch, healing may take place over night. A more severe burn may require patching for several days. Once the patch is removed, you will be using antibiotic drops and/or ointment, and perhaps a steroid as well. Follow your doctor's instructions on their use. Be sure and keep follow-up appointments.

Possible Complications

Lids: infection, scarring, trichiasis, entropion.
Cornea: infection, scarring, recurrent corneal erosion.
Other: iritis, secondary glaucoma.

Cuts—Lids

The eyelids are the eyes' first line of defense. A blink may be all that saves the eyeball itself from becoming injured. A full-thickness cut of the eyelid obviously needs to be seen by an ophthalmologist. If you are unsure whether or not a partial-thickness cut needs treatment, you should seek a medical opinion.

Lid lacerations are best repaired during the first twenty four hours following the injury. After that time there may be too much swelling to be able to put in stitches.

First Aid

Minor cuts and abrasions should be gently cleansed and antibiotic eye ointment applied. (Since any ointment you put on the lids will almost certainly get into the eye, only ointment specifically for the eye should be used.)

For cuts that require medical attention, place sterile gauze or pads *gently* on the lid. Do NOT apply pressure on the eyeball. Tape a shield over the eye and seek medical help at once.

Tests

If the eyelid laceration is the only injury, special testing is not usually ordered. However, if the cut lid is part of a more extensive injury (such as a blow to the eye, etc.), the physician may request some tests in connection with those conditions.

Treatment

Cuts involving the lower lid are especially troublesome if the tear-draining system has been damaged. If not repaired, or if not repaired carefully, the tears will not be able to drain properly.

First, the area will be gently cleansed. Before stitching, a numbing injection is given.

You will be given instructions about using antibiotic ointment. Do not get the stitches wet. Keep your appointment for follow-up exams. If the stitches seem to rub the eye, use eye ointment to ease the discomfort. If symptoms of infection develop (redness, swelling, pain, discharge, fever), contact your physician at once.

Possible Complications

Bruising, infection, chronic watering, trichiasis, entropion, ectropion.

Cuts—Conjunctiva

The conjunctiva is the membrane that covers the sclera (white of the eye) and lines the inside of the eye lids. In this section we will talk about a laceration to the scleral conjunctiva.

First Aid

Place a sterile pad or gauze *gently* over the closed eye. Tape a shield in place. Seek medical attention.

Tests

If there is no other injury, a vision test and slit lamp microscope examination will probably be all you need.

Treatment

After examination, the area will be gently cleaned. If severe, stitches may be required. The eye may be patched. You will be instructed about how to use antibiotic eye ointment. If the stitches feel scratchy, use the ointment to ease the discomfort. Some discharge will likely occur for the first twenty four hours. Be sure to keep your follow-up appointments. Contact your doctor if symptoms of infection (redness, swelling, pain, discharge, fever) develop.

Possible Complications

Subconjunctival hemorrhage, infection.

Cuts—Cornea (Corneal Abrasion)

The cornea is the clear covering over the iris (colored part of the eye). It is protected by the tears and also by the blink reflex. A corneal abrasion does not go through the cornea, but occurs when the surface layer is scratched. This abraded area can be quite painful. There may be the sensation of a foreign body lodged under the upper lid which rubs the eye during blinking. There may also be light sensitivity, redness, and watering.

First Aid

Your first impression following an abrasion is that you have something in your eye. You may not be aware that the eye is actually scratched. Using artificial tears or an irrigating solution is fine, but it won't make an abrasion feel any better. (On the other hand, if the sensation *is* caused by a foreign body, you just might wash it out.) Cover the eye gently and see your doctor.

Tests

A numbing drop may be used for comfort, then the eye is examined with the slit lamp microscope. A special dye drop is used to help the doctor see the size, location, and depth of the scratch.

Treatment

Treatment usually includes applying some type of antibiotic and a patch to the injured eye. It is important that the eye remain closed under the patch. Pain may return when the numbing effect wears off. A numbing drop is never prescribed to use at home because it will prevent the abrasion from healing. Over the counter pain reliever will usually help ease the temporary discomfort.

The outer layer of the cornea regenerates very rapidly, and is often much improved after a 24-hour period of patching. Now and then a longer length of patching will be required. When the eye no longer needs to be patched, an antibiotic drop may be prescribed for further use.

Possible Complications

Infection, scarring, recurrent corneal erosion, iritis.

Cuts—Perforation of Eyeball

Perhaps the most serious injury we will discuss is a laceration of the eyeball itself. Symptoms may include decreased vision, bleeding, an ooze of brownish black tissue from the sclera, and/or an irregularly shaped pupil.

First Aid

Have the victim lie down. DO NOT attempt to remove any foreign body. DO NOT apply gauze or shield if they will touch an object protruding from the eye. If there is no foreign object, gently apply sterile gauze or pad to the closed eye. DO NOT apply pressure. Tape a shield over the gauze. Seek medical help at once (call an ambulance if necessary).

Tests

The tests needed will depend on how severe the injury is. If practical, a vision test and slit lamp microscope examination will be performed. Other possibilities (each described in Chapter 18) include: X-ray, CT scan, ultrasonic B-scan, ultrasonic A-scan, culture, MRI, photography.

Treatment

A perforated eyeball can be such a complicated injury that we can't discuss a specific treatment. Suffice it to say that you and your doctor are engaged in a serious battle for your eye. In general, whatever can be repaired will be repaired in surgery (probably under general anesthesia). You may have to stay in the hospital for a few days. You may be given a tetanus shot. The eye may be patched.

You will almost certainly be asked to take oral antibiotics. Be sure to take them all. Follow directions carefully regarding eye drops. Do not stop using any eye medication unless your doctor tells you to. If you run out of medication, call the doctor's office (even if it's over the weekend). Keep all of your follow-up appointments.

Possible Complications

Retinal detachment, hyphema, retinal hemorrhage, corneal edema, strabismus, traumatic cataract, dislocation of the lens, subconjunctival hemorrhage, secondary glaucoma, infection, iritis.

Foreign Body—Conjunctival

The eye's first response to a foreign body is to water. This is the natural defense system at work trying to wash the foreign material out of the eye. If a foreign body becomes lodged in the conjunctiva lining the eye lid, every blink will rub the material over the eye. A foreign body could also become stuck to the conjunctiva covering the sclera.

First Aid

Do NOT rub the eye. If tearing and irrigation do not wash the particle out, seek medical help. Do NOT try to pick out a foreign body yourself.

Tests

The eye will be examined with the slit lamp microscope. An anesthetic (numbing) drop will probably be used for comfort during the exam. The physician will most likely flip the upper lid to be sure nothing is stuck on the back of the lid.

Treatment

Once the eye is numbed with drops, the foreign body will be removed. In some cases the doctor may apply eye ointment then patch the eye shut. In most instances you will be using some eye drops at home. The numbing effect of the anesthetic wears off in 15–30 minutes, so you should go home and take your favorite over-the-counter pain reliever.

Possible Complications

Subconjunctival hemorrhage, infection.

Foreign Body—Corneal

A foreign body that lodges on the cornea is often stuck on the outer tissue layer. Every time you blink, the eyelid rubs over the material. The eye is usually red, watery, light sensitive, and uncomfortable. The symptoms may not start until several hours after the foreign body enters the eye.

First Aid

Do NOT rub your eye! You may use artificial tears or an irrigating solution to try to rinse the foreign material from the eye. If irritation continues, seek medical attention.

Tests

Your eye will be examined with the slit lamp microscope. A numbing drop is used for comfort. A drop of special dye may be used to help the doctor see the foreign body.

Treatment

Once the eye is numb, the foreign body is removed. If the material was metal, a rust ring may have developed. This must also be removed. Eye ointment is applied, and the eye is patched shut. Follow your doctor's instructions about removing the patch.

Pain may return when the numbing drops wear off (about 30 minutes). Take your favorite over-the-counter pain reliever as soon as you get home.

Even though the foreign body has been removed, the eye may still feel as if there is something in it. This is because there is a raw spot on the cornea at the site of the original particle. Any such abraded area gives the sensation of something being in the eye, because the lid rubs over the wound every time you blink.

Home treatment depends in part on the type of foreign body and where it came from. In all cases, you will probably be using antibiotic eye drops. Do not stop the drops until told to by your doctor. If the foreign body came from an organic source (plant or animal matter), an oral antibiotic may be prescribed as well. Take all the tablets until they are gone.

Possible Complications

Infection, corneal scar, recurrent corneal erosion, iritis.

Foreign Body—Intraocular (Internal)

It is possible for a high-velocity particle to actually penetrate into the eyeball, perhaps causing permanent damage. These are most often caused by flying metal from grinding or cutting. In some cases there are no extreme symptoms and the patient is unaware that a foreign body has penetrated the eye.

First Aid

Do NOT attempt to remove any foreign body that is projecting from the eye, or to patch such an injury. If there is no foreign body protruding from the eye, gently apply a patch and shield. Seek immediate medical attention.

Tests

First the eye will be examined with the slit lamp microscope. A dilated exam with an ophthalmoscope will also be necessary. In addition, a B-scan ultrasound and/or an A-scan ultrasound may be ordered. These scans help locate and measure a foreign body inside the eye. X-ray or CT scan is sometimes used as well.

Treatment

Often the only treatment is surgery to remove the foreign body. (However if the foreign particle is glass or plastic, it may be left alone in certain cases.) The procedure may be done under local or general anesthesia. After surgery, the eye will be patched.

Home treatment will include eye drops or ointments. These may be antibiotic, steroid, dilation, and/or pressure reducing medications. You may also be asked to take an oral antibiotic. Do not run out of any medications or stop them without your doctor's order. If you run out, call the office (even on the weekend).

Possible Complications

Infection, subconjunctival hemorrhage, traumatic cataract, secondary glaucoma, iritis, uveitis, corneal scarring, retinal hemorrhage, retinal detachment.

Complications of Injury

The following are mentioned as possible complications of injury, but are not discussed elsewhere in the book:

1. **dislocated lens**—The lens of the eye is held in place (behind the pupil) by delicate ligaments called zonules. If the zonules are torn by injury, the lens may become misaligned or even detached. The obvious symptom is blurred vision.

   If the lens is only mildly dislocated, a change in glasses prescription to correct the vision may be all that is needed. A lens that is totally detached may drift in front of the pupil or back into the vitreous. In this case, or if the lens is still attached but severely dislocated, surgery may be required to remove it. Extracting the lens creates the situation of aphakia. Please read Aphakia, Chapter 5, to learn about treatment options for this condition.

2. **hyphema**—Blood collects inside the eye in the area between the cornea and lens. The pooled blood can sometimes be seen at the bottom of the cornea in front of the iris. Occasionally the entire front of the eye is filled.

   The classic symptom is blurred vision (which may have a red tint), especially after lying down. Vision may clear somewhat after rising, as gravity pulls the blood down and away from the pupil.

   When a hyphema occurs with an injury, you will be examined frequently with the slit lamp microscope. A B-scan ultrasound may be done if the doctor needs immediate information about the inside of the eye. Circulating blood cells may clog the drainage system of the aqueous humor, causing a rise in the eye's internal pressure (secondary glaucoma). For that reason, your pressure will be checked with a tonometer at every exam.

   There is usually no medication recommended. You will, however, probably be asked to keep your head elevated when lying down and to avoid strenuous activity for a while. In rare cases hospitalization is required. The blood generally dissolves and clears away with time.

3. **infection**—Any time tissue has been cut or torn, an entryway for germs is created. Classic symptoms of infection include pain, swelling, redness, heat, and foul drainage at the infection site. There may also be fever and a general feeling of illness.

4. **recurrent corneal erosion** (recurrent erosion syndrome, spontaneous corneal ulceration)—This problem most often occurs in an eye that has had some previous corneal injury. It is often impossible to identify the original injury, since the erosion may start months or even years later. The symptoms include awakening with a painful red eye, and sensitivity to light. This is caused by the eye lid's becoming stuck to the cornea (which has dried during the night). When the eye is opened, the lid pulls off some of the cornea's outer layer. This gives the sensation of

having something in the eye. Treatment may include patching for 24 hours followed by use of an ointment at bedtime for several months to prevent further occurrences. It is important to continue the nightly ointment as directed.

The problem tends to recur if the surface of the cornea does not heal smoothly. It is actually these "rough" areas that are sticking to the eye lid and getting torn off, leaving a new raw spot.

Sometimes minor surgery is needed. The procedure is done in the office at the slit lamp microscope after numbing drops are applied. The heaped-up tissue is gently removed and the eye is patched tight. In most cases the cornea will heal smoothly after treatment.

Sometimes a soft contact lens may be prescribed as a protective bandage in severe cases.

Here is a list of other possible complications and where to read more about them:

- angle closure glaucoma (see Chapter 14)
- allergic and bacterial conjunctivitis (see Chapter 9)
- edema, corneal (see Chapter 10)
- scar, corneal (see Chapter 10)
- double vision (see *Strabismus*, Chapter 13)
- dry eyes (see Chapter 9)
- ectropion (see Chapter 8)
- entropion (see Chapter 8)
- iritis (see Chapter 12)
- ineffective keratitis (see Chapter 10)
- retinal detachment (see Chapter 12)
- hemorrhage, retinal (see Chapter 12)
- retinal tear (discussed under *Retinal detachment*, Chapter 12)
- secondary glaucoma (see Chapter 14)
- strabismus (see Chapter 13)
- traumatic cataract (discussed under *What causes cataracts?*, Chapter 11)
- trichiasis (see Chapter 8)
- uveitis (see Chapter 12)

As you've seen in this chapter, there's a lot you can do to protect your eyes. The next chapter will give you even more helpful hints that you can use at home to keep your eyes healthy.

CHAPTER 17

Home Eye Care and Ocular Miscellany

WILLARD Marks sat with his wife in the surgery counselling office. Mrs. Marks was scheduling cataract surgery. The nurse made everything sound so easy, talking casually about eye drops, ointments, pills, and eye patches. But Willard had his doubts. *How will I be able to care for her at home?* he wondered. Then he smiled to himself and relaxed. *I can look it all up in our eye book when I get home. No problems.*

Myths

We sometimes believe some amazing things. They used to say the earth was flat, and we'd never get to the moon. How do you measure up on eye care facts? Read on and find out. (We'll also talk about myths that apply to children so you will have accurate information for your family.)

"Reading in dim light will ruin your eyes." Actually, the brightness or dimness of light coming into the eye has no effect at all on the eye's health. Heredity plays the largest part in determining whether a person needs glasses or not. Reading in poor light is difficult, but it does not make your eyes worse.

"A child with crossed eyes will probably outgrow the problem." The fact is, crossed eyes should always be checked out as soon as the problem is noticed. A crossed eye may become lazy, and not develop full vision. In addition, an eye that is crossed due to a muscle imbalance will not be outgrown. (This myth arose because an optical illusion, created by the structure of a child's face, can make it look as though an eye is crossed. As the child grows and the facial structure "stretches out," the optical illusion fades. It appears as if the child has outgrown a crossed eye.)

"It's harmful for a child to sit too close to the television." Most children love to sit close to the TV. It won't hurt them, but why do they do it? Getting closer makes the picture larger, and they feel like they're "inside" what's happening on the screen. Unlike adults, kids can focus up close without straining. True, some children sit close because they are nearsighted. But this can be corrected with glasses, and is NOT caused by the TV.

"If a child crosses his eyes, they will stick." Simply untrue.

"A cataract has to be ripe before it can be removed." With modern surgical methods, a cataract can be removed when the patient is ready . . . usually when he or she feels handicapped by failing vision. (see Chapter 11 for full details on cataracts and cataract surgery.)

"Not wearing the right glasses will damage the eyes." Wearing glasses actually has nothing to do with the health of your eyes. They simply help you see better. A lens changes the way light is focused. It does not change the eye.

"Eating carrots is good for your eyesight." Carrots are rich in Vitamin A. One of the symptoms of Vitamin A deficiency is night blindness. (see *Malnutrition,* Chapter 7.) So it would make sense that extra Vitamin A would improve sight. But it doesn't work that way. Not enough is bad, but more than enough doesn't give extra help.

"If you're not having problems, an annual eye exam is a waste of time and money." After age forty the incidence of glaucoma (see Chapter 14) and other eye diseases increases. Reading vision also gradually decreases from age forty to about sixty (presbyopia), necessitating periodic glasses changes. Vision can decrease so gradually that you're not aware of the loss. And there is no way you can tell if you have increased eye pressure (glaucoma) without being measured. In diabetes and high blood pressure, an annual dilated exam is essential to be sure no retinal problems are occurring. It's great if you're not noticing any problems. But you really need an eye exam to prove that all's well.

"People over age 60 don't need to be dilated." This rumor originated from the fact that dilation is used in young people to keep them from focusing. This is not necessary in older adults who have no capacity to focus. However, dilation is also used to hold the pupil open for retinal examination, an essential test at every age.

Eye Medications

Eye drops or ointments might be necessary for a variety of reasons. Here we'll discuss several groups of medications and guidelines for their use.

- Glaucoma: It is extremely important to follow dosage instructions when treating glaucoma. Using the drop, pill, or ointment at the specified time each day should become a habit. Forgetting a dose, or even being a few hours late, can cause the eye pressure to go up to an undesirable level. Use your medicine right on time even (especially) if you are coming in for a check-up that day.
- Antibiotics: It is important to continue using these drops until told to stop. Your symptoms may clear up and yet the infection may still be present, ready to flare up if treatment is discontinued before the germs are totally "knocked out." Don't be fooled into thinking if one drop is good, two are better. Use as prescribed!
- Steroids: They have received some bad publicity, but for the brief period usually used in treating the eye, these side effects are kept to a minimum. In using steroids it is very important that they be used only by the person for whom they were prescribed. So even if another family member develops symptoms similar to yours, they should not start using your drops! Some eye infections are made much worse by steroids, so a doctor's watchful care is necessary.
- Dilating drops: In some cases you may have to use dilating drops at home. These drops all have a red cap. The purpose of dilating is to hold the pupil still (for comfort and healing). They do not "cure" anything. Don't let anyone else use them.
- Lubricants: Dry eyes may require use of artificial tear drops frequently throughout the day. You may use them as often as necessary to make your eyes feel comfortable. (They are non-medicated and frequent use is safe.) Artificial tear ointment is usually used before going to bed at night because it blurs the vision.
- Topical anesthetic: Numbing drops are never prescribed. Although they would lessen the pain, they interfere with the healing process and can cause trouble. Rest assured that the

dose you receive for an office procedure is not harmful, but it should never be used routinely at home.

Side Effects of Eye Medications

Any medication you take can cause side effects or allergic reactions, including eye medication. Here are several you should know about.

Glaucoma

(We present a few notes here. For more detailed information, see Appendix A.)

Timoptic™ and Betagan™ occasionally cause headache, nausea, dizziness, breathing disturbances, and slowed heart rate.

Propine™ may slightly dilate the pupil, sting, cause redness, or fast heart rate.

Pilocarpine and carbachol may cause headache, decreased vision in dim light, increased blood pressure, and nausea or vomiting. Phospholine Iodide™ may also cause the same side effects, but has an additional caution as well. If you are to receive general anesthesia (be put to sleep) for any reason, you MUST notify your doctor that you are using Phospholine Iodide.

Antibiotics

These may cause an allergic reaction including rash and swelling. They may also sting when you put them in. Long term use of any one type may cause a bacteria to develop that is immune to that particular antibiotic.

Steroids

Steroids may cause elevated internal eye pressure (glaucoma) with long term use. This usually clears up once the medication is stopped. Cataracts may also develop after a long period.

Dilating Drops

May cause light sensitivity and/or blurred vision. May sting.

Lubricants

The only reaction caused by these non-medicated drops would be rash or swelling due to an allergy to a preservative or other ingredient. Unpreserved preparations are available.

Home Care

How to Give Eye Medications

The first step is always to wash your hands.

The patient is sitting or lying down comfortably with both eyes open. Ask the patient to look up. Gently pull down the lower lid. Hold the dropper close, but do not touch the eye, lid, or lashes. Dispense the drop into the pocket created by pulling the lid down.

There are several reasons why this method works so well. First, it is hard to open one eye and close the other . . . so having both eyes open relaxes the lids. Next, it is difficult to close the eyes while looking up (try it), so your patient is less likely to squeeze. Putting the drop in the pocket of the lower lid is more comfortable than having it splash on the cornea (clear front of the eye). Finally, if the patient is looking up and you happen to accidentally bump the eye with the dropper, the sclera (white of the eye) takes the blow . . . not the sensitive cornea.

Ointment is instilled in the same way. A ribbon of ointment is placed into the pocket. Don't touch the tip of the tube to the eye, lashes, or lids. The patient should then gently close both eyes (no squeezing) for a few minutes to give the ointment a chance to melt. Another method is to put the ointment on a sterile cotton swab, then gently wipe it into the pocket.

You can give yourself drops or ointments by using a similar method. Look into the mirror and pull the lid down. Put the drop or ointment into the pocket.

If the patient has difficulty opening the eyes, here's another method of giving drops. The patient lies down and gently closes both eyes. The drop is placed in the inner corner of the closed eye. Then the patient opens both eyes (or you may gently separate the lids with your fingers), allowing the drop to run in. This method also works well if you must give drops to yourself.

When treating yourself it is sometimes difficult to tell whether or not you've gotten the drop in the eye. If you keep your drops in the refrigerator, you can tell by the coolness whether or not you hit the mark.

Any medication used in the eye has the potential to affect the entire body. This is because tears drain out of the eye and eventually enter the blood stream. Two problems result. First, it creates the possibility to experience bodily side effects from eye medications. Second, if the drop is drained off the eye, it is carried away from the place where it is needed.

A very simple procedure can reduce side effects and increase eye treatment. After the drops are instilled, close the eye and gently place your forefinger against the inside corner of the eye. Keep gentle pressure in the area for several minutes. This prevents the drops from going "down the tubes." (Ointment melts slowly, so there is no need for this maneuver.)

We are often asked how close together you should use different eye drops. Waiting thirty minutes between doses is great. If that is impossible, try to wait for at least five minutes.

After using or giving an eye medication, you should wash your hands again.

How to Make A Warm Compress

Warm compresses are recommended for several eye problems. Always use a clean washcloth. Soak it in water as warm as you can stand. Do NOT make it so hot that it burns. Wring it out, then apply to the area. When it cools, reheat it again with hot water.

You can heat the cloth in the microwave. Wet and wring the cloth, then microwave it for about 15–30 seconds. (Microwave ovens vary, so you may need to adjust the time.) Be sure to test it before you place it on your skin.

You can buy a hot-pack at the drugstore. Some are used once then discarded. Others are reusable. Follow directions carefully. Never wet an electric heating pad to create "moist heat."

How to Make An Ice Pack

A plastic bag with a sealing-type closure is great. Crushed ice will be moldable to the shape of your face, but you can use ice cubes, too. Wrap the bag with a clean cloth. (A damp cloth will transmit the cold better.) Follow your doctor's directions about how long and how often to apply.

Your drug-store probably has re-usable ice packs. These are filled with gel, so are easy to mold to the area. You just chill it in your freezer.

How to Patch the Eye

If you need to patch an injured eye before seeing the doctor, please first read about the injury in Chapter 12. Some injuries should be patched lightly, others not at all.

If your eye doctor has told you to patch the eye at home, here's how. First, you will need sterile gauze or eye pads, and tape. You can get these from the drug store. (Paper tape is nice, but sometimes doesn't stick too well. Get hypo-allergenic plastic tape.) Next, instill any medications in the eye if you've been told to do so. Then have the patient close *both* eyes. Fold one pad in half and place it over the eye. Cover it with another, unfolded, pad. Tape the pads on with 5 to 6 inch strips of tape. (It usually takes five or six pieces.) The tape should run diagonally from the forehead, over the pads, across the cheek, and toward the jaw line. Don't tape into the scalp or near the mouth.

The main goal in patching is to keep the eye shut. (That's why we use two pads.) If the eye opens under the patch, you need to try again and patch tighter.

How to Tape the Eye Shut

If the eyelid does not close completely, you may be told to tape the eye shut at night. Use a four-inch strip of hypo-allergenic plastic tape. Have the patient close both eyes. Place the top edge of the tape at the crease of the upper lid. Smooth the tape down to the edge of the lid. Then gently pull the upper lid and tape down so that the lids meet. Now smooth the tape on down the cheek.

Caring for Someone Who has had Eye Surgery (Even If it's You!)

Details on any one type of surgery are covered in separate sections, so check the Contents or Index. Before the patient is released from the hospital or office, someone will give you verbal and written instructions about home care. Here we will give some basic instructions that apply to most cases. *But always follow your doctor's directions.*

The patient is often on bed-rest the day of surgery. This means it is okay to get up to go to the bathroom. If the doctor consents, the patient may be allowed to sit up and watch TV.

Make the first meal after surgery a light one. Soup and crackers are the order of the day, not steak or barbecue! Avoid alcohol since it might interact with medication. If nausea and/or vomiting occur after eye surgery, you should call the doctor's office.

Some discomfort is probably normal. Take a non-aspirin over-the-counter pain medication. If there is pain that does not go away or seems unbearable, call the doctor. (Some physicians send you home with a prescription for pain medication.)

It is normal for a wound to ooze a little during the first 24 hours. If bleeding seems excessive, notify the surgeon. Keep sutures dry.

Follow the doctor's instructions about changing dressings and applying medication. In some cases you will be told not to disturb the patch. In other cases, there is no patch. Medications may be started that same day, or the next. If you have any questions, call.

Don't drive or operate machinery on the day of surgery. Anesthesia or other medication can impair judgement.

Home Remedies

If home is where the heart is, it may also be where the healing is. There are several things you can do at home to ease common eye complaints. (If you have an injury, please check Chapter 12 for *first aid*.)

- cold compress to relieve itch of allergy
- cool wet compress to ease redness
- cool compress or ice to relieve puffiness
- specially treated sunglasses that screen out ultraviolet light exposure (lower your risk of cataracts, pterygium, corneal disease, macular degeneration)
- quit smoking to decrease the progression of cataracts, macular degeneration, and diabetic disease
- exercise (such as brisk walk) may lower eye pressure in glaucoma
- tea bags for sunburned lids. . . soak in cool water, then apply to decrease swelling and help relieve pain
- cucumber slices placed on closed lids helps to cool an itch
- a warm cloth may help unclog glands and increase lubrication for dry eyes
- eliminating allergy-causing items from the house (dust, animal dander, etc.) may decrease dark circles under the eyes caused by allergies. Food allergies (such as wheat, milk, or chocolate) may also contribute.

- warm compresses applied to a stye or chalazion may help it to come to a head and drain, or shrink in size
- focus on something at a distance (at least twenty feet away) for a minute or two after every 30 minutes of near work to help relax the eyes (this works much better than closing them)

Nutrition

Malnutrition can have a profound affect on the eyes. (See Chapter 7 for more details.) Your best defense against diet-related eye problems is to eat well-rounded meals.

Certain vitamins have been identified that especially contribute to eye health:

- Vitamin E (wheat germ, sunflower seeds, almonds, cod-liver oil, salmon) to slow down cataracts and improve retinal health
- Vitamin C (fresh orange juice, broccoli, spinach, grapefruit, strawberries, other fruit) also may help retard cataracts and improve retinal health
- Vitamin A (carrots, squash, pumpkin, brussel sprouts) is helpful in slowing macular degeneration, optimizing night vision, and relieving extreme dry eyes
- Zinc (meat, especially red meat) to improve retinal health

There are several commercially available vitamin tablets that have been specifically formulated to supply nutrients needed for eye health. These include Ocuvite™ (Storz Ophthalmics), ICaps™ (LeHaye), and Ocucaps™ (AKorn). Other companies make similar "eye vitamins." If you already take a multiple vitamin, it's easy to add enough supplements to equal the amount recommended for the eyes. Take your vitamin bottle to the pharmacy with you. Check the amount of the vitamin or mineral you wish to increase, and choose a supplement that will make up the difference. Do NOT exceed suggested amounts. Ask your pharmacist if you need help.

Travel Advice

To help your eyes perform at peak capacity, here are some tips on eye care while traveling.

Your plans for visual comfort should begin before you ever leave home. Have an eye exam to be sure your vision is up to par. Since lost or broken glasses (or contact lenses) can ruin a vacation, obtain a copy of your prescription to take with you on your trip so they can be replaced. A spare pair would be even better. You should also have a written prescription for any eye drops or other eye medications you use routinely, just in case a refill becomes necessary. For safety's sake, contact lens wearers should carry a note to that effect. In the even of emergency hospitalization, the medical staff will then be warned to remove the lenses.

Driving is the most important visual activity you will have on a trip. To reduce the glare, be sure the windshield is clean and the wipers are in good shape. Sunglasses that screen out ultraviolet rays are recommended, but be sure to take them off at dusk. Turning on your headlights at dawn and dusk increases your visibility to other drivers.

A change in scene may be accompanied by eye irritation. A dryer climate or smog may cause tearing, itching, burning, or redness. Swimming is another possible culprit causing eye discomfort. An over-the-counter artificial tear drop may give relief, but if symptoms of an infection occur (such as a discharge), you should seek professional help.

Giving in to the vacation temptation to wear your contact lenses longer than normal may produce a serious problem. Intense discomfort is the main symptom of over-wear, and your cue to find a doctor to help. Over exposure to the sun or a sun lamp is likewise very painful and necessitates medical care. Remember that light reflects off of water and sand, and limit exposure time sensibly.

Many vacation sports have potential eye hazards. Simply wearing protective glasses or goggles can greatly reduce the risk of eye injuries while playing tennis, biking, boating, etc.

Probably one of the most common accidents is simply getting something in the eye. If normal tearing or gentle irrigation does not wash out the foreign material, it will have to be removed by a doctor. If the foreign material was a chemical (bug spray, gasoline, etc.), the situation is much more urgent. Immediate flushing with water must be started, even before seeking help. This cannot be over stressed. Obviously, wearing glasses for protection, plus careful handling of chemicals, are worthy safeguards when it comes to preventing accidents.

If you should need medical attention for your eyes while traveling, simply look in the yellow pages under Optometrist or Physicians-Ophthalmologists.

Prosthesis

"Fitting a prostheses is . . . an art form," says one professional fitter. "The size and shape is important to me. But the most important thing to the patient is to have the artificial eye look like a natural eye. It's obvious that the iris [colored part of the eye] must be matched to the other eye. But most people don't realize that there are different shades of white. Also, some eyes have more visible blood vessels than others. Everything needs to match. The highest compliment I get is when someone I fit with a prosthesis comes back to my office and tells me that other people can't tell which eye is artificial."

Having an eye removed (or enucleated) is a traumatic experience. It may become necessary due to severe injury, malignancy, or a severely painful blind eye. There is no such thing as an "eye transplant." A false eye (prosthesis) is fit later to restore you to normal appearance, but it cannot restore your sight. It is normal and healthy to go through a grieving process over losing your eye. It may be wise to find a professional counselor to help you.

Enucleation surgery is done in the hospital under general anesthesia. Once the eye is removed, a round plastic implant is put in its place and the tissue is sewn closed over it. A removable plastic shell called a *conformer* is placed under the lids to help the tissues heal without caving in, so that a prosthesis can be fit later. A pressure patch is used for 1–2 days to help keep down swelling. It is normal to have a mucous discharge after surgery.

If over-the-counter pain reliever is not effective enough, your surgeon will probably prescribe something for you. The eye will be patched for 1–3 days. You will be taking antibiotics by mouth. Be sure and take them until they are gone. Follow your doctor's directions for eye drops and/or ointments.

The area beneath the lids is called the *socket*. When you pull your lids apart you will see reddish-pink tissue. This is actually the conjunctiva (membrane that covered the white of the eye). It looks similar to the tissue on the inside of your eye lid. Some of the redness will decrease as the socket heals.

When you first examine the socket after surgery, you will see the clear plastic conformer over the conjunctiva. If the conformer happens to come out and you are unable to slip it back into place, call the doctor's office. (This might be frightening to you, but it is not an emergency, or even that unusual.) Someone at the office will be able to replace it for you in a matter of seconds.

You should gradually get better. If tenderness, redness, or swelling increase, contact your physician.

About one month after surgery, you will probably be healed enough to get a temporary prosthesis. This is not the final, custom-made product, but will look more normal than a patch and allow you to begin to resume your normal life. The way your lids and socket respond to the temporary device will help the ocularist (or whoever fits you) know what details to choose for the final fit.

The modern prosthesis is made of plastic, not glass. The most common type of prosthesis is the reform prosthesis. (Another type of prosthesis, called a scleral shell, is sometimes used to hide a disfigured eye.) The base of the reform prosthesis is white plastic. A colored iris is painted on. The front of the device is covered with clear plastic. This clear over-lay has "blood vessels" imbedded in it, and is thicker in the center. Thus the reform prosthesis has a three dimensional quality. The color of white, the number and color of blood vessels, the color of the iris, and the size of the pupil are carefully chosen to match the other eye as closely as possible.

There is more than one way to fit a prosthesis. The method chosen depends on the ocularist and the condition of the socket. The ability of the lower lid to support the weight of the prosthesis, plus the anatomical shape of the bones and tissues all affect the end result.

The first element in custom prosthesis fitting is documentation. The ocularist will make notes, sketches, and photographs. Then an impression is made of the socket. One method uses dental wax, and the other dental silicone impression material. If wax is used, the ocularist "sculpts" the wax by hand to the proper shape. A silicone impression gives a "negative" of the socket contour, and no further shaping is needed. The socket is rinsed gently with saline (salt) solution before and after the impression. No anesthetic is needed.

The ocularist will show you how to insert and remove the prosthesis. Always wash your hands before handling it. While the plastic is not likely to break, it can chip or be scratched. If you remove it over a sink, line the sink with a towel.

There are commercial solutions available for lubricating the prosthesis before insertion. Artificial tear drops, saline solution, or hard contact lens conditioner can be used instead. If you must wipe the prosthesis while wearing it, wipe inward toward the nose. Wiping outward might displace or rotate the prosthesis.

Follow your ocularist's or doctor's instructions about removing the prosthesis. It is usually not necessary to remove it every day. If you leave the prosthesis in, you might clean its surface with saline and a cotton swab.

Deposits can form on the prosthesis and irritate the socket and/or lids. (You can actually have an allergic reaction to the deposits!) When you remove the prosthesis, you can clean it with contact lens cleaner, baby shampoo, mild soap, toothpaste, or denture cleaner. Rinse well before reinserting to avoid irritating the socket. Don't use alcohol because it ruins the plastic.

Always remove a prosthesis if it is causing discomfort. If cleaning and re-insertion does not relieve the problem, take the device back out and give yourself a break. If the socket continues to be uncomfortable even without the prosthesis, try hot packs for several days. If discomfort persists after that, consult your physician. Of course if the pain is severe, or you develop redness, swelling, and/or increased discharge, notify your doctor at once.

Over a period of time, the back side of the prosthesis develops fine scratches. This can irritate the tissue underneath. Have the prosthesis polished by your ocularist every 6 to 18 months as directed. He/she will also check the fit. Sometimes, as the years pass, the tissues and bone structure of the socket change. It is possible that a refit could eventually become necessary. The prosthesis itself has a life of three to seven years before needing replacement.

Coping with Loss of Vision in One Eye

Losing the vision in one eye is traumatic, and you will go through a grieving period. If you seem to have trouble making the emotional adjustments, seek the help of a professional counselor. But take heart: physically, you will learn to cope. Your brain must also adjust to being one-eyed. Be patient with yourself. All of these adaptations take time. Driving and most other activities are still possible with only one eye, as long as the vision in the remaining eye is at the legal level. (see Table 17-1 for helpful hints.)

It does not take two eyes in order to have depth perception, but you will have to learn how to judge distances all over again. Experience is on your side here. For example, you know that something in the distance appears smaller than something up close. Distant objects are gray and hazy rather than in color. Parallel lines (such as a railroad track) appear to get closer together the farther away they get. If two objects are in line but one is closer, the closer object will appear to move if you move your head to one side. (This is called parallax.) The size of familiar objects, overlapping, and shadows are other clues.

Depth perception can be developed with practice. However, a person with one eye does not have stereo vision (stereopsis), which is different from (but often confused with) depth perception. Stereopsis requires two eyes that see the same object at the same time from slightly different angles. Thus 3-D (3 dimensional) glasses, ViewMaster™ toys, and stereopticons don't work with one eye.

Your peripheral vision is decreased on the side of the blind eye. You will need to learn to turn your head to get a full view on your blind side. You should have mirrors on BOTH sides of your car.

Since you are now dependent on only one eye, you need to do everything possible to protect it. It is advisable to wear glasses with safety lenses *at all times*, even if they are not required for vision. *Always* wear safety glasses when handling chemicals, playing sports, or working around flying particles. Have an annual check up even if nothing seems wrong.

Low Vision

The term "low vision" encompasses a broad range of visual perception. In determining the level of disability, vision is measured on the standard eye chart with the best correction available. Following is a summary of vision loss and corresponding abilities:

- Normal vision is 20/15 to 20/30. With vision in this range there is no visual impairment. The person is able to function normally.
- Borderline vision loss falls between 20/40 and 20/70. The driving license is lost. Otherwise the person can get around

Table 17-1 Hints for Coping with One Eye.

Activity	Hint
Driving	• Allow more distance from the car ahead • Turn your head frequently to your blind side • Install mirrors on both sides of car • If a car along side is travelling at the same speed as you, slow down or speed up a little before judging its distance • Ask your passenger to help you judge clearance • Use caution when parking: avoid tight spaces • Use your headlights when parking in a garage: the light bounces off the wall and tells you how close you are
Walking	• Watch out for steps: you'll have a tendency to misjudge heights, especially on the last step. Be especially wary of curbs! • Turn your head frequently to your blind side, especially before turning or crossing the street
Around the house	• When reaching for an object, move your hand slowly in a direct line toward the object (be especially careful when reaching for hot drinks) • Be patient: allow extra time for detailed hobby work • Rapid head-shaking ("no-no") can simulate binocular vision and help in judging distances to close-up items • Use a needle threader • Get a range finder for your camera • Use measuring devices instead of estimating

(continued)

Table 17-1 (continued)

Activity	Hint
Sports	• Wear eye protection • Be patient: you are learning new visual skills • You will have to concentrate hard and put in more effort than before • Move a little to the side if the ball is coming straight at you (this gives you an angle and heps you judge its approach) • For shooting, you may have to switch your stace • Use a gun with an offset stock • Choose firearms that do NOT eject shells across your face • Invest in a range finder for golfing, hunting, and fishing
Social life	• To shake hands, move your hand slowly and directly toward the other person's hand; don't stop until you connect • When pouring drinks, touch the bottle or pitcher to the cup before pouring • When dining out, place your guest on your "eye side" • When dining out, beware of waiters approaching from your blind side

and function fairly well. This is a frustrating area, because the patient feels that if the glasses were just strengthened a little more, he/she would be able to see.

- Moderate low vision is from 20/80 to 20/200. The person is unable to drive, and may lose his/her job, but is still able to care for him/herself.
- Severe low vision is 20/200 to 20/400. He/she may be able to work with the help of the proper low vision aids. Traveling alone is still possible.
- Moderate blindness is vision of 20/500. Low vision aids offer limited improvement in this category. The patient may need training to learn how to get around independently.
- Severe blindness is 20/2000 or less. The patient cannot per-

form any visual functions. Non-optical aids and Braille are necessary.

Classification as being "legally blind" begins when the vision is 20/200 in the best eye. One is also legally blind if the peripheral (side) vision has closed in significantly. The "blindness" category starts at 20/500. Both of these categories are eligible for government assistance and benefits.

Vision loss can be difficult to deal with, whether it is sudden or gradual. It is normal and healthy to go through the process of grieving: denial, anger, sadness, depression, and finally acceptance. Each person's grief process is unique. Some people may adjust more quickly than others. Give yourself time. Consult professional help if you seem stuck in any one stage or need someone to talk to. Adaptation to vision loss, including learning to use visual aids, is much easier once the acceptance stage is reached.

Low Vision Aids

Seventy-five percent of those seeking low vision aids are age 65 or older. Half of all cases are due to macular degeneration. Rehabilitation of low vision depends on the cause of the loss of sight. Low vision can take several forms: the entire general vision is blurry, the central vision is blurred but the side vision is normal, there is a central blind spot, or the central vision is normal but the side vision is cut off.

A full eye exam, including a refraction is the first step in assessing what devices or adaptations may help. Your eye doctor may be skilled in prescribing low vision aids, or you may be referred to someone else. A retinal ophthalmologist often has these services available.

At the beginning of the selection process, it is important to discuss your goals with the doctor or assistant. What type of visual activities do you need or want to perform? Bring a sample of the material you hope to be able to see. How much of an improvement do you expect from a low vision aid? Having realistic expectations will help you adapt to using an aid, plus avoid disappointment. The professional who is helping you will do his/her best to suggest low vision aids that will meet your specific needs.

Another job of the low vision aid specialist is to teach you how to use the equipment. Many offices have a loan program so you can try a particular aid for a few weeks before deciding to purchase it.

Here is a brief run-down of various types of low vision aids, when they are prescribed, and what they can do.

Magnifiers: A magnifying glass may be of great help for those with macular problems, central blind spot, or central blur. They don't tend to be as useful in cases of overall haze. You must learn the best distance to hold the glass from the page. You may have to position the eye 1–2 inches above the reading material. The reading surface needs to be flat. (A clip board or reading stand works very well.) The larger the magnifying glass, the weaker the power. Thus the small magnifying glasses are the strongest.

- hand magnifiers-These are inexpensive and portable. Some have lights in the handles. A lot can be done with a simple flashlight and magnifying glass: identifying money, reading a menu, reading prices.
- stand magnifiers-The stand must be held flat on the page and the eye is placed close to stand. Some are illuminated.
- head-born devices-This category includes high-powered reading glasses, headbands, and loupes (similar to what a jeweler uses). They can be somewhat awkward, but are nice because they leave the hands free.

Telescopes: Telescopes magnify distant objects. They generally do not help those with severely restricted side vision.

The user needs steady hands for hand-held models, so those with a tremor or palsy may not be able to use them. Things "swim" when you move the eye or scope rapidly, so you must learn to move the scope slowly. Because of the magnification, things seem closer than they really are. The stronger the magnification, the smaller the area seen. Telescopes can be custom ordered, but this is expensive.

- clip-on—This type of telescope fits over your regular glasses, usually for one eye. They are inexpensive and can be focused.
- sportscope-This telescope has temples like glasses, and can be fitted for both eyes. They can be focused, but are cumbersome.

- hand-held—This portable type of telescope is merely held up to the eye.
- ring—The ring telescope is a convenient, smaller version of the hand-held model. It has a ring on it that you slip on your finger, thus the instrument is concealed in your hand. You just hold it up to your eye when you want to use it.

Closed circuit television (CCTV): This expensive system magnifies close work and projects it onto a TV screen. Contrast and brightness can be adjusted. You can switch to a "negative" image so that the letters are projected as white on black. CCTV is usually used for work or school.

Non-Optical Aids

- illumination– Most people with low vision can benefit from increased lighting. High illumination increases the contrast of light and dark, making it easier to see. Special lamps are available, or you might try a regular lamp with a 60 watt bulb. Keep the light in front of you, rather than to the side or over your shoulder.
- reduce glare—Those with generally blurred vision, central blur, or decreased side vision may have better vision if glare is reduced. This can be accomplished with tint, photogray, polaroid, or colored lenses, or anti-reflective coating.
- pinhole glasses—The opaque lenses of these glasses are full of tiny holes. They reduce scattered light rays and admit the straight-on rays that give best vision. (You need extra light to use them.)
- large print—Many people with reduced vision can benefit from large print. Books, games (such as cards and Bingo), magazines, music, phone dials, and many other items are available in large print.
- reading rectangle—This is a black card with a rectangular window. It blocks off all but a few lines of type, making it easier to keep your place when reading.
- writing aids—A writing guide is similar to a reading rectangle or a ruler. You simply write within the window or above the ridge. A check template is a check-size sheet of plastic with windows that indicate the placement of lines you must fill in. Templates can be made for other forms as well.

- talking books—Many books are available on cassette tape. Check with your local library. (See also the organizations listed at the end of Chapter 20.)

Your eye care professional can give you more information on how to care for your eyes in special circumstances. But sometimes it's not easy to diagnose a problem that needs care. In those cases, the doctor may order special tests beyond those done in a routine exam. Learn about them in the next chapter.

CHAPTER 18

Special Tests

RACHEL Hannah frowned at the papers in her hand. Scheduling cataract surgery had been easy, but the doctor had also ordered some special tests. *What in the world is a BAT?* she wondered. *And why do I need one?*

This chapter contains descriptions of tests (in alphabetical order) which may be ordered in certain circumstances. (Tests used in the routine eye exam are described in Chapter 3.)

Biopsy

For a biopsy, tissue is removed then tested to determine if a growth is malignant (cancerous). If the growth is small, the whole thing might be removed and tested. If the growth is large, only a small piece is taken for testing. The tissue is sent to a pathology lab and examined under a microscope. Your doctor will order a biopsy on any growth that might be malignant, as well as on most growths that are removed (whether they look malignant or not). Just because your doctor orders a biopsy does *not* mean that you have a malignancy.

The biopsy is often done in the doctor's office. Local anesthesia (a numbing injection) is used first to prevent you from feeling anything. The skin is cleansed, maybe a paper drape is laid around the area. The tissue is removed using sterile surgical instruments. Stitches are used if necessary. The tissue is placed in a bottle of preserving solution, labeled, and sent to the pathology lab. Your surgeon will tell you how to care for the wound.

Usually the lab is not at your eye doctor's office. Another physician, called a pathologist, evaluates and identifies the tissue. You may get separate bills from your eye doctor and your pathologist. Some surgeons include the pathologist's charge in their fee. Ask your doctor's staff what to expect.

The pathology report is generally sent to your surgeon. If the results are NON-malignant, the doctor may have his nurse or other staff member give you the good news. If the testing reveals a malignancy, the doctor may call you, or request that you come to the office to discuss the results. Some doctors ask you to make an appointment to talk about the test, regardless of the results. When given the results, be sure that you understand what you're being told. "Negative" and "positive" may mean different things to different people. The medical terms may be confusing. If you have any doubts, simply ask, "Was the tissue malignant?" A yes or no answer will make it clear.

If a malignancy is found, your surgeon will tell you what happens next. The action taken depends on the type of malignancy and whether or not the entire malignancy was removed during the biopsy. If a small piece of a growth shows a malignancy, the remainder of the growth will need to be removed. (*Cancer*, in Chapter 8, talks about skin cancer and its treatment.)

Brightness Acuity Test

* *other names: glare test*

Have you ever looked through a scratched or dirty windshield at night? Light coming through the windshield is scattered, and the glare can be horrible. It is much easier to see through the windshield in the daytime, isn't it?

A cataract can cause the same problem in the eye. Light is scattered when it hits the cataract, decreasing vision. Vision may not be too bad as long as there is no glare, but when direct sun or on-coming car lights hit you, vision may plummet to a level below legal driving.

Sometimes the cloudiest part of the cataract is in the center. If the pupil is wide, vision is better (it's like being able to see around the cataract). But if the pupil is smaller (as when bright lights hit your eyes), then you are forced to look through the cloudiest part of the cataract. So vision is worse when there's glare.

The standard vision test performed in most offices is conducted in dim lighting. There is no glare. Thus, a person with a cataract may appear not to need the cataract removed. This may be a false representation of the person's vision.

The BAT checks a person's vision in light and dark, with and without glare. The simplest way to do the test is to look at the eye chart with one eye while shining a small bright light into the other eye. This can be done twice: once in room light and again in dim light. The room light test simulates daytime glare from the sun. Repeating the test in the dark is liking meeting headlights when driving at night.

The more usual test involves looking into a machine similar to the one used to test vision for the driver's license. You are asked to read letters in bright and dim light, with and without glare.

The need to restrict driving to daylight only might be proved or disproved by the BAT. Some tests combine the contrast sensitivity test (CST, discussed later) with the glare test. The BAT, like the CST, can be used to justify cataract surgery.

Cell Count

other names: specular microscopy

This test is used to evaluate the health of the cornea (clear window over the front of the eye). The cornea must be crystal clear for good vision. While it may seem like a small part of eye, it actually has five layers. The inner-most layer, the endothelium, functions to keep the cornea clear.

The endothelium is only one cell-layer thick. (Cells are the microscopic building-blocks of the body's tissues.) Unlike some other body tissues, the endothelium does not regenerate (grow more cells to replace damaged ones). All the endothelial cells that you are ever going to have are present at birth. If some cells are destroyed, no new endothelial cells grow to take their place. The existing cells just spread thinner to cover the same area. If enough cells are destroyed, the cornea begins to get cloudy and vision decreases.

Corneal dystrophies and some kinds of eye surgery can damage the endothelium. Even procedures that do not actually destroy cells can cause stress to them. This stress may decrease the efficiency of the cells, causing cloudiness.

Observation of the endothelium can be done by using the slit lamp microscope at a high magnification. The physician can get an overview of the general health of the cornea, but counting cells this way is difficult.

The specular microscope is a high-powered magnifier capable

of seeing the tiny endothelial cells. A picture of the cells is projected onto a TV-like screen, where the cells can be counted.

Before the test, numbing drops are placed into your eye. You sit in front of the instrument with your chin and forehead in a head rest. Usually you are asked to look straight ahead (maybe at a light) and to try not to blink. Or, someone may hold your lid open. Then the probe tip of the microscope is brought forward to contact your eye. The person performing the test will make a videotape as the probe scans your eye. Since the microscope has such high magnification, even a little motion looks huge on the screen. So the assistant will encourage you to be as still as possible. The reading usually takes about a minute.

Repeating cell counts a few times a year is useful in monitoring corneal dystrophy. Also, the surgeon uses your cell count to decide if surgery is safe for your cornea. He may use it to determine what type of intraocular lens to implant during cataract surgery, or what method to use to remove a cataract.

Not everyone having cataract or other eye surgery needs a cell count. Further, a specular microscope is an expensive piece of equipment that many private practices don't have. Most cataract surgery is done successfully without cell count data.

Collagen Tear Test

Tears are made in the lacrimal (tear) gland, then drain out through the puncti (small holes in the upper and lower lids, next to the nose). In the case of dry eyes, very little tears are being produced. Unfortunately the tears that are produced quickly drain away through the puncti .

The puncti can be sealed to keep the tears on the eye. But before the surgeon closes the puncti permanently, closing them temporarily serves as a test to determine if sealing them permanently will do any good. The collagen tear plugs are placed into the puncti. They dissolve in three or four days.

Before the plugs are inserted, you will be numbed with drops to minimize discomfort. You will sit up to the microscope with your chin and forehead in the headrest. An assistant may hold your lower lids still. The physician may stretch the puncti slightly with a special instrument. Then the doctor gently pushed the plugs into the punctum.

Your lids may feel a little sore that day. On the second and third day, you should pay attention to how your eyes feel. When you return to the office, your physician will want a full report on how your eyes felt on days two and three, before the plugs dissolved. You will also be examined with the microscope. Based on this data, the doctor will decide if sealing the puncta permanently is likely to help.

Color Vision

The retina (inside lining of the eye) is made up of two types light-receiving cells: rods and cones. The cones are concentrated in your central vision and are responsible for fine detail and color vision. You've probably heard the term "color blind." This means a person cannot see certain colors as they really are. A color vision test may identify what colors a person has trouble with and/or identify the severity of the defect. In an adult, each eye is usually tested separately.

Your doctor may order this test if you are having problems with identifying colors or there is suspicion that your cones may be damaged. Some medications can alter the cones, and a color test will be done on each eye every 6–12 months to check for any deterioration. Cataracts can cause a change in color vision, but do not usually warrant a special color test. Some jobs (military, police, some industries) may require a color test as part of the requirements to get or keep a job.

Isochromatic Plates

This is one of the most common tests, and involves looking at a series of plates. Each plate has a number made up of colored dots inside a circle of other colored dots. A normal eye can identify the number. A person with a color defect may see a different number or no number at all. Some tests have lines or figures instead of numbers, but it still works the same way. The plates may be on cardboard pages, in a viewer, or on a screen. This test is often used as a screening device and identifies the presence of a defect but does not tell its severity. Some of these tests only screen for blue/green defects and no other colors. It takes about a minute to do both eyes. Some form of this test will be available at most every optometric and ophthalmic office.

Hue Tests

These tests may take five minutes or longer. You are given plastic caps with colored tops and asked to arrange them in order of closest matching color. The first cap is chosen for you so that you have a starting place. The length of the test depends on whether or not each eye is tested separately, and on how many caps there are. Your answers are recorded on a special graph or grid. The pattern of your response shows what type of defect exists and how severe it is. Some private offices may not have this test, most university clinics will.

Computerized Tomography

* other names: CT scan, CAT scan

The CT scan uses X-rays and computers to show a cross-section. (A cross-section is what you see when you cut something in half). A regular X-ray shows a one-dimensional image with the bones in front super-imposed over those in the back. Tissues such as muscle cast a shadow on regular X-ray pictures. The CT scan, however, uses fan-shaped X-ray beams to X-ray a slice instead of an entire structure. That way there are no super-imposed structures or shadows.

A CT of the head, which includes the eyes and the bones and structures around them, can be very useful. A CT might be ordered in case of suspected tumor, fracture, or inflammation.

During a CT scan, you lie down in a sort of tunnel or tube while the pictures are taken. Patients with claustrophobia may be given medication to help them relax. Overweight patients may not be able to have the scan if they cannot fit into the tube. A CT of the head takes 20-40 minutes. During that time you will hear humming and clicking noises.

Dye can be injected into a vein in the arm during a CT. The dye will show up in certain tissues on the X-ray. The contrast created by the dye can help in diagnosis. CT scans are generally done in a hospital.

Contrast Sensitivity Test (CST)

Think about the regular eye chart for a moment. It has dark black figures on a bright white background. There is high contrast between the figures and the background. This high-contrast chart is the standard for determining vision.

Now think about the world around you. Most of what we look at is not high contrast—it is shades and shadows: light objects against light backgrounds, dark objects against dark backgrounds. Because the eye chart is high contrast and the real world is a mixture of contrasts, the vision from an eye chart is often much better than actual vision. This difference between vision on the chart and "real" vision is especially important when you have cataracts. Vision must drop to a certain level before insurance will consider surgery to be necessary.

Mrs. Bennett has a cataract. "I just can't see!" she tells her doctor. Her doctor checks her vision on the eye chart. "I'm sorry, Mrs. Bennett. Your vision is 20/40. Medicare won't pay to remove your cataract yet." Mrs. Bennett is unhappy. She is having trouble recognizing faces and seeing road signs, but she doesn't "qualify" for the surgery that would help her. It doesn't make sense.

If Mrs. Bennett had a contrast sensitivity test, it would show that her true vision is very poor—low enough to justify surgery. Medicare will accept a failed CST as grounds for cataract surgery.

A CST can also be helpful in detecting and/or monitoring glaucoma, macular degeneration, and other problems.

Corneal Sensation

The cornea (clear covering over the eye) has very sensitive nerve endings. This sensitivity is a protective device so you will blink instinctively if something touches your cornea. You can also tell if there is something in eye, or if your eye feels dry.

Some corneal diseases, as well as long-term contact lens wear, can damage the cornea's sense of feeling. If the cornea is numb and you rub your eye, you may scratch your cornea. Or you may not notice that your eye is dangerously dry. Either of these situations may cause an infection to set up in the eye. If you have a disease process that affects the corneal nerves, your doctor may order a corneal sensation test to determine if damage has occurred.

The simplest way to perform this test is to touch the cornea with a wisp of cotton. (DO NOT try to do this to yourself!) If you can feel the cotton, you will blink involuntarily.

This test gives a rough "Yes/No" answer, and does not tell how much damage may have occurred. There is an instrument, called an anesthesiometer, which can actually give a measurement of the cornea's sensitivity. It has a fine nylon thread on a handle. The thread is gently touched to the cornea. At first the touch is so gentle it is not felt. The reading is taken by noting the length of the thread when you can first feel it touch. This test is only slightly uncomfortable.

Corneal Topography

Have you ever seen a topographical map? Such a map shows the elevations and depressions of an area. A topograph of the cornea shows the curvatures of the entire cornea. Such a "map" is useful before cataract surgery if astigmatism is going to be corrected at the same time. It is also used before refractive surgery, which alters the way light is focused in the eye (see *Refractive Surgery,* Chapter 6). Keratoconus, a disease of the cornea, can also be measured by topography.

The part of the topograph instrument that you see looks like a small screen with circles on it. The eye that is not being tested may be patched. You will be asked to place your chin and forehead in the headrest. Try to keep your eye open and still (but you may blink if you have to). Once the assistant has aligned the machine with the eye, the measurement takes only a few seconds. There is no pain or any kind of sensation.

Any of the cases mentioned above can be handled without topography. It is a new, expensive instrument that is likely to be found in university and large clinic settings.

Electroencephalography (EEG)

The EEG detects electrical changes in the brain. Twenty electrodes (sticky pads with wires connected to them) are placed about the head and face. If there is a lot of hair at the spot where an electrode must be placed, that tiny area might be shaved. The test is painless, and takes anywhere from 10 to 30 minutes. Certain conditions, such as epilepsy, cause changes in the brain waves that an EEG can detect. In eye care, an EEG might be used to find the cause of increased pressure in the skull. Such increased pressure can cause changes in the optic nerve.

Electromyography (EMG)

Electromyography is used to evaluate the function of the muscles that move the eye. It is used to identify paralyzed and weak muscles.

A slim needle, which is attached to a monitoring instrument, is inserted into one muscle at a time. (A numbing drop is used to minimize discomfort.) If the muscle can function, it creates a blip on the screen, as well as a noise. A paralyzed muscle creates no blip or sound. A weak muscle does not cause as strong a response as a healthy one. Electromyography can be repeated every so often to monitor muscle weakness in cases of myasthenia gravis and certain muscle diseases.

Electronystagmography (ENG)

Eye muscle response can also be evaluated by use of ENG. In this test, small sticky pads with wires attached are stuck to the skin beside the eye. The test is painless. You are asked to watch a rotating drum with stripes on it. The instrument measures the movement of your eyes as you try to track the stripes.

Another use of ENG is to measure nystagmus, an involuntary jerking of the eyes.

Electrooculography (EOG)

The function of the retina (inside lining of the eye) may be evaluated using an EOG. It may be ordered in cases of macular degeneration, retinitis pigmentosa, Vitamin A deficiency, or retinal detachment. Eye movements may also be evaluated by EOG. It is not a common test, and is used mostly in universities.

The EOG is painless. Small electrodes (flat little sticky-pads smaller than a dime and attached to wires) are placed around one or both eyes. The pads do not touch the eye itself. Readings are taken in room light and again in the dark.

Electroretinography (ERG)

ERG tests the function of the retina (inside lining of the eye), and shows whether or not poor vision is caused by a retinal problem. It is used to help diagnose and evaluate hereditary retinal disease such as retinitis pigmentosa, severe color blindness, and severe night blindness. It is also used to evaluate the retina when there are circulation problems either in the eye itself or in the carotid artery.

A numbing drop is placed in the eye to be tested. A contact lens, which has several wires connected to it, is placed on the eye. (The wires do not touch the eye.) Blinking may feel odd or uncomfortable, although not really painful. When the test begins, the assistant will flash a light into the eye. The instrument records the electrical response of the retina to the flash of light. It is not a commonly used test, and thus found mainly in university settings.

Exophthalmometry

The exophthalmometer is used to measure eye protrusion. There are several reasons the eyes might protrude (push out further than normal). The most common is overactive thyroid.

There are several different kinds of exophthalmometer. With the most common type, the instrument is held up to your face. The edges of the instrument fit right to the outer corners of your eyes. You will be asked to look straight ahead. The doctor or assistant looks into a gauge on either side of the instrument and takes a reading. The test is painless and takes less than a minute. Readings may be repeated every few months to see if the eye(s) protrude more and more.

Fluoresceine Angiography (FA)

Like the rest of the body, the eye is nourished by blood vessels. The blood supply must be good in order for the eye to be healthy. If the flow of blood to the eye is reduced, there may be problems.

The FA test shows how the blood vessels of the retina are functioning. Dye is injected through an IV in the arm or hand. Then, photographs are taken as the dye enters the blood vessels of the eye. (Although the camera uses special filters, this in NOT an X-ray, laser, or radiation.) The filters cause the dye to glow, giving a dramatic picture of the blood vessels. From the photographs, the physician can detect areas of leakage, blockage, and degeneration.

Someone will explain the procedure, and you will probably be asked to sign a consent form. If you have ever had a reaction to injected dye, be sure to let them know. Your eyes will be dilated. Before the dye is injected, you will be asked to sit up to the camera. Your head and chin will be leaning into a head rest. A few photos will be taken before the dye is started. You will be asked to look straight ahead, or perhaps at a small light. You may blink now and then, but try not to blink constantly. The light from the camera will be bright, and someone may have to help hold your eyelids open. When the photographer is ready, the dye is injected. There is usually no reaction, but some may feel a brief wave of nausea. Unless you feel very ill, try to remain still at the camera. Photos will be snapped every second or so for about a minute, then you may be allowed to sit back and rest. A few more pictures may be taken at later intervals over the next ten or fifteen minutes. From dilation to finishing photos, the entire process lasts about an hour. The actual photography takes maybe twenty or thirty minutes. If you normally have trouble driving while dilated, you may want to have someone drive you home.

The FA can also be done to evaluate the blood vessels of the iris (colored part of the eye). If this is done, you will not be dilated.

The dye enters the blood stream of your entire body, not just the eye. Your skin may have a sallow or yellow cast to it and your urine will be bright yellow for 24 to 48 hours as the dye leaves the body.

Ask the assistant how long it will be before you get the results. Often your doctor will schedule an appointment and will discuss the results at that time.

There are many reasons why a doctor might order an FA. The most common is diabetic retinopathy. In this case, the doctor is looking for hemorrhages, leakage, and neovascularization (growth of new abnormal blood vessels). The FA may be used to decide if you need laser and if so, where.

The FA may also be useful in patients with high blood pressure, macular degeneration, and other retinal conditions.

Many ophthalmologists have a camera in their office. Some use a camera at the hospital or university clinic.

Gonioscopy

Aqueous (the watery fluid inside the eye) is constantly being formed then drained out of the eye. If the aqueous does not drain properly, pressure builds up in the eye. When the pressure gets high enough to damage the optic nerve, it is called glaucoma (see Chapter 14).

The aqueous drains out of a very specific part of the eye, between the cornea (clear covering over the eye) and the iris (colored part of the eye). This area is called the "angle" of the eye. The angle cannot be seen with the regular slit lamp microscope. A special lens, with prisms and mirrors in it, must be used with the microscope to allow the doctor to see into the angle.

First, your eye will be numbed with drops because the gonio lens touches the eye. You will sit with your head and chin in the headrest of the microscope. The doctor will hold your lids open and place the gonio lens against your eye. It is very important for you to keep BOTH eyes opened. You will be asked to look straight ahead. It is okay to blink now and then. When you blink, you will probably feel the lens against your lids. While that may feel funny, it shouldn't hurt. If you can keep from squeezing your eyes, you should be comfortable during the entire test. It only takes a minute or so to look at an eye.

Using the gonio lens, the doctor can see if the draining area of the angle is open or closed. Pressure can quickly build up if the draining area is closed. Sometimes eye drops can be used to open the angle. If a large portion of the angle is closed, your doctor may decide to do a laser iridotomy (discussed under *Angle closure glaucoma*, Chapter 14) to provide more drainage.

Interferometer

The interferometer is used before cataract surgery to estimate what your vision will be after the cataract is removed. It uses laser or other light beams to project a series of parallel lines into the eye. (Although it may use laser, this is NOT a treatment, nor does it alter the eye in any way.) The instrument may be held in the assistant's hand, or it may be attached to a slit lamp microscope. If attached to the microscope, you will sit with your chin and forehead in the headrest. The assistant will ask you if you see the lines. If you do, you will be asked if the lines are vertical, horizontal, or tilted to the left or right. The test is painless and takes only a minute or so per eye.

Keratometery

*   other names: K readings, K's, ophthalmometry*
The keratometer measures the curvature of the cornea (clear window of the eye). The cornea may be curved the same amount

in every direction (like a marble). Or it may be more curved in one direction than in another (like the back of a spoon). Taking a reading with the keratometer tells the steepness and direction of the cornea's curvature.

To have a K reading, you will sit up to the instrument with your chin and forehead in a head rest. You will be asked to look straight ahead, perhaps at a small light. As long as you don't flutter your eyelids, it's okay to blink. The machine may take the reading automatically, but the most common type requires an assistant to take the reading manually. It takes a minute or less to read each eye. The instrument does not touch the eye, and there is no pain.

K readings are used in fitting contact lenses. In this case, the doctor orders a lens with a curve that matches the curve of your eye.

Some corneal diseases can change the shape of the cornea. Frequent K readings are used to monitor the progression of the disease prcess.

K readings are especially important before and after refractive surgery. Refractive surgery is done to change your vision by altering the shape of the cornea. It is most often used in cases of nearsightedness or asigmatism.

Corneal transplant surgery is another example of surgery that changes the cornea's shape. In this case, K readings are often taken at every visit after surgery. The cornea's curvature changes during the healing process. Once the K readings indicate that the curvature is stable, the doctor will be ready to prescribe glasses.

In those over 40, the most common need for keratometry is prior to cataract surgery. Before surgery, K readings are taken. The readings are used to decide what power of implant to place in the eye. After surgery, K readings are often used to determine when the eye is stable. Once the eye is stable, glasses can be prescribed. The K readings may also be used to help find the correct glasses prescription. If stitches were used to close the wound during cataract surgery, the physician uses the K readings to decide if sutures need to be removed, and if so, which ones.

Keratoscopy

The keratoscope is used to estimate the contour of the cornea. It does not give a numerical measurement, but rather an idea of how the cornea curves. This is useful in keratoconus and high astigmatism. The keratoscope has a camera attached to it. The photos provide a permanent record that can be compared from one exam to the next.

The part of the keratoscope that you see looks like a screen with circles on it. A photograph is taken as you look at the circles. This photo shows the reflection of the rings on your cornea. There is no pain or other sensation.

Macular Photostress Test

This simple test gives a rough idea of macular function. (The macula is the part of the retina that gives you fine central vision.) This test may give the early indication of macular degeneration.

First, your vision is checked on the eye chart. Then, a flashlight is held very close to the eye for ten seconds. When the flashlight is turned off, the assistant counts how many seconds until you can see the eye chart again. (It may take a minute or more.) Some offices may have a special instrument for this test, which may be part of the routine eye exam .

Magnetic Resonance Imaging (MRI)

MRI testing is fairly new on the scene. The MRI is not radiation, but uses a combination of radio and magnetic waves to create an image on a screen. It is used to view soft tissues such as the eye and brain. Bones don't show up on the MRI at all, as they do in X-rays and CT scans. So the MRI is ideal for looking at soft structures surrounded by bone, especially at the base of the brain. In eye care, an MRI is used to examine swelling, tumors involving blood vessels, and nerve conditions.

Because of the strong magnetic field, people with pacemakers, metal implants, or embedded metal (such as shrapnel, or a metallic foreign body inside the eye) cannot have an MRI. Otherwise, there is no known risk.

During an MRI, you lie down in a tunnel or tube. If you are claustrophobic, you may be given medication to help you relax. A scan of the head takes 20-40 minutes. During that time you will hear some noises as the machine works. MRI is available in most medical centers.

Nasolacrimal Evaluation

"Nasolacrimal" refers to the system that drains tears OUT of the eye. Tears drain through tiny holes in the lids into tubules leading to a sac, called the nasolacrimal sac. From this sac, tears drain through more tubules and into the back of the throat. Several tests can be done to see if the drainage system is open.

1. Fluoresceine dye evaluation— Several drops of fluoresceine (a yellow dye that glows when a blue light shines on it) are placed into the eyes. The drops may sting a little for a few seconds. About five minutes later, the assistant looks into your nose with a blue light. If the drainage system is open, the dye can be seen inside the nostrils. In another version of the fluoresceine test, the dye is inserted directly into the nasolacrimal sac. An alternative is to have you blow your nose and checking the tissue for fluoresceine.
2. Irrigation test— After numbing with drops, saline (salty) fluid is placed directly into the punctum (opening in the lid). If the nasolacrimal system is open, you will taste the saline. If the system is not open, the saline will just run down your face. This test is sometimes used as a procedure to rinse out a known blockage.
3. X-ray evaluation— In this test, a substance that shows up on X-ray is injected into the sac. X-rays are taken to find the location of the blockage. The test is painless.
4. Photographic evaluation— For this technique, a radioactive drop is placed in the eye. A camera with a special filter is used to take photos as the drop drains out of the eye. There is no discomfort.

Ophthalmodynamometry

This test gives information about the pressure in the main arteries of the retina. After the pupils are dilated, the doctor looks into the eye with an ophthalmoscope. Pressure is applied to the eye with the ophthalmodynamometer, which is a small spring-loaded device. (Numbing drops are used to minimize discomfort, but you will feel some pressure.) The reading is taken when the increasing pressure causes the blood vessel to collapse. The blood vessel recovers as soon as the pressure is released. Each reading takes about 5 seconds, and is usually repeated several times.

This test may be important in evaluating blood flow to an eye that has been experiencing vision "black outs".

Pachymeter

* other names: pachometer, pac

The cornea (clear cover over the front of the eye) may seem small and thin, but it is actually five layers thick. The cornea is thinnest in the middle and thicker at the edges. The pachymeter is an instrument used to measure corneal thickness.

Some A-scan ultrasound units and specular microscopes have a built-in pachymeter. Other pachymeters are separate instruments.

A numbing drop is placed in the eye, so the test is painless. Try to keep both eyes open and look where the assistant tells you. Someone may hold your lids open for you. The probe tip may be attached to a slit lamp microscope and you'll put your chin and forehead in a head rest. Or the assistant may hold the probe-tip by hand. The tip is gently touched to different parts of the cornea as readings are taken of the tissue's thickness. The readings may take about a minute per eye.

Pachymetry provides very useful information prior to corneal transplant surgery or refractive surgery. Generally, a pac is not necessary before cataract surgery. The physician may want a pac reading to monitor corneal dystrophy (breakdown of the cornea) or other diseases that can cause the cornea to thin.

Photography

The eye is an amazing structure. It is the only organ of the body that we can look into without having to cut (or put in a scope). Because of this, photography plays a big role in eye care.

External Photos

External photos may be taken with a regular camera. Some offices put a picture of each patient in the patient's medical record to aid in identification. Regular photos may also be needed before eyelid surgery of many kinds to show the need for surgery. Your insurance company may require photos before they will approve payment for certain procedures. Pictures may also be taken before strabismus surgery (surgery to straighten the eyes). You may be asked to sign a release allowing the photos to be used in medical journals or for other purposes. If you do not wish your pictures to be seen by anyone, you should not sign the release.

Slit Lamp Photography

Magnified photos of the eye's exterior can be made using a camera mounted on a slit lamp microscope. These photos may be used to monitor growths for a change in size or appearance from one visit to the next. Or, they may be used to document the presence and appearance of a growth prior to surgery. You will sit with your chin and forehead in a headrest. The photographer will tell you which way to look. It is okay to blink now and then. Keep both eyes open unless told to close them. An assistant may hold your lids. The slit lamp light and flash may be bright, but there is no pain and nothing touches the eye.

Retinal Photographs

Pictures of the eye's interior require a special camera called a fundus camera. (The fundus is the back of the eye.) The fundus camera is used to take pictures of the retina (inside lining of the eye), optic nerve, and retinal blood vessels.

Your pupils are usually dilated for this type of photography because the camera light would cause your pupil to constrict (get smaller), creating a tinier opening to photograph through. With the pupil dilated, the pupil is help open wide enough to get a good view.

You will sit up to the camera with your chin and forehead in the headrest. You will need to keep both eyes open. Usually you are asked to look straight ahead at a small light. During the photography session, the assistant may move the light and/or have you look in other directions.

The camera does not emit X-rays, radiation, or laser. It does not touch the eye. You may find the bright light somewhat uncomfortable. You may blink occasionally. If you are unable to keep your eye open, an assistant will hold your lids for you.

It usually takes only a few minutes for routine photos. More extensive photo studies will take longer.

Some examples of when and why fundus photos may be ordered include:

1. Glaucoma—Photos are taken of the optic nerve, often once a year. These pictures provide a permanent visual record to assist in judging whether or not the nerve is being damaged.
2. Diabetes—Pictures provide a record of any hemorrhages, leakage, and neovascularization (growth of new abnormal blood vessels). They also show laser work, often done to prevent further damage.
3. Hypertension (high blood pressure)—Annual pictures show if the eye's blood vessels are being distorted, squeezed, or blocked. Photos also record any hemorrhages or leakages.
4. Growths, freckles, and other retinal lesions can be recorded on film to document changes in size and/or appearance.
5. Other diseases, trauma, and conditions commonly photographed: macular degeneration, retinal detachment, retinal tears and holes.

Placido Disk

The Placido disk is used to evaluate the cornea's curvature. The disk itself looks like a big lollipop: a circle about 9 inches across on a handle. The front of the disk has rings printed on it in wide black and white bands. There is a small hole in the middle. The assistant holds the disk close to you, and looks at the disk's reflection on your cornea. He or she will make a few notes in your chart about what the reflection looks like. The test is painless and takes only half a minute or so. The Placido disk is useful in cases of disease that can alter the cornea's shape, astigmatism, and corneal transplant surgery (before and after). Most offices will have a disk.

Potential Acuity Meter (PAM)

The PAM is a device used to estimate what your vision could be if a cataract was removed, similar to the interferometer, described earlier. The instrument projects an eye chart onto the back of your eye. All you have to do is read the letters or numbers. The level of letters you are able to see gives a good idea of what you would see if you had no cataract. The test is very important to your doctor if there is any doubt about your present vision and/or the health of your eye.

Ashley Sanders has cataracts and macular degeneration. His vision on the regular eye chart is 20/200. His PAM test is 20/40. His doctor tells him, "Mr. Sanders, based on my tests, removing your cataract should help you see a lot better. Now because you also have some macular degeneration, I don't expect you'll have 20/20 vision. But I think the improvement you'll get is worth doing surgery."

Bonnie Aleshire has a cataract in her right eye. But the right eye has also been lazy and weak all her life. Like Mr. Sanders, she also sees 20/200 on the regular eye chart. Her PAM test is 20/100. "Mrs. Aleshire," her doctor says, "Removing your cataract might help some, but not a lot because that's always been a weak eye. If the cataract gets worse, then it might be worthwhile to remove it. But let's just keep an eye on it for now."

Schirmer's Tear Test

* other names: tear test, basal tear test

Most of the tears that bathe the eye come from the lacrimal (tear) gland. Tears are important because the eye must be kept moist.

The Schirmer's tear test measures tear production. Small strips of filter paper (paper-thin and about the size of a cardboard match) are used. About 1/4 inch of the strip is placed between the lower lid and the eye. The rest of the strip hangs outside over the lower lid.

In the most common type of test, your eyes will be numbed with some drops first. The strips are inserted and left in place for five minutes. During that time it is best if you look up, rather than straight ahead. You may blink if you need to. (If the strips were put in properly, blinking should not cause them to fall out.) As the five minutes passes, your tears wet the test strips. At the end of the test, the strips are removed. The amount of wetting down the strip is measured in millimeters with a ruler. Twelve millimeters or more is considered normal.

Sometimes the test is done without numbing drops. In this case, the doctor usually wants to find out how much your eyes tear when irritated. This may be useful to know if you are being fitted for contact lenses.

A tear test can help the doctor diagnose dry eyes. Also, some physicians want a tear test done prior to eyelid surgery. (Dry eye symptoms can worsen after surgery, although this may be only temporary.) A tear test may be done before and after procedures to close the punctum (opening in the lids where tears drain out of the eye).

Stereo Testing

Do you remember the stereopticon or the stereo viewer? Cards or disks are inserted into these gadgets, producing pictures that appear to be three dimensional—to most people. To others, they just look like flat pictures. The difference is stereo vision.

In order to have stereo vision (or stereopsis), the eyes must be straight (that is, looking at the same thing at the same time) and the vision has to be about equal in each eye.

Stereo testing gives the physician an idea of how well your eyes are working together. As with many eye tests, there are several types of stereo tests.

In the most usual type, you wear your bifocals or reading glasses (if you use them). Another pair of glasses (these are slightly shaded) are put *over* your glasses. You must keep both eyes open. The assistant shows you some figures in a folder or on a board, or you may look into a machine. Some of the figures look flat, others look as if they are raised up, floating off the page. The number of "floating" figures you can identify is the grade of your stereo vision.

Stereo testing may be done before and after surgery for strabismus (crossed eyes) to document improvement. (Crossed eyes do not have stereo vision because they do not look at the same thing at the same time.) Stereo testing may also be required for disability tests and some jobs. Since a cataract can cause blurred vision in one eye, it can cause a decrease in stereopsis.

Stereo vision is not the same as depth perception, however. A person with one eye does not have stereo vision, but does have depth perception.

Tonography

The aqueous (watery fluid inside the eye) is constantly being formed and drained out of the eye. Tonography measures the rate that the aqueous leaves the eye.

The test uses a tonometer (instrument that measures eye pressure) that is hooked up to a graph machine. First, numbing drops are placed in the eye. The assistant gently holds the lids and applies the tonometer. It is best to keep both eyes open and look straight up (the test is done lying down). There should be no pain. The tonometer is held in place for four minutes, then removed from the eye.

Tonography is used mainly by glaucoma specialists in university settings.

Ultrasound

* other names: A-scan, B-scan

The eye is the only organ of the body that we can look into without having to cut or insert a scope. But sometimes we need more information than what we can merely see.

Ultrasound is high-speed sound energy. Submarines use ultrasound to send sound waves toward the ocean's bottom. A map of the ocean floor is made by receiving the echoes as they bounce back from the sea bottom. In ocular ultrasound scanning, sound waves are used to create a picture or graph of the eye on a screen.

Ultrasound is especially useful if the physician cannot actually see into the eye. The cornea (clear covering over the front of the eye) may be scarred, there could be a thick white cataract, or there could be bleeding inside the eye. But an ultrasound can still penetrate the eye in any of these situations.

Basically there are two types of ultrasound: A and B. We will discuss each.

A-Scan

The A-scan is used primarily to measure the length of the eye. The length of the eye is used in a mathematical formula to determine the power of intraocular lens implant (IOL) used in cataract surgery. This formula is run separately on every eye the cataract surgeon does. An A-scan can also be used to evaluate the eye's interior for tumors or foreign bodies.

There are several types of A-scan, but the procedure is about the same with each. Your eye will be numbed with drops. You will be asked to keep both eyes open and look straight ahead (or, someone may hold your lids open). The assistant touches the probe tip of the A-scan to your eye. (The probe may be attached to a slit lamp microscope, or the assistant may hold it by hand.) Several readings are usually taken. The measurement is painless, and generally takes about a minute per eye.

An A-scan unit is found in most ophthalmology offices.

B-Scan

The B-scan shows a computerized cross-section of the eye. (A cross-section is what you'd see if you cut an object in half.) This is especially helpful when the physician cannot see into the eye.

The probe-tip is usually held in the operator's hand. The test may be done sitting or reclining. The probe-tip may be placed on the closed lid or directly on the eye. If the probe touches the eye, you will be given numbing drops to keep you comfortable. You will feel vibration and pressure from the probe, but it should not hurt. The assistant will tell you where to move your eyes. (In many other tests we have discussed, you are asked to look only straight ahead; with the B-scan it is important that the operator scan many parts of your eye.)

If the probe tip contacts your eye, you will probably be lying back during the test. The operator may put a thick liquid on the probe tip. This "goo" helps conduct the ultrasound waves, and may be a little messy.

During the scan, a TV-like monitor shows a computer image of the parts of the eye. The probe is turned one way, then the other, as well as applied to different locations on the eye. Now and then the operator will "freeze" the picture and take a photograph of the screen. This gives a permanent record of the scan.

Among the structures that can be seen are the cornea, lens, retina, eye muscles, optic nerve, and fat behind the eye. Abnormalities that can be detected include blood, foreign bodies, dislocated lens or intraocular lens, retinal tear or detachment, and growths.

Amy Cole slowly went blind several years ago, but never sought medical care. Last month her daughter took her to an ophthalmologist, who told her that her cataracts were so thick that he couldn't see through them. "Mrs. Cole," he explained, "I can't tell if the retina, or lining inside the back of your eye, is healthy or not. For example, if your retina is detached, then removing the cataract won't help your vision. But I can't see back there to tell."

The doctor ordered a B-scan. "Good news!" he said after the test. "The scan seems to indicate that your retina is fine. I don't know exactly how good your vision will be after cataract surgery, but I think it's worthwhile to go ahead." Eight weeks after surgery, Mrs. Cole agrees, too. Her vision has improved to driving level. She is planning on having the other eye done soon.

The B-scan may be available in some private practices and clinics, but is generally found in specialty (retinal) practices and universities.

Visually Evoked Response (VER)

* other names: visually evoked potential (VEP)

The flow of light from the eye to the brain can be tested using the VER. It is especially useful in patients who cannot speak, or those who cannot co-operate with regular vision testing. The VER can help distinguish whether or not blindness is due to a problem with the eye or is psychological.

A VER test is painless. Small electrodes (flat pads smaller than a dime, with wires attached) are placed over the "bumps" at the base of the skull. The electrodes are sticky like tape, and the area may have to be shaved to get good contact. The other end of the wires is attached to an instrument. A light is flashed into the eyes, and the electric response of the brain is recorded by the instrument. It is not a commonly used test, and is found mostly in university settings.

Visual Field Testing

* other names: peripheral vision test, side vision test

Visual field tests check your peripheral vision—what you see around and to the sides that you're not looking directly at. For example, focus on the period at the end of this sentence. You are using your central vision to look at the period. But you still see much more than just the period. As you look at the period, you can still see that there are words all around it. You can tell what the closest letters are without looking directly at them. The letters that are further away are visible, but not clear enough to recognize. You are probably also aware of the edges of the book. (Maybe you can also see your feet over the top of the book, propped up on your coffee table.) Perimetry measures your ability to see the things "on the edges."

Several different diseases and conditions can cause a loss in the visual field. In fact, some diseases cause specific patterns of loss. Thus a visual field test can be essential in diagnosing some eye problems.

There are a number of ways to test the peripheral vision. Confrontation visual fields, described in detail in Chapter 3, is a rough screening test that is often part of every complete eye exam. The next three sections will talk about more specialized visual field tests.

Amsler Grid

This test checks only a small area around your central vision. You will wear your bifocals or reading glasses if you have them. Each eye is tested individually, so one eye is covered at a time. The assistant shows you a grid which is held at your normal reading distance. You should focus on the dot in the center of the grid. As you look at the dot, the assistant will ask you some questions:

1. Do you see the central dot?
2. As you look at the dot, are you aware of all four corners?
3. Are all the lines straight and square? Or do some appear to bow, bend, or wave?
4. Do you see all the lines? Are some areas blotted out, faded, or missing?

If you do see any blobs or distortions, you may be asked to sketch them right on the grid. This becomes part of your record.

The Amsler grid test may be used if you have told the doctor or assistant that you have any of the following symptoms:

1. a veil or curtain over part of your vision
2. straight lines appear curved or broken
3. a blob or cloud in one area of your vision
4. parts of words seem to disappear when you read.

The grid may be used to help diagnose macular degeneration, floaters, and retinal tear or detachment. Often patients with macular degeneration are given a grid to check themselves at home. To do the self-check, look at the grid while covering one eye. The main purpose of this test is to detect any *changes* in central vision. If you notice any new distortions, blobs, or missing areas, notify your doctor at once. The Amsler grid, often printed on cards or as a tablet, is found in every eye doctor's office.

Marion Veal, 63, had noticed that some letters seemed distorted while she was reading. Her ophthalmologist checked her with an Amsler grid. The test showed that some lines, near the center, were distorted. The doctor dilated her pupils and examined the back of her eye. "Mrs. Veal, you have a little degeneration in your eyes. That's what is causing your problems with reading. I want you to check yourself with this grid several times a week. When you look at the grid, you will still see these central squiggly lines, just as you did today. What I want you to look for is any CHANGE: a larger area is distorted, or new areas of wiggly lines appear. As long as things stay as they are now, you don't need to call me and I'll see you again in six months. But if you notice any changes, call me right away."

Tangent Screen

The tangent screen is used to check the central thirty degrees of the visual field. This covers a larger area than the confrontation field or Amsler grid. The tangent screen itself is a 4 foot by 4 foot piece of black felt. Circles and lines are sewn into the screen with black thread. There is a small white button in the center of the screen.

One eye is tested at a time, the other eye is patched. Usually the test is done without your glasses on, unless your vision without glasses is very poor. You will sit about 3 feet from the screen. Your job during the entire test is to look at the central white button. The assistant will move another white dot from the outer edge of the screen toward the center. When you first see the assistant's white dot, you give some signal to indicate that you see it. The assistant maps out your responses on the screen using black-tipped pins. The pattern of the map shows the doctor the outer limits of your peripheral vision and any blind spots inside those limits.

Your physician will explain the test results to you. You will be interested to see your blind spot on the map. (Each eye has a blind spot representing the place where the optic nerve enters the eye.)

The tangent screen is a quick way to map out peripheral vision. Perimetry, described next, takes a good bit more time. Your doctor may order a tangent screen if he feels you might not be able to tolerate the longer testing time needed for perimetry.

A tangent screen test can be used in most of the situations described in the next section. This method has been around for a long time, and has generally been replaced by computerized perimeters. Some newer offices may not have a tangent screen, but most established offices and clinics will.

Perimetry

Perimetry is the most sophisticated way to map out peripheral vision. The procedure is similar to that of the tangent screen, but perimetry maps out a much larger area. The test is done using a perimeter, which may be operated by hand or computer. A basic screening test may take only a couple minutes per eye. More detailed testing may take ten to twenty minutes per eye, sometimes more. The test is painless, but can be tedious and fatiguing.

Before starting, the assistant will explain the test to you. One eye is patched. You will sit up to the machine and place your chin and forehead in the head rest. The inside of the perimeter is white and may be round, like part of a bowl. Once you are seated and in position, you will notice a small circle or dot in the bowl straight in front of you. This is where you will look for the entire test.

While you look at the center dot, a light will flash on somewhere in the bowl. When you see the light come on, you will press a button on a hand-held buzzer. This lets the assistant (or computer) know that you saw the light. Try to push the button as soon as you see the light.

It is very important that you always look at the center dot. If you start looking around the bowl trying to see where the next light is coming from, you will invalidate the test. The assistant is watching to be sure you continue to look at the dot. He or she may remind you to look straight ahead if your eye wanders.

It is best if you can relax during the test. No one sees every light. At times you may go for a while without seeing anything. Don't worry. Just wait, and continue to look straight ahead. Eventually you will see a light again. At other times you may think you see the light, but you are not sure. Go ahead and press the button. Whether operated by computer or human, each area is checked more than once. If there is any question about a response, it will be double-checked.

Be sure to blink your eye often during the test. If you stare, your eye may get dry. This can cause blurred vision, and the eyes may water and burn. Let the assistant know if you are uncomfortable. Usually the chair and/or perimeter can be adjusted so that your back and neck are relaxed. If you get unusually tired, sleepy, or cramped, ask to take a break. The test can be paused for a moment while you stretch.

The results of the test will be interpreted by your physician. The test reveals how far out your side vision extends. Your "blind spot" (caused by the area where the optic nerve enters the eye) is mapped out, too. Any blank areas in the side vision, enlargement of the blind spot, or patterns of loss in the side vision are visible on a well-done test. Some of the patterns are typical of certain diseases or conditions. By examining the pattern of the visual field, the doctor can diagnose glaucoma, lid droop, optic nerve disease, even certain brain disorders.

Perimetry is often repeated once a year (especially in glaucoma) to see if any change is occurring. In the case of lid droop, a copy of the test results may be sent to your insurance company to show the need for lid-lifting surgery when applying for prior approval.

Most ophthalmology offices (private, clinic, and university) will have some type of perimeter. Many optometrists and neurologists have them as well.

X-rays

Conventional X-rays, which are pictures of bony structures, are sometimes used in ophthalmology. They may be used to identify bone fractures, foreign bodies, and tumors.

In most cases, you will lie face-down on the X-ray table. The assistant may immobilize your head by using a headband or sandbags. In some instances, you may be asked to lie on your side or in some other position. If you are uncomfortable, tell the assistant. He or she may be able to use pillows to support your back or neck. X-rays are not painful. The time required will depend on the number of pictures and positions needed. Your physician or a radiologist (doctor whose specialty is reading X-rays) will interpret the photos and tell you the results. The answers may be available in minutes, or several days depending on the urgency of your case and the developing process required. X-rays are usually done at a hospital facility.

There are certainly are a lot of special tests, aren' there? You may be wondering, *How does anybody pay for all that?* We'll talk about finances and insurance in the next chapter

CHAPTER 19

Financing Eye Care

The cost of health care rose 5.9% from 1992 to 1993. And whether you are in the 40–64 age bracket or are now covered by Medicare, health care and insurance probably takes up a good part of your personal budget. Then there are the out-of-pocket expenses . . . .

Charges and Fees

There is so much variation in charges that the best we can do here is to give a few generalities.

Your first step in financial planning is to talk to the cashier before you ever have your eye exam. Find out: How much is the exam? What services does the exam fee include? Under what circumstances could the fee go up? (For example, the doctor needs to run extra tests.) Will someone tell me if I need testing done that is not covered by the exam fee?

Most offices expect payment when the services are rendered, especially for eye exams. (For surgery they often file insurance first, see next section.) If paying for the exam is a problem for you, make arrangements *before* your visit. Talk to the office manager or financial secretary about making payments. You may be asked to sign a financial agreement to pay a certain amount over a period of time. If you owe money (for surgery, for example) and an unexpected situation arises making payment suddenly difficult, contact the office.

The charge for a full eye exam usually includes visual acuity testing, muscle evaluation, simple peripheral vision check, pupil evaluation, slit lamp exam, pressure check, and dilated retinal exam. The fee may or may not include the refraction. (See Chapter 3 for a full description of each of these tests.) Most of the tests in Chapter 18 carry an additional charge.

If you have tests done outside your eye doctor's office, the facility where you have the test done will probably bill you separately from your eye doctor. If you have a test that has to be interpreted by another physician, you may be charged by the clinic for the test and *also* by the doctor giving the interpretation. (Examples include a pathologist who examines tissue from a biopsy, or a radiologist who reads X-rays.) If you are having surgery, you may get a bill from the anesthesiologist.

It is often impossible to tell exactly what your charges will be until the exam, testing, and treatment are all over.

Another area where the office staff can help is when you have questions about charges or your bill. At the end of each exam, you will probably receive an itemized bill. This bill lists common exam types, procedures, and diagnoses with their codes. The codes are used by the office as well as insurance companies to control charges and collect information. Here are some terms you may see which relate to the type of exam performed:

- comprehensive—a "full" eye exam which includes history, vision, confrontation visual fields, muscle testing, pressure check, microscopic exam, dilated exam, and some special tests
- emergency—an unforeseen visit made for a special, sudden problem; charges will vary according to problem and special testing or procedures required
- established—means you have been seen by this doctor before (within the past 3 years, time limit may vary)
- intermediate—a shorter eye exam that includes history, vision, external exam, and some special tests (example: a 6-month dilated exam for diabetes)
- limited—a short exam that includes history, vision, and special tests that pertain only to a certain problem (example: routine pressure check in glaucoma)
- new—means this is your first appointment (within 3 years, time limit may vary) with this doctor
- refraction—the "glasses check" portion of the exam

If you are having surgery, charges can be estimated before the procedure is done. Circumstances that require the doctor to use additional equipment or supplies will probably increase the fee. Also, find out if you will be billed separately for any items or services (such as operating room time, the cost of any implants, nursing staff, etc.).

You may be able to economize a little by having more than one procedure at a time, if that is appropriate. Going into the operating room once is always cheaper than twice! Ask your doctor if having the two procedures together is possible, and if this will save you any money. An example would be having a lower lid blepharoplasty done at the same time as the uppers. Or suppose you are scheduled for cataract surgery, and have a growth on your eyelid that you want removed. Ask the surgeon to remove the growth at the same time as the cataract.

When you are making financial plans for surgery, find out how much follow-up time is included in the surgeon's fee. This usually depends on the procedure (for example, a cataract extraction would have more follow-up time than a growth removal).

Insurance in Brief

Okay, we'll admit it. Both authors are more comfortable talking to you about medical things. But since you need to know about insurance, we asked the experts: the ladies who do the actual filing day in and day out. In this section we'll examine their best advice.

First, you must understand that your health insurance is a contract between you and the insurance company. It is not the responsibility of the doctor's office to "get the company to pay." The job of the doctor's office is to report an expense and *request* payment. It is up to *you* to be sure that the insurance company holds up their part of the bargain. It is important that you know your policy. No company will pay for a procedure that is not covered by your contract, and no doctor's office can convince them that they should.

There are so many companies and different policies out there that no insurance clerk can be familiar with them all. Only your insurance company representative who is familiar with *your* policy can tell you for certain whether an item will be covered or not.

The good news is that most every office is familiar with Medicare. If Medicare is your primary (main) insurance, filing is fairly cut and dry. The world of secondary (supplemental) insurance can be confusing.

More good news is that the doctor's office will often file your insurance for you. Be sure to ask before your appointment. If the office files for you, you MUST provide them with:

1. your CURRENT (up-to-date) insurance card
2. the address of the insurance company
3. a signed release giving the doctor's office permission to release records to the insurance company

There may be certain circumstances where you must file for yourself. Filing procedures may vary from one company to the next, but usually all you need to do is:

1. obtain a copy of the company's claim form
2. fill out the patient portion (name, address, policy number, etc.)
3. attach a copy of the doctor's itemized bill

Insurance Payment

Usually the insurance payment goes right to the doctor's office, where it is credited to your account. However, in some cases the check may come directly to you. In this instance, it is very important that you take the check (and any letter that may have come with it) to the doctor's office. You must sign the check over to the doctor as payment of your medical bill. Some people are confused, thinking that the insurance company is sending them a check for their personal use. They cash the check and make the mortgage payment with the money. In reality, the check was issued to the patient for paying the doctor. The doctor's office receives a notice from the insurance company that the patient has been sent the check, so the money can always be traced. This type of misunderstanding can be very embarrassing! Don't let it happen to you.

What Insurance Approves vs. What Insurance Pays

This is another concept that is very important to understand, especially with Medicare.

What insurance "approves" is the insurance company's idea of the charge for a service. For example, suppose the doctor's fee for a special test is $100.00. Now imagine that your insurance company only approves a charge of $60.00 for the test.

But that doesn't mean that the company will pay the $60.00. The insurance company will only pay a percentage of its approved charge. The percentage varies according to your policy. Suppose your policy will cover 80% of the approved charge. In our example, then, insurance would pay $48.00 on the $100 test. That leaves a balance of $52.00 owed the doctor.

As this book goes to press, physicians who are Medicare providers have agreed to accept what insurance approves and write off the rest. This creates misunderstandings of its own. This is NOT an agreement for the doctor to accept only what insurance actually pays. So in the above example:

> $100.00 physician's fee
> −$60.00 approved charge
> $40.00 doctor writes off (looses)

$60 X 80%= $48.00 insurance payment

> $60.00 approved charge
> −$48.00 insurance payment
> $12.00 approved but not paid by insurance (payment comes out of your own pocket, termed "co-payment")

Procedures that are not approved at all by insurance are charged to you. An example is the refraction (glasses check), for which Medicare does not approve payment. This is billed directly to the patient.

Common Terms

Insurance jargon can be confusing. Here's a glossary of common insurance terms and what they mean.

- accept assignment—the office will accept the amount that your insurance approves
- accept what insurance approves—same as accept assignment
- accept what insurance pays—an illegal practice in which the physician accepts insurance payment and writes off the balance
- allowable (or approved) charges—the amount a company will allow for a certain procedure that is covered under your policy
- coinsurance (or co-payment)—the payment you make out of your pocket to cover the difference between what insurance approves and what insurance pays
- covered procedures—those tests, exams, and surgery that your policy will help pay for (read your policy)
- deductible—a set amount of money that you must pay (usu-

ally per year) before your insurance will begin making payment, even for some covered charges

- Medicaid—provides medical care for the indigent ("welfare"); the dollar amount paid for medical services varies with the recipient's income
- Medicare—government-issued insurance for those over 65 or disabled
- Medicare part A—covers hospital services; there is no premium
- Medicare part B—covers physician services, lab and testing, and other services; it is voluntary, and there is a premium
- non-covered procedures—those tests, exams, and surgery that your policy will NOT help pay for (read your policy)
- participating physician—a doctor who has agreed to file insurance for patients using a specific insurance company
- premium—your payments to the insurance company to "buy" your policy
- primary insurance—if you have more than one policy, the primary is always filed first
- prior approval (also called preauthorization and precertification)—a requirement by the insurance company that you notify them BEFORE having certain services (such as surgery), otherwise they may not make payment
- release of information—you agree, by signature, that the doctor's office can release your medical information to the insurance company in order to obtain payment
- second opinion—a requirement by the insurance company that you see another doctor about your condition before the company will agree to pay for certain services (such as surgery)
- secondary (supplemental) insurance—if you have secondary insurance, it is filed second, after the primary insurance has paid
- superbill—a detailed receipt from your physician which you can use to file insurance yourself
- write-off—the difference between the doctor's charges and what insurance approves (the physician takes this as a loss)

Other Financial Assistance

There are many clubs and organizations that offer financial help to those in need of eye care. Your local Lions or Lioness Clubs may be able to provide some assistance with low vision aids or other materials. Knights Templar usually directs their funds toward eye surgery.

If you cannot afford your eye medications, tell your doctor. The office may have samples you can have. Also, some drug companies have a program to make medications available to those who need financial assistance. Someone in your doctor's office should be able to register you. The medications will come to the office and be given to you from there.

Sometimes the needed assistance isn't financial. You might be in a position to guide someone who is visually impaired. Plus, there are many companies and groups that offer aid of one sort or another. Read the next chapter to learn more!

CHAPTER 20

Help: How to Give It, How to Get It

THE whole family held their breath while Dr. Jackson removed the bandage from Eileen Britton's right eye. Both eyes had been blind for several years because of corneal disease. But yesterday Mrs. Britton had a corneal transplant. The patch was off. Everyone waited.

"I can see!"

Suddenly everyone was laughing and talking at once.

Several days later, at home, Mrs. Britton sighed.

"What's the matter, Mom?" asked her daughter.

"I was thinking of my new cornea. It came from someone else, you know . . . a young man who was killed in a car wreck. What a tragic loss of life."

Her daughter nodded, but took her mother's hand and squeezed it. "I do feel bad for his family. But I'm so grateful for their generosity. Mom, they gave life back . . . to you!"

Organ donating is only one way to help others. In this chapter we will look at helping others and finding help for yourself when visual problems occur.

Disability

The term "disability" refers to a person who has a handicap that limits normal function. The disability might be physical (such as loss of a limb), sensory (such as low vision), or mental.

Your local Social Security office and/or social worker can help you learn what benefits you might be entitled to and how to go about getting them. To find a social worker, call your local Department of Family and Children's Services.

If you have worked for a certain period of time, you may be eligible for Social Security Disability Income. The amount of this monthly income depends on how long you worked and what your salary was. If you are visually impaired and have dependent children, they may be eligible for benefits, too. Another type of income, Supplemental Security Income, is available to low-income visually impaired persons based on the income of the immediate family. You may also qualify for health care benefits from Medicare or Medicaid. Regulations for these funds and services change periodically, so check with your social worker.

Your social worker will help you apply for the services you need. Often a letter or form is sent to your physician requesting information about your condition. The agencies will specifically want to know your diagnosis, your vision, the extent of your disability, the length of your disability, how your disability affects your life, and any prospect of improvement.

Other assistance that may be available includes financial assistance for buying special equipment, tax benefits (exemptions and deductions), rent subsidy, food stamps, scholarships, and telephone directory assistance. You may even qualify for handicapped parking for the person who drives for you (as long as you are with them).

If your visual disability is temporary, you may still qualify for some help. This might include disability pay, temporary credit suspension, and other services.

Donating

"Organ donation" makes most folks think of the highly dramatic donations of hearts and kidneys. Some organ gifts may seem small, but have tremendous impact on those who receive them. Eye donation is one of those. In 1990 alone, some 1132 eye surgeries were performed in Georgia using donated eye tissue, usually the cornea. Today, up to 30 such surgeries may be scheduled in one week.

A person of any age can be an eye donor, and most eyes are acceptable. The Georgia Eye Bank reports that of the 50,000 deaths in that state each year, some 49,000 of them would be usable donations. It doesn't matter if a person wears glasses or contacts. Even someone who has glaucoma, has had cataract surgery, or has other eye problems can be a donor.

All you have to do to be an eye donor is sign the back of your driver's license or an eye donor card. There is never any cost to the family of a donor, and all donated eyes are used in the fight to prevent blindness.

How to Guide the Blind/Partially Sighted

The Golden Rule in helping the visually disabled is to ASK if they need help. If you are guiding a blind person, don't push them ahead of you. Let them take your elbow and walk beside or slightly behind you. Give the person a description of where you are going as you walk. For example, suppose a blind woman is visiting your church and you are guiding her to your classroom: "Mrs. Earl, I'm so glad you're visiting us today. May I go with you to your classroom?"

"Yes, thank you, and please call me Judy. I do fine in places I'm familiar with, but a new place is always a challenge!"

"I understand. Would you like to take my arm? We'll go down this hallway to our left . . . now we take the hall to the right. Here's a doorway. Our class is the first door on the right. Here we are, another doorway. The chairs are set up on either side, with an aisle leading from the door. Do you prefer to sit in any particular spot?"

"I like to sit on the aisle with the door behind me to my left."

"That's fine. Here we are. The chair is on your right."

"Thanks so much! I was a little nervous about coming to a new place. You're a great guide!"

"Oh, you're welcome! I have to go back to the welcome station now, but this is my class, too. I'll be back a few minutes after the bell rings. We can go into the sanctuary together after class. Let me introduce you to our teacher . . ."

If you must negotiate stairs, first give a verbal warning. Stop at the edge of the first step. You will stay one step ahead each time. When you get to the bottom, pause again.

Other Ways to Help

Here are some other suggestions: Don't talk louder! Speak directly to the person, not to others around or with him/her. Let the person know when you've come into the room and when you leave. A blind person can't see you smile, but can hear it in your voice. Give any directions from the blind person's point of view (such as "on your right" or "on your left"). If you've brought him to an unfamiliar place, describe where he is, especially where the exits are. Tell where food is on a plate (*only* if asked!) by giving clock positions (for example, "meat at twelve o'clock, potatoes at four, and beans at eight").

If you are writing to a partially sighted person, use a black marker and make your letters two or three lines tall. For gifts to the visually impaired, you might consider a large print address book, crossword puzzle book, or cook book. Books on tape are also an excellent choice, as is a good reading lamp.

There are many other ways to help the blind and partially sighted. For example, some of the organizations listed at the end of this chapter accept donations or offer memberships. Others may be able to lead you to volunteer agencies where you could help. Recording books on tape is another way to contribute.

Finding Information

There are many places you can go to for information on organizations, companies, and agencies that help the blind and partially sighted. Your local public library is a good place to start. The reference section should have some books that can help you find publications and organizations.

A medical or hospital library may be able to help, too. Even if the library doesn't carry specific lists of agencies, it probably has access to such a list. Many medical library computers are connected to MedLine (a computer pathway to the National Library of Medicine). Within the MedLine link is a special service to find organizations. The search is done by topic (such as "blindness") and by state. Thus you can get specific information on agencies that help the blind in your state. The print-out includes name, address, phone number, and a description of services.

You should also contact your state's Commission for the Blind. Some states have a printed resource guide listing the different agencies and services available in the state as well as nationally.

We have compiled a list of some of the agencies that might be able to help. Name and phone number (plus address and description when available) are given. Some of the organizations listed are research facilities that are working on ways to prevent blindness. Others are service agencies, or provide information.

Publications

* the following information is subject to change.

- *Directory of Services for Blind and Visually Impaired Persons in the United States.* Write to the American Foundation for the Blind, 11 Penn Plaza, Ste. 300, New York, NY 10001 (or call 1-800-232-5463)
- *Living With Low Vision: A Resource Guide for People with Sight Loss* by Fran A. Weisse and Susan L. Greenblatt. Write to Resources for Rehabilitation, 33 Bedford St., Ste. 19A, Lexington, MA 02173

A free list of National Institute of Health publications can be obtained by writing: Editorial Operations Branch, NIH; Bldg 37 Room 2B03; Rockville, MD 20892

For information on health services, write: Office of Communications; Health Resources and Services Administration; 5600 Fishers Lane; Rockville, MD 20857

The following can be obtained from Superintendent of Documents, US Government Printing Office, Washington, D.C. 20402 (or call the order desk at 202-783-3238); prices and availability subject to change:

- *Self-Care and Self-Help Groups for the Elderly: A Directory.* National Institute on Aging. 1984. 128 pages. NIH Publication # 84-738. S/N 017-062-00134-1. HE20.3852:E12. $4.25
- *Directory of State and Area Agencies on Aging.* Committee Publication # 99-490. Y4.Ag4/2:Ag4/9/985.
- *Nutrition and Your Health: Dietary Guidelines for Americans.* Home & Garden Bulletin 232. S/N 001-000-04248-3. A1.77:232. $2.25
- *Directory of Living Aids for the Disabled Person.* Veterans Administration 1982. S/N 051-000-00158-3. VA1.2:D63/3. $7.50
- *Directory of National Information Sources on Handicapping Conditions and Related Services.* 3rd ed. Office of Special Education and Rehabilitation Services. S/N 065-000-00142-0. ED1.202:H19/2. $8.00
- *Diabetes and Your Eyes.* NIH Publication # 83-2171. HE20.3002:D54/4/983.

- *Pocket Guide to Federal Help for the Disabled Person.* Dept. of Education. S/N 065-000-00227-2. ED1.8:D63/985. $1.00
- *Recreation and Leisure for Handicapped Individuals: Information, Resources, Funding Guide, Publications Available from Federal Resources.* S/N 065-000-00076-8. ED1.8:R26/2. $5.50
- *Address List: Regional and Sub-regional Libraries for the Blind and Physically Handicapped.* LC19.17:983.
- *Braille Books.* LC19.9/2:982.
- *Braille Scores Catalog. Pt. 1–Classical, Music and Musicians. Pt. 2–Popular, Music and Musicians.* LC19.2:M97/13/pt.1,2.
- *Cassette Books.* LC19.10/3:983.
- *Historical Fiction.* LC19.11:H62.
- *Talking Books: Adult.* LC19.10/2:982-83.

Other Books of Interest:

The International Low Vision Directory by Anne Yeadon. Write to Institute for the Visually Impaired, Pennsylvania College of Optometry, 1200 W. Godfrey Ave., Philadelphia, PA 19141.USA

Guide to Popular US Government Publications by LeRoy C. Schwarzkopf (reference section of your local library)

What to do When You Can't Afford Health Care by Matthew Lesko. Published by Information USA (reference section of your local library)

Organizations

* the following information is subject to change.

Encyclopedia of Associations by Gale Research, Inc. This book may be in the reference section of your local library. Look up organizations by using key words such as eye, eyes, blind, blindness, vision, visual, visual impairment, visually impaired, visually handicapped, and sight.

American Academy of Ophthalmology
P.O. Box 7424
San Francisco, CA 94120
phone 415-561-8500
(ask for brochures on eye care available to public)

American Council of the Blind (ACB)
1155 15th St. NW, Ste. 720
Washington, DC 20005
phone 1-800-424-8666
(information, referral, legal consultation, membership)

American Foundation for the Blind
11 Penn Plaza, Ste. 300
New York, NY 10001
phone 1-800-232-5463
(job index, low vision clinic, aids, training, more)

Associated Services for the Blind
919 Walnut St.
Philadelphia, PA 19107
phone 215-627-0600

Association for the Education & Rehabilitation of the Blind and Visually Impaired
206 N. Washington St., Ste. 320
Alexandria, VA 22314
phone 703-548-1884
(a membership organization, 2 newsletters)

Association for Macular Disease
210 E. 64th St.
New York, NY 10021
phone 212-605-3719
(newsletter and hotline for those with macular disease; non-profit, accepts donations)

Braille Institute
741 N. Vermont Ave.
Los Angeles, CA 90029
phone 213-663-1111
(braille and talking books at no charge, but you must apply)

Council of Citizens with Low Vision
1400 N. Drake Rd., No. 218
Kalamezoo, MI 49007
phone 1-800-733-2258

Fight for Sight, Inc.
160 E. 56th St., 8th Floor
New York, NY 10022
phone 212-751-1118
(research, referrals, information)

Foundation for Glaucoma Research (FGR)
490 Post St., Ste. 830
San Francisco, CA 94102
phone 415-986-3162
(educational material, informal non-medical counselling network, *Gleams* newsletter)

Guide Dog Foundation for the Blind
371 E. Jericho Tpke.
Smithtown, NY 11787
phone 516-265-2121
(accept applications, provide brochures and training)

Knights Templar Eye Foundation
P.O. Box 579
Springfield, IL 62705-0579
phone 217-523-3838
(eye treatment and hospital care for the needy)

Lions Clubs International
300 22nd St.
Oak Brook, IL 60521
phone 708-571-5466
(call to find a local group near you; local organizations offer rehabilitation,
aids, and devices)

National Association for the Visually Handicapped
22 West 21st St.
New York, NY 10010
phone 212-889-3141
(membership organization: counselling, education, lending library,
large print books, low vision aids)

National Braille Association
#3 Town Line Circle
Rochester, NY 14623-2513
phone 716-427-8260
(free catalog in print or on cassette, braille books, music, text books,
transcribing, education/seminars)

National Braille Press
88 St. Stephen St.
Boston, MA 02115
phone 617-266-6160
 (free brochures and catalog, books and tapes such as crafts, cooking,
computers)

National EyeCare Project
P.O. Box 429098
San Francisco, CA 94142-9098
phone 1-800-222-EYES
(Sponsored by the American Academy of Ophthalmology, this helps
provide medical eye care for the elderly, especially the needy. Call
or write for a fact sheet and information.)

National Eye Institute
Bldg. 31 Room 6A32
31 Center Dr. MSC 2510
Bethesda, MD 20892-2510
phone 301-496-5248
(provides resources, journal articles, refers to organizations that study particular eye problems, refers to clinical studies looking for patients)

National Eye Research Foundation
910 Skokie Blvd., No. 207A
Northbook, IL 60062
phone 708-564-4652
(public information center on eye care)

The National Federation of the Blind
1800 Johnson St.
Baltimore, MD 21230
phone 410-659-9314
(tapes, braille, and large print materials dealing with the emotional and legal aspects of visual impairment; *Braille Monitor* magazine)

National Library Service for the Blind and Physically Handicapped
Reference Section
Library of Congress
1291 Taylor St., NW
Washington, DC 20542
phone 1-800-424-8567
(library service, information on blindness, bibliographies)

National Society to Prevent Blindness
500 E. Remington Rd.
Schaumburg, IL 60173
phone 708-843-2020
(information on eye disease and injury)

Recording for the Blind
20 Roszel Rd.
Princeton, NJ 08540
phone 609-452-0606, 1-800-221-4792
(lends taped educational books to student of all ages and adults in business and the professions)

Vision Foundation
818 Mt. Auburn St.
Watertown, MA 02172
phone 617-926-4232
(self-help organization, buddy phone network, Visually Impaired Elders project, information, resources)

Xavier Society for the Blind
The National Catholic Press and Library for the Visually Handicapped
154 East 23rd St.
New York, NY 10010
1-800-637-9193
(Provides braille, large print, or cassette materials, primarily spiritual material)

Additional Sources of Products

* the following information is subject to change.

American Printing House for the Blind
P.O. Box 6085
Louisville, KY 40206
phone 502-895-2405
(catalog of educational materials, supplies, books, aids, etc.)

Associated Services for the Blind
919 Walnut St.
Philadelphia, PA 19107
phone 1-800-876-5456
(retail and catalog sales)

Independent Living Aids, Inc.
27 E. Mall
Plainview, NY 11803
phone 516-752-8080

Lighthouse Low Vision Products
36-02 Northern Blvd.
Long Island City, NY 11101
phone 1-800-453-4923
(free catalog, consumer items, publications)

Science Products for the Blind
Box 888
Southeastern, PA 19399
phone 1-800-888-7400
(free catalog)

Computer Adaptations and Software

* the following information is subject to change.

American Foundation for the Blind
11 Penn Plaza, Ste. 300
New York, NY 10001
phone 1-800-232-5463
(information, reading machine)

American Printing House for the Blind
P.O. Box 6085
Louisville, KY 40206
 phone 502-895-2405
(catalog, software, hardware)

American Thermoform Corporation
2311 Traverse Ave.
City of Commerce, CA 90040
phone 213-723-9021
(printer that produces braille and ink on same copy)

Digital Equipment Corporation
P.O. Box CS 2008
Nashua, NH 03061-2008
phone 1-800-344-4825
 (speech sythesizer)

HumanWare
6245 King Rd.
Loomis, CA 95650
phone 1-800-722-3393
(lap top computer with speech)

Recording for the Blind
phone 1-800-221-4792
(taped references about computers)

Telesensory Systems, Inc.
455 N. Bernardo Ave.
Mountain View, CA 94043
phone 415-960-0920
(speech synthesizer, braille display, print to tactile image conversion)

Vision Research and Care

* the following information is subject to change.

Eye Bank Association of America
 1001 Connecticut Ave., NW, Ste. 601
Washington, DC 20036-5504
phone 202-775-4999
(promotes donor programs)

Fight for Sight, Inc.
160 E. 56th St., 8th Floor
New York, NY 10022
phone 212-751-1118

Lions and Lioness Clubs
check your local phone directory for group in your area

Myopia International Research Foundation
1265 Broadway: Room 608
New York, NY 10001
phone 212-684-2777
(research on nearsightedness, funded by private donations)

Recording for the Blind
20 Roszel Rd.
Princeton, NJ 08540
phone 609-452-0606, 1-800-221-4792
(needs volunteers to make recordings)

APPENDIX A

Glaucoma Medications

The numbers in parenthesis following the strength of eye drops is the size bottle(s) available (*ml* means milliliters; there are about 20 drops in one ml). In addition to the actual medication, these drugs also contain various carriers, buffers, and preservatives. Thus an allergic reaction might be due to the preservative or other component, and not to the drug at all. Side effects listed here are those that the drug itself might cause. Symptoms of mild allergic reaction include rash and itching. Serious allergic reaction might be indicated by shortness of breath and/or tightness in the chest. Contact your physician or pharmacist if you seem to be allergic to your medication.

Drug interactions are another area of concern. Make sure that the physician who prescribes your glaucoma medications knows about ALL other medicines you take, *even over-the-counter-ones*. Also inform your medical doctor about your eye medications.

Location Key

To look up your medication, locate the trade name and find the drug name. The medications are listed in alphabetical order by drug name.

Trade name	Drug name
Eye drops:	
AKarpine	pilocarpine
Betagan	levobunolol
Betoptic	betaxolol
Betoptic-S	betaxolol
Epifrin	epinephrine
E-Pilo	pilocarpine/epinephrine combination
Eppy/N	epinephrine

Trade name	Drug name
Eye drops (continued):	
Glaucon	epinephrine
Humorsol	demarcarium
Iopidine	apraclonidine
Isopto Carbachol	carbachol
Isopto Carpine	pilocarpine
Ocu-Carpine	pilocarpine
Ocupress	carteolol
OptiPranolol	metapranolol
PE	pilocarpine/epinephrine combination
Phospholine iodide	echothiophate iodide
Pilagan	pilocarpine
Pilo	pilocarpine
Pilocar	pilocarpine
Pilostat	pilocarpine
Propine	dipivalyl epinephrine
Timoptic	timolol
Ointments:	
Eserine	physostigmine
Floropryl	isoflurophate
Pilopine gel	pilocarpine
Eye inserts:	
Ocusert	pilocarpine
Oral medications, tablets and pills:	
Diamox	acetazolamide
Neptazane	methazolamide
Oral medications, liquids:	
Glyrol	glycerin
Osmoglyn	glycerin
IV fluids:	
Diamox	acetazolamide
Osmitrol	mannitol
Ureaphil	urea

Drug Listing

Eye Drops

Drug name: apraclonidine
Trade name(s): Iopidine
Strength(s): 1% (Comes in bullets of 0.1 ml, two bullets in each foil pouch. Also comes in bottle.)
Purpose/action: Decreases aqueous formation.
Side effects: May cause decreased blood pressure, slow heart rate, sleeplessness, irritability, impotence.
Notes: Used in the office before and after certain laser treatments to prevent a pressure rise in the eye. May be used at home for a short period of time. Protect drops from light.

Drug name: betaxolol
Trade name(s): Betoptic, Betoptic S
Strength(s): Betoptic S = 0.25% (2.5, 5, 10, 15 ml); Betoptic = 0.5% (2.5, 5, 10, 15 ml)
Purpose/action: Selective beta blocker, believed to decrease aqueous production.
Side effects: Does not appear to affect breathing as much as others in this group. May rarely cause nausea, vomiting, diarrhea, impotence, loss of appetite, sleeplessness, slow heart beat, dizziness, headache, lack of energy. May sting.
Notes: After instilling drop, close eyes and gently press fingers against inner corners of eyes for about one minute. If using Betoptic S, gently shake bottle before use. May need to gradually decrease use if general anesthesia is planned.

Drug name: carbachol
Trade name(s): Isopto Carbachol
Strength(s): 0.75%, 1.5%, 2.25%, 3% (All come in 15 and 30 ml bottles except for 2.25%, which comes in 15 ml bottle only.)
Purpose/action: Believed to increase outflow of aqueous by pulling open the drainage meshwork.
Side effects: Pupils are made very small. May blur vision. May decrease night vision, may decrease side vision. May cause sweating, salivation, nausea, vomiting, diarrhea, weakness and fatigue, decreased blood pressure, tremor.
Notes: May sting. May cause headaches when first started, this

usually decreases with use. Often prescribed instead of pilocarpine when pilocarpine is ineffective or not usable. Not usually used in patients with heart failure, asthma, active peptic ulcer, hyperthyroid, Parkinson's disease, recent stroke, or high or low blood pressure.

Drug name: carteolol
Trade name(s): Ocupress
Strength(s): 1% (5, 10 ml). Bottle has white cap. Label has blue letters.
Purpose/action: Beta blocker, believed to decrease aqueous production.
Side effects: Slowed heart beat, heart palpitations, lowered blood pressure, shortness of breath, nausea, vomiting, diarrhea, impotence, loss of appetite, sleeplessness, confusion.
Notes: Not usually used in patients with lung disease (asthma or emphysema, for instance) or heart disease (such as congestive heart failure, slow heart beat, heart block, and low blood pressure). Thought to have less effect on cholesterol. After instilling drop, close eyes and gently press fingers against inner corners of eyes for about one minute. May sting. May need to gradually decrease use if general anesthesia is planned.

Drug name: demecarium
Trade name(s): Humorsol
Strength(s): 0.124%, 0.25% (5 ml)
Purpose/action: Believed to increase outflow of aqueous by pulling open the drainage meshwork.
Side effects: Pupils are made very small. May blur vision. May decrease night vision, may decrease side vision. May cause sweating, salivation, nausea, vomiting, diarrhea, abdominal cramps weakness and fatigue, decreased blood pressure.
Notes: Not used in angle closure glaucoma. After instilling drop, close eyes and gently press fingers against inner corners of eyes for about one minute. May sting. May cause headaches when first started, this usually decreases with use. Wash hands after use.
Interactions: Must be discontinued if general anesthesia (using succinylcholine) is needed.

Drug name: dipivalyl epinephrine
Trade name(s): Propine
Strength(s): 0.1% (5, 10, 15 ml). Has purple top.
Purpose/action: May increase aqueous outflow through blood vessels, also decreases aqueous production.
Side effects: Elevated blood pressure, rapid heart beat, headache. May sting, eye may get red, may cause allergic reaction in eye.
Notes: Similar to epinephrine, but side effects are not as strong. Not used in angle closure glaucoma.

Drug name: echothiophate iodide
Trade name(s): Phospholine iodide
Strength(s): 0.03%, 0.06%, 0.125%, 0.25% (5 ml dropper bottle with green cap and black bulb)
Purpose/action: Believed to increase outflow of aqueous by pulling open the drainage meshwork.
Side effects: Pupils are made very small. May blur vision. May decrease night vision, may decrease side vision. May cause headaches when first started, this usually decreases with use. May cause iris cysts, cataracts, retinal detachment, sweating, salivation, nausea, vomiting, diarrhea, abdominal cramps, weakness and fatigue, decreased blood pressure.
Notes: Must be kept refrigerated. May sting. Not used in angle closure glaucoma. After instilling drop, close eyes and gently press fingers against inner corners of eyes for about one minute.
Interactions: Must be discontinued before use of general anesthesia.

Drug name: epinephrine
Trade name(s): Epifrin, Eppy/N, Glaucon
Strength(s): 0.25%, 0.5%, 1%, 2% (Bottle size varies among manufacturers. 7.5 and 10 ml size is common. Epinephrine 1:1000 comes in 12 ml droperettes.)
Purpose/action: May increase aqueous outflow through blood vessels, also decreases aqueous formation.
Side effects: Dilates pupils. May cause rapid heart beat, heart palpitations, headache, fainting, increased blood pressure.
Notes: Not usually used in patients with heart problems. Not used in patients who have had cataract surgery WITHOUT intraocular lens implant. Not used in angle closure glaucoma. After instilling

drop, close eyes and gently press fingers against inner corners of eyes for about one minute.

Drug name: levobunolol
Trade name(s): Betagan
Strength(s): 0.25% (5, 10 ml), 0.5% (5, 10, 15 ml)
Purpose/action: Beta blocker, believed to decrease aqueous production.
Side effects: Slowed heart beat, decreased blood pressure, shortness of breath, nausea, vomiting, diarrhea, impotence, loss of appetite, sleeplessness, headache.
Notes: Not usually used in patients with lung disease or heart failure. After instilling drop, close eyes and gently press fingers against inner corners of eyes for about one minute. May sting. If you miss a dose, don't try to catch up by using two drops instead of one.
Interactions: May need to gradually decrease use if general anesthesia is planned.

Drug Name: metapranolol
Trade name(s): OptiPranolol
Strength(s): 0.3% (5, 10 ml). Bottle has a white cap. Label has blue and black letters.
Purpose/action: Beta blocker, believed to decrease aqueous production. May slightly increase drainage.
Side effects: Slowed heart beat, heart palpitations, headache, altered blood pressure, shortness of breath, nausea, vomiting, diarrhea, impotence, loss of appetite, sleeplessness, confusion.
Notes: Not usually used in patients with lung disease or congestive heart failure. After instilling drop, close eyes and gently press fingers against inner corners of eyes for about one minute. May need to gradually decrease use if general anesthesia is planned.

Drug name: pilocarpine
Trade name(s): Akarpine, Isopto Carpine, Ocu-Carpine, Pilagan, Pilo, Pilocar, Pilostat
Strength(s): 0.25%, 0.5%, 1%, 2%, 3%, 4%, 5%, 6%, 8%, 10% (Bottle size varies according to manufacturer. 15 and 30 ml seem standard.) All have a green top.
Purpose/action: Believed to increase outflow of aqueous by pulling open draining meshwork.

Side effects: Pupils are made very small. May blur vision. May decrease night vision, may decrease side vision. May cause sweating, salivation, nausea, vomiting, diarrhea, weakness and fatigue, altered blood pressure, tremor, fast heart beat.

Notes: May sting. May cause headaches when first started (this usually decreases with use).

Drug name: pilocarpine/epinephrine combination
Trade names(s): PE, E-Pilo
Strength(s): This preparation has 1% epinephrine. The strength of the pilocarpine varies: 1,2,3,4, and 6% are available.
Purpose/action: Reduces aqueous production and increases outflow.
Side effects: Difficulty in dark adaptation. Eye irritation, headache, heart palpitations, irregular heart beat.
Notes: Not used in angle closure glaucoma. Used with caution in those with hypothyroid, high blood pressure, heart disease, and bronchial asthma. Protect drops from light.
Interactions: May need to discontinue prior to use of general anesthesia.

Drug name: timolol
Trade name(s): Timoptic, Timoptic XE
Strength(s): 0.25% (blue top), 0.50% (yellow top). Both strengths available in 2.5, 5, 10, 15 ml. Preservative free preparations in both strengths are available in single-dose vials (0.45 ml). 0.5% has yellow tag, 0.25% has blue tag.
Purpose/action: Beta blocker, believed to decrease aqueous production.
Side effects: Slowed heart beat, heart palpitations, lowered blood pressure, shortness of breath, nausea, vomiting, diarrhea, impotence, loss of appetite, sleeplessness, confusion.
Notes: Not usually used in patients with lung disease (asthma or emphysema, for instance) or heart disease (such as congestive heart failure, slow heart beat, heart block, and low blood pressure). After instilling drop, close eyes and gently press fingers against inner corners of eyes for about one minute.
Interactions: May need to gradually decrease use if general anesthesia is planned.

Eye Ointments

Drug name: isoflurophate
Trade name(s): Floropryl
Strength(s): 0.0215% (3.5 g tube). Label is blue and white.
Purpose/action: Believed to increase outflow of aqueous.
Side effects: Pupils are made very small. May blur vision. May rarely cause sweating, salivation, nausea, vomiting, diarrhea, weakness and fatigue, decreased blood pressure.
Notes: Wash hands after use. May cause headaches when first started, this usually decreases with use.
Interaction: Must be discontinued before use of general anesthesia.

Drug name: physostigmine
Trade name(s): Eserine
Strength(s): 0.25% (3.5 g tube). Tube is green and white.
Purpose/action: Believed to increase outflow of aqueous.
Side effects: Pupils are made very small. May blur vision. May decrease night vision, may decrease side vision. May cause headaches when first started, this usually decreases with use. May cause sweating, salivation, nausea, vomiting, diarrhea, weakness and fatigue, decreased blood pressure. Allergic reaction in the eye is common.

Drug name: pilocarpine
Trade name(s): Pilopine gel
Strength(s): 4% (5 gram tube)
Purpose/action: Believed to increase outflow of aqueous.
Side effects: Pupils are made very small. May blur vision. May decrease night vision, may decrease side vision. May cause headaches when first started, this usually decreases with use. May cause sweating, salivation, nausea, vomiting, diarrhea, weakness and fatigue, decreased blood pressure.
Notes: Convenient because it only has to be used once daily. If used at bedtime, any blurred vision occurs during sleep.

Eye Inserts

Drug name: pilocarpine
Trade name(s): Ocusert
Strength(s): 20, 40 (box of 8)
Purpose/action: Believed to increase outflow of aqueous.

Side effects: Pupils are made very small. May blur vision. May decrease night vision, may decrease side vision. May cause headaches when first started, this usually decreases with use. May cause sweating, salivation, nausea, vomiting, diarrhea, weakness and fatigue, decreased blood pressure.

Notes: Convenient because the insert is replaced every seven days. Wash hands before and after placement. It is best to replace at bedtime. Check for the presence of the insert before and after sleep.

Oral Medications

Tablets and Pills

Drug name: acetazolamide
Trade name(s): Diamox
Strength(s): 125 mg (white tablet), 250 mg (white tablet); 500 mg (orange sustained-release capsules)
Purpose/action: Blocks formation of aqueous.
Side effects: Tingling or numbness in hands or feet, weakness, fatigue, drowsiness, nausea, vomiting, weight loss, loss of appetite, impotence, kidney stones.
Notes: Not used if patient is allergic to sulfa. Not combined with high doses of aspirin.

Drug name: methazolamide
Trade name(s): Neptazane
Strength(s): 25 mg (square white tablet), 50 mg (round white tablet)
Purpose/action: Decreases aqueous production.
Side effects: Numbness and tingling in hands and feet, drowsiness and fatigue, nausea and vomiting.
Notes: Not used if patient is allergic to sulfa. Not combined with high doses of aspirin. Not usually used in patients with kidney disease. Not used in patients with severe lung obstruction. In case of stomach problems, take over-the-counter antacids.

Liquid

Drug name: glycerin
Trade name(s): Osmoglyn, Glyrol
Purpose/action: Increases sugar content of blood, causing aqueous to be filtered out.

Side effects: Nausea, vomiting, headache.

Note: Used on an emergency basis to quickly reduce pressure in angle closure glaucoma attack. May be used to lower pressure before eye surgery.

Note: Not usually used in diabetic patients.

IV fluids

Drug name: acetazolamide
Trade name(s): Diamox
See above under Tablets and Pills.

Drug name: mannitol
Trade name(s): Osmitrol
Purpose/action: Draws aqueous fluid out of the eye.
Side effects: Altered blood pressure, chest pain, headache, blurred vision, dizziness, nausea, vomiting, diarrhea, dry mouth, thirst.
Note: Used on an emergency basis to quickly reduce pressure in angle closure glaucoma attack.

Drug name: urea
Trade name(s): Ureaphil
Purpose/action: Draws aqueous fluid out of the eye.
Side effects: If medication leaks into skin at injection site, may cause phlebitis and sloughing in that area.
Note: Used on an emergency basis to quickly reduce pressure in angle closure glaucoma attack.

APPENDIX B

Drugs Affecting the Eyes

THE *Physician's Desk Reference of Drug Side Effects* lists over 160 different types of drugs with side effects involving the eye. These include oral medications, eye medications, and injected medications. Those listed below are the drugs which were found to have a certain side effect 3% or more of the time. Those drugs not listed were reported to cause eye or vision problems less than 3% of the time. If you are taking any drug and experience any disturbance in your vision or eyes, contact your physician or pharmacist. This list is arranged alphabetically according to trade name (which are registered trademarks).

A/T/S—eye irritation (17 out of 90)
Accutane capsules—conjunctivitis (2 in 5), corneal opacities (5 in 72)
Anestacon solution—blurred vision, double vision
Artane—blurred vision (30–50%)
Asendin tablets—blurred vision (7%)
Bentyl—blurred vision (27%)
Buprenex injectable—small pupil (1–5%)
Cesamet pulvules—visual disturbances (13%)
Cordarone tablets—light sensitivity (4–9%), visual disturbances (4–9%)
Dilantin—jerking motions of eyes
Disopyramide phosphate CR capsules—blurred vision (3–9%), dry eye (3–9%)
Enkaid capsules—blurred vision (3.4%), visual disturbances (3.4%)
Extended phenytoin sodium—jerking motions of eyes
Intron A—visual disturbances (up to 7%)
Limitrol—blurred vision
Ludiomil tablets—blurred vision (4%)
Marplan tablets—blurred vision
Mexitil capsules—blurred vision (5.7–7.5%), visual disturbances (5.7–7.5%)

Naprosyn—visual disturbances (less than 7%)

Norpace—blurred vision (3–9%), dry eyes (3–9%)

Novantrone—conjunctivitis (0–5%), eye disorders (2–7%)

Orthoclone tablets—light sensitivity (4–9%)

Permax—visual disturbances (5.8%)

Quarzan capsules—blurred vision

Riduara capsules—conjunctivitis (3–9%)

Roferon-A injection—visual disturbances (5%)

Tambocor tablets—blurred vision (15.9%), visual disturbances (15.9%)

Tegison capsules—corneal changes (10–25%), double vision, dry eye (1–10%), eye disorders (50–75%), retinal disorder (10–25%), tearing (1–10%), visual disturbances (10–25%)

Tonocard tablets—blurred vision (1.3–10%), visual disturbances (1.3–10%)

Wellbutrin tablets—blurred vision (14.6%)

Xanax tablets—blurred vision (6.2%)

Oral contraceptives (birth control pills)

use of oral birth control can have the following effects on the eyes:

1. changes in the cornea-contact lens fit may change
2. increased risk of retinal vein occlusion - (see page 240)
3. increased risk of retinal artery occlusion - (see pages 236-237)
4. increased risk of optic neuritis - (see pages 231-233)
5. increased risk of ischemic optic neuropathy - (see pages 223-224)
6. "blind spots" associated with migraine headaches -
   (see pages129-130)

APPENDIX C

Medications Containing Aspirin

MOST of the medicines listed here are named by their registered trademarks. Some are over-the-counter, and some are prescription drugs. While as complete as we could make it, there are other aspirin-containing medications not on this list. Check with your physician or pharmacist.

Alka-Seltzer tablets
Alka-Seltzer Plus Cold
   Medicine
Anacin capsules and tablets
APC tablets
APC with codeine (Tabloid
   brand)
Anacin Maximum Strength
   capsules and tablets
Arthritis Pain Formula (by
   the makers of Anacin
   tablets)
Arthritis Strength Bufferin
Ascodeen-30
Ascriptin
Aspergum
Aspirin
Aspirin suppositories
Bayer Aspirin
Bayer Children's Chewable
   Aspirin
Bayer Children's Cold tablets
Bayer Timed-released Aspirin
BC powders

Buff-A-Comp tablets
Buffadyne
Bufferin
Butalbital
Cama Inlay-Tabs
Cheracol capsules
Congespirin
Coricidin D decongestant
   tablets
Coricidin for children
Coricidin Medilets tablets
Coricidin tablets
Darvon with A.S.A.
Darvon-N with A.S.A.
Dristan decongestant
Duragesic
Ecotrin tablets
Emprazil, Emprazil tablets
Empirin, Empirin with
   codeine
Emprazil-C tablets
Equagesic
Excedrin
Fiorinal, Fiorinal with codeine

4-Way Cold Tablets
Gemnisyn
Goody's Headache Powders
Indocin
Measurin
Midol
Momentum Muscular
    Backache Formula
Monacet with codeine
Norgesic, Norgesic Forte
Norwich Aspirin
Pabirin Buffered Tablets
Panalgesic
Pepto Bismal
Percodan, Percodan Demi
    tablets
Persistin
Quiet World Analgesic/
    Sleeping Aid

Robaxisal tablets
SK-65 Compound
St. Joseph Aspirin for
    Children
Sine-Aid
Sine-Off Sinus Medicine
    tablets (aspirin formula)
Stendin
Stero-Darvon with A.S.A.
Supac
Synalgos capsules
Synalgos-DC capsules
Tolectin
Triaminicin tablets
Vanquish
Verin
Viro-Med tablets
Zorprin

Non-Retinal Laser Surgery

Problem	Procedure	Reference
Dry eyes	Seal drainage ducts (Argon)	page 170
Angle closure glaucoma	Iridotomy (YAG or Argon)	page 263
Open angle glaucoma	Trabeculoplasty (Argon)	page 257
Open angle glaucoma	Cycloablation (laser microendoscope)	page 260
Cloudy posterior capsule after cataract surgery	Capsulotomy (YAG)	page 215

APPENDIX E

When to Call Your Doctor

Any case of:

- a sudden shower of new floaters
- flashes of light
- vision blacks out
- sudden loss of vision
- a "curtain" seems to come over your vision
- "blind spots" in your vision
- vision loss that comes and goes
- red and painful eye (with or without decreased vision)
- sudden double vision
- a new difference in the size between the pupils where one eye is red and light sensitive
- a skin growth that changes in size or appearance

If you have macular degeneration:

- increased or new distortion on the Amsler grid

If you have had cataract surgery:

- pain that does not go away
- irritation that is not relieved by using prescribed ointment
- drastically decreased vision after vision had begun to improve
- flashes of light
- new, large floaters or a sudden shower of floaters
- curtain over vision or vision blacks out

If you have had retinal laser:

- flashes of light
- new, large floaters or a sudden shower of floaters

- curtain over vision or vision blacks out

If you have had an accident:

- a foreign body in the eye
- the eye is painful
- an object has penetrated the eye (do NOT attempt to remove it yourself)
- the vision decreases
- chemicals splash in the eye (irrigate for 15 minutes immediately, then call)
- a wound becomes red, hot, swollen, and angry
- the pupil shape has changed
- you can see blood inside the eye in front of the iris
- you later develop any of the symptoms in the first category above

If you have had a corneal transplant:

- after improving, the eye begins to get worse (discomfort, red, light sensitive, watering, decreased vision)

If you have had a YAG laser capsulotomy:

- flashes of light
- new, large floaters or a sudden shower of floaters
- curtain over vision or vision blacks out

If you have had plastic surgery:

- the wound becomes angry, red, hot, and tender
- any sutures break
- an allergic reaction (rash, itching, shortness of breath, etc.)

Check Lists

Surgery Preperation Chart

Do you need:	Yes	No	Date
a preoperative exam by your surgeon			
a physical			
lab work			
to make prepayment			
to make arrangements for payment			
preregister at hospital/clinic			
obtain pre-authorization from insurance			
a second opinion			
Other instructions:			

Before surgery are you to:	Yes	No	Date
bathe and wash your hair			
use eye medications			
discontinue any eye medications			
stop eating and drinking after midnight			
leave out contact lenses			
discontinue medications containing			
aspirin			
discontinue blood thinners			
begin taking vitamin tablets			
Other instructions:			

On surgery day are you to:	Yes	No	Date
leave dentures or partials at home			
wear a button-up-the-front shirt			
take your regular medication			

take insulin or diabetic medication
have someone to drive you home
have someone to stay with you overnight
leave off any make-up
Other instructions:

After surgery are you to:	Yes	No	Date
remove the eye patch			
sleep on side opposite the operated eye			
sleep with head elevated			
use eye medications			
avoid straining			
avoid stooping			
return to the surgeon's office			
use over-the-counter pain medication as needed			
avoid aspirin-contining products			
Other instructions:			

When can you:	Yes	No	Date
drive			
wear make-up			
resume aspirin-containing products			
resume blood thinners			
go back to work			
resume all normal activities			
Other instructions:			

Medication Recording Chart

Medication name:				Dosage: right eye				Dosage: left eye			
Time:											
Day 1											
Day 2											
Day 3											
Day 4											
Day 5											
Day 6											
Day 7											

Medication name:				Dosage: right eye				Dosage: left eye			
Time:											
Day 1											
Day 2											
Day 3											
Day 4											
Day 5											
Day 6											
Day 7											

Vision Recording Chart

Date	Right Eye	Left Eye	Date	Right Eye	Left Eye

Pressure Recording Chart

Date	Right Eye	Left Eye	Date	Right Eye	Left Eye

APPENDIX G

Home Testing Items

Vision Testing Chart

To test your vision, hold this chart about two feet in front of you. Test each eye separately.

Chart 1: Row number 8 is 20/20 vision. If you can't read line 5, it's time for an eye exam!

Chart 2: This is a test for astigmatism. Are one or two lines darker, sharper, easier to see than the rest of the lines? If so, you probably have astigmatism in that eye.

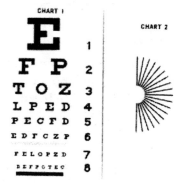

Amsler Recording Chart

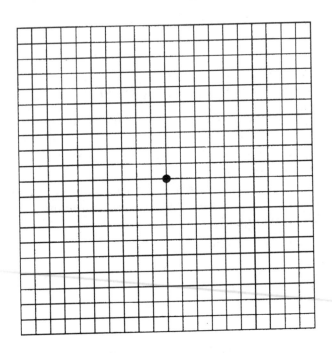

Questions to Ask Yourself:

1. Do you see the dark spot in the center of the squared chart?
2. Looking at the spot, can you see the four sides of the square?
3. Do you see the whole square? Are the holes or spots blurred anywhere
4. Do you see all the lines up & down? Are they equal?
5. Can you see anything else such as a movement, vibration, or waving, shining color, etc.?
6. How many small intact squares do you find between the blur or distortion.

GLOSSARY

A-scan—a type of ultrasound used to measure the length of the eye

amblyopia—a "lazy eye" that has poor vision from childhood

analgesic—medication to relieve pain

anesthetic—medication to prevent or block pain

angle—the interior portion of the eye between the cornea and the iris, where the aqueous drains out

angle closure glaucoma—glaucoma caused by the iris pushing into the angle and cutting off aqueous drainage

anisocoria—unequal pupil size

anterior chamber—the inside portion of the eye between the cornea and iris

aphakia—having no lens inside the eye

aqueous—watery fluid inside the eye, circulated between the cornea and lens

arcuate keratotomy—method of refractive surgery used to reduce or eliminate astigmatism

arcus senilis—a benign, creamy ring around the outer edge of the iris, caused by fatty deposits and occurring later in life

astigmatism—irregularly-curved cornea, results in blurred vision

atrophy—deterioration of a tissue

B-scan—type of ultrasound used to create a computer picture of the inside of the eye

benign—not cancerous

bifocal—a lens with two focusing points

binocular—pertaining to two eyes

binocular vision—quality of vision in which both eyes work together; the eyes focus on the same object and fuse the images together

biopsy—taking a sample of tissue for lab analysis

blepharitis—infection of the lids

blepharoplasty—surgery to repair baggy eyelids

blepharospasm—lid twitch ("tic")

blind spot—a naturally-occurring area with no vision, at the point where the optic nerve enters the eye

canaliculitis—infection of the canaliculus

canaliculus—tear-draining tube (plural, *canaliculi*)

capsule—envelope encasing the lens of the eye

cataract—clouding of the lens of the eye

cellulitis—inflammation of tissues

cerebrospinal fluid—fluid surrounding the brain and spinal cord

chalazion—inflammation and infection caused by a stopped-up gland in the eye lid

choroid—layer of blood vessels that lies beneath the retina

chronic open angle glaucoma—(see open angle glaucoma)

ciliary body—a structure at the root of the iris, responsible for aqueous formation

ciliary muscle—muscle that focuses the lens

claustrophobia—fear of being closed in

cones—light receptor cells in the retina that are responsible for color and finely-detailed vision

congenital—present at birth

conjunctiva—clear membrane that lines the inside of the lids and covers the sclera

cornea—clear window over the front of the eye

cryotherapy—treating tissues by use of a cold probe

dacryocystitis—infection and inflammation of the nasolacrimal sac

depth perception—ability to tell an object's position

dermatochalasis—baggy eyelids

diabetic retinopathy—retinal disease caused by diabetes

dilate—to open

diplopia—double vision

disc—the "head" of the optic nerve, visible when looking into the eye with an ophthalmoscope

ectropion—out-turned eyelid

edema—swelling caused by excess fluid

endophthalmitis—inflammation of the entire eye

entropion—in-turned eyelid

enucleation—removal of the eyeball

epikeratophakia—procedure in which donated corneal tissue is "ground" to a prescription then sewn onto the recipient's cornea

episclera—layer of fibers and blood vessels covering the sclera

episcleritis—inflammation of the episclera

exophthalmometer—instrument used to measure the protrusion of the eyeball

exophthalmus—protrusion of the eyeball(s)

farsighted—refractive error where there is an inability to focus up close (hyperopia)

filtering procedure—glaucoma surgery that creates a new drainage space for the aqueous

floaters—specks in the vision caused by the shadow of clumps of protein and other debris in the vitreous

fluoresceine angiography—a photographic procedure involving the injection of fluoresceine dye; the blood vessels of the retina and iris are studied as the dye enters them

fluoresceine dye—a dye that glows in blue light; may be used as an eye drop to evaluate the cornea, or injected (as in fluoresceine angiography) to evaluate blood vessels

focal photocoagulation—laser treatment of a small area of the retina

fovea—central area of macula that gives fine, detailed, central vision

fundus—the inside back of the eye that is visible with an ophthalmoscope

glaucoma—build up of pressure inside the eye that causes nerve damage and/or loss of side vision

gonioscopy—examination of the angle of the eye using a special lens

Herpes simplex—the virus that causes cold sores

Herpes zoster—the virus that causes shingles

hordeolum—medical term for a stye

Hruby lens—lens used to view the fundus

hyperopia—farsighted; unable to focus at near

hypertensive retinopathy—retinal disease caused by high blood pressure (hypertension)

hyphema—blood in the aqueous

intraocular—inside the eye

intraocular lens implant (IOL)—plastic lens implanted inside the eye to take the place of the eye's natural lens

intraocular pressure (IOP)—the pressure inside the eye, caused by the force of the aqueous

iridectomy—removal of a wedge of iris to allow aqueous drainage

iridotomy—cutting a hole in the iris (with laser) to allow aqueous drainage

iris—colored part of the eye

iritis—inflammation of the iris; also known as anterior uveitis

keratitis—inflammation or infection of the cornea

keratoconus—type of corneal dystrophy where the cornea becomes elongated and cone-shaped

keratometer—instrument used to measure corneal curvature

keratometry—the act of measuring the cornea with a keratometer

lacrimal gland—the main tear gland

laser—high-energy light beam used in treating the eye

lazy eye—one eye that is weak from childhood; amblyopia

legal blindness—vision that is worse than 20/200 in the best eye (even with glasses), or a significant loss of side vision

lens—focusing mechanism of the eye, lies behind the pupil

lensometer—instrument used to read the prescription of glasses lenses

leukemia—cancer of the blood cells

low-pressure glaucoma—condition where the intraocular pressure is normal, yet the nerve is being damaged or the side vision is being lost

macula—portion of retina used for fine central vision

macular degeneration—deterioration of the macula causing loss of reading vision, commonly in the later years

malignant—cancerous

miosis—constriction of the pupil

monocular—pertaining to one eye

monovision—correcting one eye for distance vision and the other eye for near vision

myopia—nearsighted; unable to focus at distance

nasolacrimal duct—tube leading from nasolacrimal sac to the nasal cavity

nasolacrimal sac—sac where draining tears collect

nearsighted—a refractive error where one can see up close but not at a distance (myopia)

neuritis—inflammation of a nerve

nevus—a mole that you're born with

nuclear sclerosis—a cataract produced by the hardening and yellowing of the lens

nystagmus—jerking ("dancing") eyes

ocular hypertension—condition where eye pressure is elevated but the nerve is not being damaged

ocularist—professional who fits prosthetic (artificial) eyes

oculist—ophthalmologist

open-angle glaucoma—most common type of glaucoma in which the aqueous drainage is NOT blocked, yet is not adequate (causing a rise in the eye's pressure)

ophthalmologist—a medical doctor (M.D.) who has specialized in the eye and is licensed to do exams, prescribe medications, and perform surgery

ophthalmometer—another name for keratometer, an instrument used to measure corneal curvature

ophthalmoscope—instrument used to view the inside of the eye

optic nerve—the nerve that runs from the brain to the back of the eye

optic nerve head—the portion of the optic nerve that can be seen when looking into the eye with an ophthalmoscope

optic neuritis—inflammation or degeneration of the optic nerve

optician—eye professional who makes and fits glasses

optometrist—eye doctor who has attended a special college for eye care and is licensed to do exams, fit contacts, and prescribe glasses; in some states may prescribe medications

orbit—the bony socket of the eye

pachymeter—instrument used to measure corneal thickness

panretinal photocoagulation—laser spot-treatment of the entire retina

papilledema—swelling of the optic nerve head

papillitis—inflammation of the optic nerve head

phacoemulsification—technique of cataract removal using ultrasonic vibration to break the cataract into small pieces

photocoagulation—treatment involving the absorption of light (usually laser) by the tissues and the conversion of that light into heat energy

photophobia—sensitive to light

pinguecula—small benign growth on the conjunctiva

posterior chamber—the interior portion of the eye between the iris and the lens

presbyopia—loss of the ability to see to read, usually starting around age forty

prism—special lens that bends light in such a way that seems to shift an object's location; used in strabismus and double vision

prosthetic eye—an artificial eye

pseudophakia—an eye with an intraocular lens implant

pterygium—benign wedge-shaped growth that extends from the conjunctiva onto the cornea

ptosis—sagging or drooping of a structure

punctum—opening in the lid where tears drain into the canaliculi (plural, *puncti*)

pupil—opening in the iris that adjusts to let light into the eye

radial keratotomy—surgery in which linear incisions are made in the cornea to correct myopia

refraction—testing with lenses and use of clinical judgement to arrive at a glasses prescription

refractive error—condition where light coming into the eye is not focused on the retina, resulting in a blurred image

refractive surgery—surgery performed to correct or change the refractive error of the eye

refractometry—testing with lenses to measure a refractive error

refractor—instrument containing rotating lenses, used to measure the refractive error of the eye

retina—the lining of the inside of the eye; contains light receptor cells responsible for sight

retinoscope—instrument used to evaluate refractive errors

rods—light receptor cells in the retina responsible for night vision

Schermer's tear test—a measurement of tear production

sclera—the white of the eye

scleritis—inflammation of the sclera

second sight—the ability, caused by cataracts, to read up close without glasses when one needed them before

secondary glaucoma—glaucoma caused by a secondary source, such as injury, medications, inflammation, etc.

slit lamp microscope—specialized microscope used to examine the eye

socket—the tissue-lined orbit that remains after an eye has been removed

strabismus—crossed eyes

stye—lid swelling caused by infection of the lash follicle

systemic—involving the entire body

tarsorrhaphy—surgery to close or partially-close the eyelids—may be temporary or permanent

thermal—refers to heat

tonography—test to measure the outflow of aqueous

tonometer—instrument used to measure the pressure inside the eye

topography—map of the cornea's contours

trabecular meshwork—the tissue in the angle that filters the aqueous

trabeculectomy—surgical removal of a portion of the trabecular meshwork in order to increase the drainage of aqueous

trabeculoplasty—laser treatment of the trabecular meshwork in order to increase aqueous drainage

trichiasis—in-turned eyelash

trifocal—a lens with three focusing points

ultrasound—high-frequency sound waves

ultraviolet light—invisible, harmful light rays

uvea—collective term for the iris, ciliary body, and choroid

uveitis—inflammation of the uvea

visual field test—mapping out of the peripheral vision

vitrectomy—surgical removal of the vitreous

vitreous—jelly-like substance inside the eyeball, behind the lens

vitreous cavity—portion of the eye from the lens back, that is filled with vitreous

zonules—tiny ligaments that hold the lens of the eye in place

REFERENCES

Adler's Textbook of Ophthalmology, Eighth Edition. Published in 1969 by W.B. Saunders Company in Philadelphia.

"Alternative draping technique for claustrophobic patients," by Johnny L. Gayton, Tammy S. Tesseniar, and Janice K. Ledford. Published in *Ophthalmic Surgery,* September 1990.

An Atlas of Head and Neck Surgery, Vol. 1, 2nd Edition, by John M. Lore, Jr., M.D. Published in 1973 by W.B. Saunders Company, Philadelphia, Pa.

"Combined cataract and strabismus surgery," by Johnny L. Gayton and Janice K. Ledford. Published in *Annals of Ophthalmology,* August 1993.

"Combined phacoemulsification and trabeculectomy," by Johnny L. Gayton and Janice K. Ledford. Published in *Annals of Ophthalmology,* January/February 1995.

Disease Free, by Matthew Hoffman, William LeGrow, and the editors of Prevention Magazine Health Books. Published in 1993 by Rodale Press, 33 East Minor St., Emmaus, Pa.

The Doctors Book of Home Remedies, edited by Debora Tkac of Prevention Magazine Health Books. Published in 1990 by Rodale Press, 33 East Minor St., Emmaus, Pa.

Duanes's Clinicial Opthalmology, edited by William Tasman, MD, and Edward Jaegar, MD. Revised in 1991 and published by JB Lippincott Company, Philladelphia, PA.

Exercises in Refractometry, by Janice K. Ledford. Published in 1990 by SLACK, Inc., of Thorofare, New Jersey.

"Fresh tissue Mohs surgery and reconstruction of oculofacial lesions," by Janice K. Ledford, in *The Surgical Technologist,* July 1991.

General Ophthalmology, Eleventh and Thirteenth Editions, by Daniel Vaughan and Taylor Asbury. Published in 1986 and 1992 by Lange Medical Publications, Los Altos, California.

High-Speed Healing, by the editors of Prevention Magazine Health Books. Published in 1991 by Rodale Press, 33 East Minor St., Emmaus, Pa.

"Immediate periorbital reconstruction following Mohs surgery:

three case studies," by Johnny L. Gayton, David Kent, and Janice K. Ledford in *Journal of the Medical Association of Georgia*, February 1991.

Manual of Ocular Diagnosis and Therapy, Second Edition, edited by Deborah Pavan-Langston, M.D. Published in 1985 by Little, Brown and Company of Boston.

Manual of Ophthalmic Terminology, by Harold A. Stein, Bernard J. Slatt, and Penny Cook. Published in 1982 by the C.V. Mosby Company, 11830 Westline Industrial Dr., St. Louis, Missouri 63141.

The Merck Manual, Fifteenth Edition, edited by Robert Berkow. Published in 1987 by Merck Sharp & Dohme Research Laboratories, Rahway, N. J.

Orthoptics and Ocular Examination Techniques, edited by William Scott, Denise D'Agostina, and Leslie Lennarson. Published in 1983 by Williams and Wilkins of Baltimore.

Ophthalmic Technology: A Guide for the Eye Care Assistant, edited by Stephen Rhode and Stephen Ginsberg. Published in 1987 by Raven Press of New York.

Ophthalmic Medical Assisting: An Independent Study Course, edited by the American Academy of Ophthalmology. Published in 1991 by the Academy.

Opticianry, Ocularistry and Ophthalmic Technology, by Basil Blair and others. Published in 1990 by SLACK, Inc., of Thorofare, New Jersey.

"Side approach effective in reducing preoperative against-the-rule astigmatism," by Johnny L. Gayton and Janice K. Ledford. Published in *Phaco & Foldables* in January/February 1993.

A Singular View: The Art of Seeing With One Eye, by Frank B. Brady. Published in 1979 by Medical Economics Company, Oradell, New Jersey 07649.

INDEX

Books by Starburst Publishers

(Partial listing—full list available on request)

The Crystal Clear Guide to Sight for Life

—Gayton & Ledford

Subtitled: *A Complete Manual of Eye Care for Those Over 40*. **The Crystal Clear Guide For Life** makes eye care easy-to-understand by giving clear knowledge of how the eye works with the most up-to-date information available from the experts. Contains more than 40 illustrations, a detailed index for cross-referencing, a concise glossary, and answers to often-asked questions. This book takes much of the guesswork out of eye problems, alleviating fear and apprehension often experienced by patients when medical problems develop.

(trade paper) ISBN 0914984683 **$15.95**

Migraine—Winning The Fight of Your Life   —Charles Theisler

This book describes the hurt, loneliness and agony that migraine sufferers experience and the difficulty they must live with. It explains the different types of migraines and their symptoms, as well as the related health hazards. Gives 200 ways to help fight off migraines, and shows how to experience fewer headaches, reduce their duration, and decrease the agony and pain involved.

(trade paper) ISBN 0914984632 **$10.95**

Health, Happiness & Hormones   —Arlene Swaney

Subtitled: *One Woman's Journey Toward Health After a Hysterectomy*. A frightening and candid look into one woman's struggle to find a cure for her medical condition. In 1990, when her story was first published in *Prevention* magazine, author Arlene Swaney received an overwhelming response from women who also were plagued by mysterious, but familiar, symptoms leading to continuous misdiagnoses. Starting with a hysterectomy Swaney details the years of lost health that followed as she searched for an accurate diagnosis. Her story is told with warmth and compassion.

(trade paper) ISBN 0914984721 **$9.95**

Stay Well Without Going Broke   —Gulling, Renner, & Vargas

Subtitled: *Winning the War Over Medical Bills*. Provides a blueprint for how health care consumers can take more responsibility for monitoring their own health and the cost of its care—a crucial cornerstone of the health care reform movement today. Contains inside information from doctors, pharmacists and hospital personnel on how to get cost-effective care without sacrificing quality. Offers legal strategies to protect your rights when illness is terminal.

(hardcover) ISBN 0914984527 **$22.95**

Dr. Kaplan's Lifestyle of the Fit & Famous   —Eric Scott Kaplan

Subtitled: *A Wellness Approach to "Thinning and Winning."* A comprehensive guide to the formulas and principles of: FAT LOSS, EXERCISE, VITAMINS, NATURAL HEALTH, SUCCESS and HAPPINESS. More than a health book—it is a lifestyle based on the empirical formulas of healthy living. Dr. Kaplan's food-combining principles take into account all the major food sources (fats, proteins, carbohydrates, sugars, etc.) that when combined within the proper formula (e.g. proteins cannot be mixed with refined carbohydrates) will increase metabolism and decrease the waistline. This allows you to eat the foods you want, feel great, and eliminate craving and binging.

(hardcover) ISBN 091498456X **$21.95**

The World's Oldest Health Plan   —Kathleen O'Bannon Baldinger

Subtitled: *Health, Nutrition and Healing from the Bible.* Offers a complete health plan for body, mind and spirit, just as Jesus did. It includes programs for diet, exercise and mental health. Contains foods and recipes to lower cholesterol and blood pressure, improve the immune system and other bodily functions, reduce stress, reduce or cure constipation, eliminate insomnia, reduce forgetfulness, confusion and anger, increase circulation and thinking ability, eliminate "yeast" problems, improve digestion, and much more.

(trade paper-opens flat) ISBN 0914984578 **$14.95**

Allergy Cooking With Ease   —Nicolette M. Dumke

Subtitled: *The No Wheat, Milk, Eggs, Corn, Soy, Yeast, Sugar, Grain, and Gluten Cookbook.* A book designed to provide a wide variety of recipes to meet many different types of dietary and social needs and, whenever possible, save you time in food preparation. Includes: Recipes for those special foods that most food allergy patients think they will never eat again; Timesaving tricks; and Allergen Avoidance Index.

(trade paper-opens flat) ISBN 091498442X **$12.95**

The Low-Fat Supermarket   —Judith & Scott Smith

Subtitled: *A Guide to Weight-Loss, Cholesterol Control and Good Nutrition* for the Entire Family. A comprehensive reference of over 4,500 brand name products that derive less than 30% of their calories from fat. Information provided includes total calories, fat, cholesterol and sodium content. Organized according to the sections of a supermarket. Your answer to a healthier you.

(trade paper) ISBN 0914984438 **$10.95**

Parenting With Respect and Peacefulness   —Louise A. Dietzel

Subtitled: *The Most Difficult Job in the World.* Parents who love and respect themselves parent with respect and peacefulness. Yet, parenting with respect is the most difficlult job in the world. This book informs parents that respect and peace communicate love—creating an atmosphere for children to maximize their development as they feel loved, valued, and safe. Parents can learn authority and control by commonsense, interpersonal, and practical approaches to day-to-day issues and situations in parenting.

(trade paper) ISBN 0914984667 **$10.95**

Books by Starburst Publishers—cont'd.

From Grandma With Love —Ann Tuites

Subtitled: *Thoughts for Her Children Everywhere.* People are taught all kinds of things from preschool to graduate school, but they are expected to know instinctively how to get along with their families. Harmony within the home is especially difficult when an aging relative is involved. The author presents personal anecdotes to encourage caregivers and those in need of care. Practical, emotional and spiritual support is given so that all generations can learn to live together in harmony.

(hardcover) ISBN 0914984616 **$14.95**

A Woman's Guide To Spiritual Power —Nancy L. Dorner

Subtitled: *Through Scriptural Prayer.* Do your prayers seem to go "against a brick wall?" Does God sometimes seem far away or non-existent? If your answer is "Yes," *You* are not alone. Prayer must be the cornerstone of your relationship to God. "This book is a powerful tool for anyone who is serious about prayer and discipleship."—Florence Littauer

(trade paper) ISBN 0914984470 **$9.95**

Winning At Golf —David A. Smith

Addresses the growing needs of aspiring young golfers yearning for correct instruction, positive guidance, and discipline. It is an attempt not only to increase the reader's knowledge of the swing, but also sets forth to inspire and motivate the reader to a new and rewarding way of life. **Winning At Golf** relays the teachings of Buck White, the author's mentor and a tour winner many times over. It gives instruction to the serious golfer and challenges the average golfer to excel.

(trade paper) ISBN 0914984462 **$9.95**

Purchasing Information

Listed books are available from your favorite Bookstore, either from current stock or special order. To assist bookstore in locating your selection be sure to give title, author, and ISBN #. If unable to purchase from the bookstore you may order direct from STARBURST PUBLISHERS. When ordering enclose full payment plus $3.00 for shipping and handling ($4.00 if Canada or Overseas). Payment in US Funds only. Please allow two to three weeks minimum (longer overseas) for delivery. Make checks payable to and mail to STARBURST PUBLISHERS, P.O. Box 4123, LANCASTER, PA 17604. Credit card orders may also be placed by calling 1-800-441-1456 (credit card orders only), Mon-Fri, 8 AM-5 PM Eastern Time. **Prices subject to change without notice.**

1-96